RECYCLING THE DISABLED

MANCHESTER
1824

Manchester University Press

DISABILITY HISTORY

Series editors

Dr Julie Anderson, Professor Walton Schalick, III

This new series published by Manchester University Press responds to the growing interest in disability as a discipline worthy of historical research. The series has a broad international historical remit, encompassing issues that include class, race, gender, age, war, medical treatment, professionalisation, environments, work, institutions and cultural and social aspects of disablement including representations of disabled people in literature, film, art and the media.

Already published

Deafness, community and culture in Britain: leisure and cohesion, 1945–1995
Martin Atherton

Destigmatising mental illness? Professional politics and public education in Britain, 1870–1970
Vicky Long

Framing the moron: the social construction of feeble-mindedness in the American eugenics era
Gerald V. O'Brien

Worth saving: disabled children during the Second World War
Sue Wheatcroft

RECYCLING THE DISABLED

ARMY, MEDICINE, AND MODERNITY IN WWI GERMANY

Heather R. Perry

Manchester University Press

Published by Manchester University Press
Altrincham Street, Manchester M1 7JA, UK
and Room 400, 175 Fifth Avenue, New York, NY 10010, USA
www.manchesteruniversitypress.co.uk

Distributed in the United States exclusively by
Palgrave Macmillan, 175 Fifth Avenue, New York,
NY 10010, USA

Distributed in Canada exclusively by
UBC Press, University of British Columbia, 2029 West Mall,
Vancouver, BC, Canada V6T 1Z2

British Library Cataloguing-in-Publication Data
A catalogue record for this book is available from the British Library

Library of Congress Cataloging-in-Publication Data applied for

ISBN 978 0 7190 8924 4 hardback

First published 2014

Typeset in 10/12pt Arno Pro by
Servis Filmsetting Ltd, Stockport, Cheshire
Printed in Great Britain by
TJ International Ltd, Padstow

Contents

List of figures

Series editors' foreword

You know a subject has achieved maturity when a book series is dedicated to it. In the case of disability, while it has co-existed with human beings for centuries the study of disability's history is still quite young.

In setting up this series, we chose to encourage multi-methodologic history rather than a purely traditional historical approach, as researchers in disability history come from a wide variety of disciplinary backgrounds. Equally 'disability' history is a diverse topic which benefits from a variety of approaches in order to appreciate its multi-dimensional characteristics.

A test for the team of authors and editors who bring you this series is typical of most series, but disability also brings other consequential challenges. At this time disability is highly contested as a social category in both developing and developed contexts. Inclusion, philosophy, money, education, visibility, sexuality, identity and exclusion are but a handful of the social categories in play. With this degree of politicisation, language is necessarily a cardinal focus.

In an effort to support the plurality of historical voices, the editors have elected to give fair rein to language. Language is historically contingent, and can appear offensive to our contemporary sensitivities. The authors and editors believe that the use of terminology that accurately reflects the historical period of any book in the series will assist readers in their understanding of the history of disability in time and place.

Finally, disability offers the cultural, social and intellectual historian a new 'take' on the world we know. We see disability history as one of a few nascent fields with the potential to reposition our understanding of the flow of cultures, society, institutions, ideas and lived experience. Conceptualisations of 'society' since the early modern period have heavily stressed principles of autonomy, rationality and the subjectivity of the individual agent. Consequently we are frequently oblivious to the historical contingency of the present with respect to those elements. Disability disturbs those foundational features of 'the modern'. Studying disability history helps us resituate our policies, our beliefs and our experiences.

Julie Anderson
Walton O. Schalick, III

Preface and acknowledgements

This book is based on ideas I first developed in my doctoral dissertation. I have since then significantly revised and expanded those concepts in order to include substantially new research and historiographical developments. My dissertation was written under the wise and genial tutelage of James Diehl at Indiana University. I have many fond memories of Bloomington and am grateful for the superb education that I received there. My dissertation carries the imprint of the rigourous discussions I had with Jim, Anne Carmichael, Carl Ipsen, Dror Wahrman, Mark Roseman, Jeanne Peterson, Ellen Dwyer, Bill Cohen, and Elisabeth Domansky, and echoes of those conversations can be found in this book, as well. I am lucky to have had such great role models and friends while I was there. Jason Crouthamel, Brian Els, Andy Evans, Tim Pursell, Jude Richter, Jeremy Rich and Lynn Sargeant could always see the humour in studying history. My dissertation research was supported by fellowships from the Max Kade Foundation, the History Department at Indiana University, and the German Academic Exchange Service (DAAD), but I would not have completed it without the support of a position as Editorial Assistant at the *American Historical Review*. I learned much about the professional side of the discipline through working with Mike Grossberg and Maureen Coulter and I thank them for that.

My past and present colleagues at the University of North Carolina Charlotte have been engaging and supportive of my research since the day I arrived. Karen Cox, Christine Haynes, Melissa Feinberg, Jim Hogue, Steve Sabol, John Smail, John David Smith, and Peter Thorsheim provided valuable comments on early versions of chapters I presented at our departmental seminars and other venues. The additional research necessary for revising my dissertation into this book was supported by a Brooke Hindle Post-Doctoral Fellowship from the Society for the History of Technology (SHOT), a Faculty Re-Invitation grant from the DAAD, a Faculty Research Grant, a Dean's Grant, and a Junior Research Leave from the College of Liberal Arts and Sciences at UNC Charlotte as well as a Francis Lumsden Gwynn award.

Librarians, archivists, and staff at institutions in both Germany and the United States have been invaluable in finding the materials upon which this research is based. In Berlin the staff at the Bundesarchiv in Lichterfelde, the Bundesarchiv Filmarchiv, and the Staatsbibliothek Preussischer Kulturbesitz were always prompt and efficient. In Freiburg the staff of the Bundesarchiv-Militärarchiv found almost everything I requested – sometimes more than once. The archivists at the Bayerisches Haupstaatsarchiv-Kriegsabteilung were surprisingly amiable and much warmer than the cold winter I spent in Munich. The archivists at Siemens in Munich and in Dresden at the Hygiene Museum and Library, the Hauptstaatsarchiv, and the Dresdner Stadtarchiv pointed me in many new directions to sources I would have never found on my own. To all of them I am thankful for their help and patience and to their institutions for allowing me the use of their materials. In the United States, Arlene Shaner at the New York Academy of Medicine helped me navigate the Douglas McMurtrie collection as we both discovered new things there. At the National Library of Medicine, Stephen Greenberg was generous with help, advice-and a tripod! Ann Davis, the head of the Interlibrary Loan Department at the Atkins Library at UNC Charlotte has been an indefatigable champ at hunting down books and pamphlets and convincing libraries around the world to send them to us. I could not have accessed many of the rare materials this research is based upon without their expertise and assistance. This book includes images reprinted from medical textbooks and newspapers from the period. In every instance, I have made the best effort to trace and acknowledge the copyright holder.

Over the years, I have presented my ideas at dozens of conferences and other intellectual venues including the AHA, GSA, AAHM, SSHM, SSHA, EAHMH, AAA, the Max Planck Institute for the History of Science in Berlin, the European University Institute in Florence, the Centre for the History of Science, Technology, and Medicine in Manchester, and the Institution for Historical Research in London. The comments and feedback I received on each of those occasions helped me to refine and improve my arguments. In some cases, those meetings led to other fruitful collaborations as well. I'd like to thank particularly Wolfgang Eckart, Leo van Bergen, Ana Carden-Coyne, Lynne Fallwell, Chris Fischer, Michael Gross, Karen Hagemann, Hans-Georg Hofer, Heather Jones, Tait Keller, Thomas Kühne, Beth Linker, Cay-Rüdiger Prüll, Erika Quinn, Jeff Reznick, Lutz Sauerteig, Walt Schalick, Thomas Schlich, Bob Whalen, and Helen Valier. I'm particularly indebted to Roger Chickering, not only for his stalwart encouragement, but also for his valuable feedback on an early draft of the entire manuscript at a critical stage. The anonymous readers for Manchester University Press challenged me to place some of my ideas in comparative perspective and the book is all the better for that. Since our very first meeting Julie Anderson has been supportive of this project and I thank her for her unwavering faith in it. Emma Brennan at Manchester University Press has been lovely to work with and exceedingly patient. Rachel Evans put forth meticulous effort in copy-editing the manuscript and John Noble indexed it with great care and for that I thank them both. Despite the input of all these good people, any errors or mistakes that remain are of my own making.

My friends and family have stood by me and this book for a very long time. My parents have never doubted me. Tracy Luedke and Lynn Sargeant have been unstinting in their friendship, advice, and good cheer. Finally, Andy Boram did not know he was signing up for the war when we met, but he has steadfastly and lovingly sustained me through the final push. To them I dedicate this book.

A note on language

Unless otherwise noted, all translations in this work are my own. The reader will notice that in some instances I have used words that to modern ears might sound insensitive. The words 'cripple', 'cripple-care', and even 'the disabled' are widely understood today as pejorative or insensitive terms, but during the time period which this study examines, they were not just common social and medical parlance, they were considered particularly important denotative terms. As other linguistic markers evolved during the war, many amputees fought loudly to *retain* the label of 'war-cripple' [*Kriegskrüppel*] because they resented being subsumed into the larger and less explicit category of 'war damaged' [*Kriegsbeschädigte*] or 'war invalid' [*Kriegsinvalide*]. To men who had lost their arms or legs, being 'lumped together' with the blind or the tubercular or the psychologically damaged was considered an insult and an elision of the significant bodily sacrifice that they had endured and which set them apart from other war disabled soldiers. 'War cripple' was a label that many claimed proudly and insisted upon being called. Out of respect for them, where appropriate, I have not modernised the instances in which this language was used for especial denotative purposes. In other instances, I have retained the more accurate, though perhaps anachronistic sounding, translations of 'the disabled' [*Schwerbeschädigte*] or 'the maimed' [*Versehrte*], when the language itself is revealing of historical attitude or phenomenon under discussion. Moreover, in translations of titles, names, organisations, and other official organs, I have also tried to remain historically true to the actual language that was used.

Introduction

WAR AND MEDICINE IN WORLD WAR I GERMANY

> Due to the desperate circumstances, the exploitation of all manpower – even the slightest – is hereby ordered. Therefore all war-disabled soldiers who are capable of even the slightest amount of useful work are being commandeered for duty. Even those who have been labelled as 'severely injured' that is, evaluated at a medical disability of 50% or more, are still capable of work. Moreover, every public and private workplace must be informed that severely injured workers are better than none at all. … The war-disabled must be informed that he is not being healed out of pity, but rather because his labour is crucial for the collective good. (General Hermann von Stein, German War Ministry, 1918)[1]

The science and technology of the First World War simultaneously destroyed and re-created the male body. Military historians have detailed minutely how technological innovations fundamentally changed the nature of modern warfare between 1914 and 1918.[2] Not only did new weapons such as chemical gas, machine guns, and exploding artillery shells impact on operational strategies and battlefield tactics, they also created radically new kinds of injuries to the human body.[3] For instance, chlorine gas not only blinded its victims, but also triggered fluid production in their lungs, causing a soldier's slow and painful death by 'drowning' on dry land.[4] High-powered rifles could shoot bullets through the air at speeds of up to 2500 feet per second, releasing up to 7200 horsepower of energy. Whereas 'slower' bullets might shoot through the body or simply remain embedded within it, bullets released with this much energy could cause the explosion or even disintegration of body parts.[5] One 1917 German army study found that 75 per cent of all wounds came from artillery shells which had developed into formidable weapons of destruction.[6] Male bodies were invaded with bullets, shrapnel from grenades, or other uncontrollable flying debris whose trauma caused as many internal injuries as external ones. Those who did not die were often horribly and permanently wounded, requiring in many cases not just immediate care but also long-term convalescence.

Surprisingly, however, much less attention has been paid to how innovations in human medicine and science responded to these injuries. In fact, while the armaments industry had been steadily inventing new weapons of mass destruction, innovations in surgery and trauma care enabled doctors to save the lives of many of those gravely injured. Others invented new devices and therapies for healing battle injuries during the conflict itself. It is this parallel development in medical care which partly explains why there was such a preponderance of disabled soldiers left in the wake of World War I: those who would have died of their wounds in previous wars might now recover.[7] These survivors placed increasing demands on war-time medical services – both military and civilian. Some were returned to battle while others were left permanently disabled. Ironically, given the rate at which soldiers were both injured and healed, one could argue that the advanced technology of the First World War resulted in the industrial production of not just war, but also disabled men.

The casualties of the First World War were unprecedented in Imperial Germany. Between 1914 and 1918 13.2 million men shuffled through the German armed forces.[8] Although statistics vary, most historians agree that some 2,037,000 men were killed in battle while another 5,687,000 were wounded. The number of wounded is somewhat hard to determine as some soldiers were wounded, healed, and were then wounded again. Thus some may have been counted more than once as 'wounded'.[9] Studies of German war veterans have estimated the number of permanently disabled at 2.7 million[10] and the number of amputees at 67,000.[11] Although this number may seem small when contrasted with the casualties of the Second World War, when compared to German casualties of previous wars, this number was astronomical. For instance, in the Franco-Prussian War (1870–1871) a total of 88,488 men were wounded, while just 28,208 fell on the battlefields.[12] Comparatively in the second of Germany's wars of unification, the Austro-German War of 1866, the Prussian Army lost just 2,931 soldiers and those German states and principalities aligned with Austria lost a mere 1,147.[13] When one considers that in the First World War the number of men wounded and killed *per day* eventually well-exceeded these figures, it is easy to see how the high casualties of war quickly became overwhelming.[14]

This high casualty rate – the numbers of wounded and killed – posed multiple problems for the war-time state. The majority of Germany's soldiers were between the ages of eighteen and thirty-four, that is, young healthy men on whom both the German military and labour economies placed a high premium.[15] As both sides in the armed conflict settled into a war of attrition with the 1916 slaughters at Verdun and the Somme, battle strategies that focused on mutually 'bleeding the enemy white' posed a constant drain on the manpower resources of the German military; healthy, able-bodied men were in steady demand to replenish the supply of cannon fodder at the front.[16] At the same time, however, the empire's armed forces were exerting pressure on munitions factories to speed up the production of war materiel in order to meet the demands of the new technological war; requests for exemption from military service steadily increased as the pool of available labour failed to meet the requirements of industry.[17] In addition to the competing manpower demands of the German army, the military-industrial complex itself was steadily draining labour from the countryside – whether through military draft or the high factory wages negotiated by German labour representatives. The subsequent dearth of workers on German farmland, combined with the Allied blockade during the war, contributed directly to the food shortage which seemed to paralyse the home front during the terrible 'turnip winter' of 1916–1917. Keeping labour available for the agricultural sector of the German economy gained increasing importance as both the war and the Allied supply blockade continued.[18] Finally, in addition to the growing crisis in manpower plaguing the war-time state, perhaps an even greater dilemma posed by the high number of battle casualties was the question of what was to become of these permanently injured men *after* the war – when they could no longer support themselves or their families by returning to their pre-war civilian jobs. The overwhelming casualties of the First World War, then, did not only contribute to a manpower crisis *during* the war, but also to one which loomed threateningly over the post-war horizon. Whether Germany won or lost the war, the question remained: what would the empire do with its disabled soldiers?

Thus, the 'disabled question' was on the minds of many Germans during the war years. In addition to the fears that these injuries produced among the wounded and their families, military leaders, health professionals, insurance officials, bourgeois philanthropists, entrepreneurial businessmen, church congregations, trade unions and veterans' organisations all became equally concerned with the fate of the disabled soldier during the war. At a time, then, when manpower was already at a premium, the emerging claims of a small group of German doctors – orthopaedists – that they could physically restore these men and their bodies appeared to serve not just the immediate interests of the war-time state, but also those of its post-war future, as well. Ironically, convinced that they were winning the war, most Germans predicted that post-war economic rebuilding and territorial expansion would require even more available workers. Thus, in the midst of 'total war', the possibility of healing and re-fashioning these severely injured soldiers into what they considered to be 'useful', 'productive', and self-sufficient members of the national economy – that is, to 'recycle' them as they termed it – appeared to hold for many contemporary Germans the answer to all of the empire's war-time military, social, and economic problems.

This book examines the medical, cultural, and military processes which ultimately made it possible for Hermann von Stein, the Prussian Minister of War, to order the mobilisation of Germany's severely disabled soldiers. As the quote at the beginning of this introduction makes clear, by late 1918 the manpower shortage had become so severe that the German Army was demanding that even soldiers categorised as being 50 per cent disabled, that is, having lost a limb or more, were to be re-deployed in the service of the fatherland. More than a history of military medicine, this is a study about the increasingly entwined relationship between medicine and war in the waning stages of the German Empire. Specifically it traces the 'medicalisation of war' under the conditions of total mobilisation from 1914 to 1918. This process of medicalisation included both the militarisation of medicine as well as the militarisation of the disabled body in Germany's first 'total war'. Fundamental to these two developments, however, was the growing participation of medical professionals – in this instance orthopaedists – in the organisation of the modern 'war machine'. As this book demonstrates, the so-called 'recycling of the disabled' was a direct result of the convergence of multiple war-time processes.

Medicine and war

Given the centrality of medical care for wounded soldiers from 1914 through to 1918, it is surprising that for decades few studies of medicine – German or otherwise – during this period existed. Indeed only recently have historians begun to approach the topic of medicine in war from any serious academic standpoint. Military historians of the war have largely ignored both soldier care and the medical corps in their scholarship. Until the 1990s, most histories of war-time medicine consisted primarily of either the military medical department reports, the memoirs or amateur histories written by doctors who had served in war and later recorded their personal experiences, or studies of social programmes and pension politics of war veterans – studies which generally focus on the *post-war* experiences of soldiers.

The limited research available on German war-time medicine reflects this general scholarly trend. During and after the war, several medical accounts of the conflict appeared in print, but these are largely sanitation reports that: recorded and categorised the casualties of the war; recorded the general organisation of the medical services; and summarised medical developments observed by doctors in the field. For instance, *Die deutschen Ärzte im Weltkrieg: Ihre Leistungen und Erfahrungen*, published in 1920, detailed the significant diseases, injuries, and medical conditions observed during the war and described how the empire's military and civilian medical personnel responded to them, while the colossal ten volume, multi-authored chronicle of Germany's war experience, *Der grosse Krieg*, included chapters on military medicine within the German army and navy.[19] And, although these reports offer good general summaries of how medical services were organised or the types of wounds that soldiers experienced, they lack both the historical distance and contextualisation central to academic scholarship. Studies of the medical department or military medical organisation are rare among the many histories of the Prussian and other German Armies in the Great War.[20] A few medical personnel who enlisted or were drafted into the conflict have left behind records of their experiences – some of which, such as the war diary of Hugo Natt, have only recently come to light and been published.[21] But the lack of general enthusiasm or respect for any serious medical history of the German Army in the Great War is best evidenced in the response to a dissertation written on the subject at the Free University of Berlin in 1968. Christian Kliche's thesis entitled 'The Situation of German Military Doctors in the First World War' was included in *Der Spiegel* magazine's list of 'worthless dissertations' completed between 1966 and 1968 – and its scant 67-page length suggests even Kliche could find little to include in the analysis fifty years after the conflict.[22]

Studies of Germany's wounded soldiers from this war have received somewhat greater scholarly attention – although this attention has not come from medical historians. Rather, social and political historians have examined the government pension and demobilisation programmes instituted for ex-servicemen[23] or the post-war politics of veterans.[24] Robert Whalen's seminal work, *Bitter Wounds*, documents well the dissatisfaction and protests of wounded soldiers regarding their aftercare and the pension reforms passed in response to these demands.[25] In her book, *The War Come Home*, Deborah Cohen offers a comparison of the state programmes and private philanthropic efforts that emerged in Great Britain and Germany for disabled soldiers of the Great War. But Cohen's goal is to explain why British veterans were more supportive of their post-war government than German veterans were of theirs – despite the fact that the social welfare benefits emanating from London paled when compared to those coming from Berlin. Thus, although Cohen includes a brief examination of rehabilitation medicine, hers is really a study of how the social welfare which was developed for disabled soldiers impacted on veterans' politics and attitudes after the war.[26] In an effort to understand the 'outsider' position of Germany's WWI veterans and their lack of support for democracy in the fledging Weimar Republic, both of these studies have argued that disabled soldiers were dissatisfied with their service pensions, felt forgotten in the larger post-war economic and social crises of the new state, or simply rebelled against an unwanted liberal government in the violent manner they had 'learned' during the war.[27] Thus, while medical historians have been researching the development of soldier care and veteran rehabilitation programmes within the United States, Great Britain, and other member-nations of the Allied forces in the Great War, historians of Germany have been primarily concerned with the post-war political voice of the disabled soldier – using him as a prism for understanding why Germany's first experiment with democracy ended with the Nazi seizure of power. Indeed for decades, most academic studies examining German war-time medicine or soldier health during this war focused on the *psychological* trauma experienced by soldiers – as if shellshock, its diagnostic 'discovery', and subsequent treatment were the only major medical concerns of military or civilian authorities in the Great War.[28]

It was not until the 1990s that social historians of medicine began to take more seriously the topics of medicine and health in war time, and several important essay collections have emerged on this topic.[29] Since then historians of medicine have been examining more closely the impact of the First World War on developments in modern medicine. Studies have pointed to the ways in which war provided an experimental laboratory for developments in such fields as pathological research, typhoid vaccinations, venereal disease, and pulmonary conditions.[30] At first, this research concentrated primarily on war-related developments in British and American military and civilian medicine, but this is beginning to change. Susanne Michl's published dissertation, *Im dienste des Volkskörpers: deutsche und französische Ärzte im Ersten Weltkrieg*, offers a discursive analysis of how doctors in war-time France and Germany perceived themselves and their medical work. Through an examination of medical journals published on both sides of the western front, Michl argues that medical experts envisioned themselves as health authorities whose work was crucial not only for individual survival, but also for the survival of the 'national body' (*Volkskörper*). Michl's reliance on war-time medical journals and the words of professional elites written from the safety of the desk, however, results in a study which seems to miss the opportunity to examine the impact or lived experience of these attitudes on the population.[31] One cannot help but wonder: how did the self-perceptions of these doctors translate into medical, military, or social policy towards others? What material impact did this medical discourse have on civilians, on soldiers, on military organisation? The recent collection *War, Trauma, and Medicine in*

Germany and Central Europe (1914–1939) focuses specifically on how the war impacted on the practice, experience, and development of military medicine in the armies of the Central Powers. The essays in this book offer readers a glimpse into ways that the German and Austrian responses to trauma not only differed from those in Great Britain or America, but even from each other – thus reminding readers that soldiers in Central Europe did not have a uniform experience of injury or injury care.[32] Daniela Angetter has examined Austrian military medicine and its evolution on the southern battle front once Italy entered the war; however, her study concentrates on how the terrain, climate and geographical location of battles on the Isonzo and in the Alps influenced medical and organisational practices specific to the Habsburg Army and not Germany.[33] Leo van Bergen's comparative book on soldiers' experiences of the Great War synthesises a wide variety of primary and secondary sources which illuminate the horrors and suffering that Germans and others nationals endured on the Western Front, but these are presented more as episodes or vignettes than deep analyses or discussions of military medicine.[34]

In addition to describing how war encouraged medical discovery or practice, medical historians also began looking at this relationship from another angle by trying to determine how modern medicine might have influenced the conduct or course of war. In studies which described how medical developments improved military efficiency, transformed military medical units, bettered battle conditions, or increased survival rates, these medical historians were describing ways in which modern medicine had facilitated military goals.[35]

By the turn of the twenty-first century, medical historians began thinking more theoretically about the relationships between the structures and institutions of both the military and medical 'spheres' during war. Roger Cooter questioned the very foundations upon which these supposedly causal relationships rested by casting significant doubt on the widely accepted historical dictum that war was 'good' for medicine. He challenged the notion that war has acted as a handmaiden to medical progress by pointing out several instances wherein the upheaval of war had impeded or slowed down medical discovery, not advanced it.[36] Medical historians began to question what Cooter termed the perceived 'goodness of war for medicine'.[37] Mark Harrison further complicated these relationships by adding in a third variable: modernity and the pressures of modernisation. He urged historians to look at how the Weberian forms of modernisation – centralisation, rationalisation, and the relentless quest for efficiency – had created the conditions in which doctors and medical care became significant components in the successful 'management of modern warfare'.[38] These ideas have been particularly fruitful, and his recent scholarship has revealed the importance of modern military medicine to British military strategies and victories in both the First and Second World Wars.[39] But these developments have yet to make a significant impact on historical scholarship on medicine and war in Germany, with perhaps one exception: the period under National Socialism.[40]

Alongside this growing interest in social and cultural history of war-time medicine, scholars became increasingly curious about how modern societies had dealt with and reacted to the disabling of an entire generation of soldiers – not once, but repeatedly over the course of the twentieth century. In the wake of each mass slaughter, not only did individual soldiers require healing, but so, too, did state economies, national psyches, and definitions of family, gender, and sexual roles. Both Joanna Bourke and Seth Koven have examined how the image of the severely injured serviceman's body shaped both public attitudes and memories of the Great War in Britain.[41] Jeffrey Reznick's book on the organisation of medical care for wounded British soldiers demonstrates how these services healed not just individual soldiers, but helped to mend an entire nation through what he called the 'culture of care-giving'.[42] Sabine Kienitz's anthropological study of disabled veterans in the Weimar Republic examines how the body of the wounded soldier took on multiple symbolic meanings for a nation rebuilding – politically, economically, and physically – after the war, but it has found little audience among non-German readers.[43] Ana Carden-Coyne's work examines how citizens reconciled the victory of war with what seemed to be the permanent destruction of male bodily integrity. Through artistic, commercial, and architectural re-presentations of the male body as whole, virile, and classically beautiful, post-war societies were able to cope with the aftermath of war.[44] Marina Larsson has demonstrated how the rehabilitation and pension programmes developed for disabled members of the Australian and New Zealand Army Corps (ANZAC)s operated alongside public commemorations to re-integrate these soldiers – and their families – into post-war Australian society, even if it was not always successful.[45] And finally, Julie Anderson and Beth Linker have demonstrated how the medical attitudes and public responses towards disabled servicemen from the Great War, as well as state policies for them, ultimately shaped the treatment of those permanently injured in subsequent wars. Anderson's study of disabled Britons reveals how rehabilitation programmes and policies developed for injured soldiers and war workers from both the First and Second World Wars had significant influence – sometimes positive, sometimes negative – on the civilian disabled population within the nation, while Beth Linker has argued that among the long-term legacies of US involvement in the Great War, one must not forget the establishment of a 'rehabilitation ethic' and the Veterans

Administration – both of which continue to guide the aftercare of wounded soldiers in America to this day.[46] Yet for all the vast wealth of information about disabled soldiers, national health, and military medical care that we glean from these works, they focus primarily on Britain, Australia, and the United States – Anglophone nations that not only won the war, but dictated the terms of the peace after it as well. Historical studies which describe and analyse the rehabilitation goals, culture, and experience in war-time Germany continue to lag behind. This is surprising – not only because the German armed forces experienced significantly higher casualties than *all of these nations combined* (and thus had far more bodies to heal), but also because the limited research which does examine German medical experiences from this war has consistently pointed out how substantially *different* war-time medical developments in Germany were from those in Allied nations.[47]

This book marks an attempt to think more critically about the relationships between war, medicine, and modernity in World War I Germany. It is neither an exhaustive account of military medicine during the war nor an examination of the entire breadth and scope of medical practice in that time. What it does do is examine how the pressures of modern war impacted medical development, military organisation, and socio-cultural perceptions of the physically disabled body. In doing this, and by considering aspects of these phenomena that were uniquely German, the book aims to broaden what has been a predominantly Anglo-American conversation and perspective.

The book begins with an examination of orthopaedics in Germany and outlines how the war prompted its practitioners to re-orient their field – a re-orientation that resulted not only in their medical specialisation, but also catapulted them significantly into the public's and the military's eyes. It follows with a look at how the high rates of injury to extremities among the nation's soldiers inspired a revolution in medical care and prosthetic technology. In recounting these developments, this study demonstrates that in the cases of orthopaedic specialisation and the development of modern artificial limbs the war was indeed 'good for medicine'. Next, this book turns to the practice and organisation of rehabilitation medicine in Germany in order to show how these war-time medical developments quickly influenced both military and civilian treatments for physically wounded soldiers. Then it examines the deeper impact of these medical advances on the social, cultural, and military spheres of war-time Germany. In tracing the medicalisation of disability during the war, this book reveals a significant shift in popular perceptions and expectations of the permanently injured body – one which persisted into the post-war period and helped shaped the new social order of Weimar Germany. Finally, the book concludes with a look at the impact of all these developments on the medical re-organisation of German society, industry, and military for 'total war' and ultimately facilitated the recycling of the empire's disabled soldiers.

This recycling rested upon the convergence of three simultaneous historical developments: specialisation, militarisation, and medicalisation. And though the historical details of these processes are outlined in the following chapters, it might benefit the reader to clarify the terms themselves in advance. Medical specialisation is largely understood as the increasing division of labour among medical practitioners which took place over the course of the eighteenth century through to the twentieth century. While historians can generally agree on when modern specialisation emerged, there are diverse explanations for what drove this process. According to some it was a response to the exponential growth of scientific knowledge while to others it represented the rationalisation of patients, disease, and health care in the increasingly bureaucratised nation-state of the nineteenth century. Specialisation might be usefully contrasted with professionalisation, which was a process occurring at roughly the same time and which was driven by the desire of trained, academic elites to distance themselves from lay competitors. Unlike professionalisation, however, specialisation was largely a competition *between* trained elites trying to differentiate themselves from one another and establish their expertise in particular medical fields.[48]

Although the definition of militarisation can vary among scholars, I use it to denote the 'process in which civil society organizes itself for the production of violence'.[49] In this sense my understanding of militarisation draws heavily on the work of Michael Geyer who has argued that militarisation should be understood as the manner by which 'societies remake themselves and their social-political orders for the purposes of organizing destruction'.[50] When considering the process of militarisation in WWI Germany, one must examine how the re-organisation of German society for 'total mobilisation' was also promoted and organised by civic leaders and civilian authorities. It was not solely a military process. Unlike nineteenth-century 'militarism' which can be understood as the forced imposition of military values or culture upon civilians, militarisation during the First World War involved various segments of the civilian population rushing to participate voluntarily in the mass re-organisation of German society for war. What is important to this understanding, therefore, are two central tenets. Firstly, that militarisation was a process driven as much by forces from below as it was from above. And secondly, that militarisation was an on-going process which required constant modifications as the conditions for the continued 'production of violence' during the war changed.

Medicalisation is equally important to this study and thus important to define. Most scholars understand medicalisation to be the process by which human behaviours or bodily conditions are re-defined and treated as 'medical problems'. This process is usually, although not always, led by medical experts who use their authority as the basis for facilitating this reorganisation of bodily knowledge. One might thus understand the medicalisation of society as the process by which social conditions are re-defined according to medical ideas or by which societies are re-organised according to medical values. In this study, I use medicalisation in two ways. First, I use it to describe the process by which a body perceived as 'permanently crippled' was transformed into one 'temporarily injured' and which could be healed via medical intervention. This can be understood as the 'medicalisation of disability'. Secondly, I am interested in how German orthopaedists used their medical expertise to become authorities in the re-organisation of the empire for 'total war'. This process is denoted as the 'medicalisation of war'.[51]

Organisation of the study

Chapter 1 examines how the First World War transformed the practice of orthopaedic medicine. It begins with a discussion of pre-war attempts by orthopaedists to professionalise, while also outlining the limits which prevented their efforts. As the war forced many orthopaedists to modify existing treatments or invent wholly new ones, these doctors began to argue that their medical expertise could offer the German state that which no other health professionals could – the full restoration of the severely wounded soldier and his re-insertion into the economic fabric of the nation. In arguing that they were uniquely qualified to heal the disabled, orthopaedists began to carve out their own specialised sphere of medicine and slowly distance themselves from their professional competitors. As chapter 1 ultimately points out, the Great War had a far more significant impact on the professional and social trajectories of orthopaedics in the German Empire than it did in other nations.[52]

In order to return the disabled to work, however, orthopaedists needed to re-invent several aspects of their field. These innovations are the subjects of chapters 2 and 3. Chapter 2 examines the revolution in prosthetic design and demonstrates how the new project of rehabilitating the disabled soldier necessitated the development of a wide variety of new artificial limbs. Therefore orthopaedists joined ranks with engineers and 'scientists of work' to develop prosthetic devices which more closely replicated the functions rather than the form of the human body. This 'functional revolution' in artificial limb technology – and its correlation to deeper war-time fears about class, gender, and the body – is the subject of chapter 2.

Rehabilitating the disabled soldier required more than simply re-inventing his body through sturdy technology, however. Returning these men to the workplace also required the creation of new rehabilitative treatments, therapeutic institutes, and social programmes. Therefore orthopaedists expanded the scope of their expertise to include developing broader programmes of re-membering (*Wiedereingliederung*) the disabled soldier back into society. The social re-membering included not just the physical rehabilitation of his body, but also the post-convalescence management of the ex-serviceman through a system of *Berufsberatung* which could include career counselling, vocational training, additional secondary education, geographical relocation, and even job placement. Indeed, as chapter 3 demonstrates, the reinsertion of the wounded warrior into the socio-economic fabric of the Empire was ultimately guided with as much attention to the crumbling social order of war-time Germany as it was to the individual needs of the permanently maimed.

Chapter 4 looks at how orthopaedists expanded their work to include the re-education of contemporary Germans about the disabled body. Many Germans rejected the notion that the permanently injured body was capable of rejoining the workforce – or that disabled soldiers especially should be expected to do so. Therefore orthopaedists undertook an 'enlightenment campaign' designed to shift popular perceptions of the injured body. This re-education was designed not only to prove to Germans that the disabled body could be re-enabled through medical technology and returned to work. It also aimed to gain the support and help of the public by demonstrating ways in which the average citizen could help in this project. Through this medicalisation of disability, that is, the re-casting of it as a medical condition which could be cured, orthopaedists argued that the permanently injured citizen should no longer be financially reliant upon the state, but rather should remain an economically self-sufficient member of society.

Chapter 5 examines how the rehabilitated soldier was recycled within the war-time economy of the German Empire. It traces how the healing of the disabled was incorporated into the national re-organisation of labour once the shortage of manpower reached desperate proportions in 1916. First it demonstrates how German industrial leaders began re-using the disabled for the production of war materiel. Then it shows how the military, too, re-organised itself in order to harness more effectively the labour of these newly restored workers. Through two case studies – the Siemens factory in Berlin and the Deputy War Office in Dresden (Saxony) – I show how both industry and army became major proponents of 'recycling the disabled'. All of these subsequent developments, however, were fundamentally dependent upon war-time innovations in orthopaedics and rehabilitation medicine. Therefore the story of how German disabled soldiers were recycled must begin there.

Notes

1 BArch R1501/113089. Letter from General Hermann von Stein, German War Ministry (Minister of War) to all Deputy War Generals, all Deputy War Economic Offices, the Navy, Ministry of the Interior, Ministry for Trade, and all Occupation Armies. September 6, 1918.

2 The vast literature on the military history of the First World War is too abundant to list here. Some good sources for the implications of technology and battle include Holger Herwig, *The First World War: Germany and Austria-Hungary, 1914–1918* (New York: Arnold, 1997), 58–60, 188–92; Dennis Showalter, 'Mass Warfare and the Impact of Technology', pp. 73–93 in Roger Chickering and Stig Förster, eds, *Great War, Total War: Combat and Mobilization on the Western Front, 1914–1918* (New York: Cambridge University Press, 2000).

3 Robert Weldon Whalen, *Bitter Wounds: German Victims of the Great War, 1914–1939* (Ithaca: Cornell University Press, 1984), 50–3.

4 Martin Gilbert, *The First World War: A Complete History* (New York: Holt and Company, 1994), 143–4.

5 Whalen, *Bitter Wounds*, 50.

6 Friedrich Ring and H.W. Hackenberg, *Zur Geschichte der Militärmedizin in Deutschland* (Berlin: Deutsche Militärverlag, 1962), 219–20. Showalter, 'Mass Warfare', 75.

7 [Reichsarbeitsministerium]. *Deutsche Sozialpolitik 1918–1928: Erinnerungsschrift des Reichsarbeitsministeriums* (Berlin: Mittler und Sohn, 1929), 208.

8 Whalen, *Bitter Wounds*, 39.

9 There are discrepancies regarding the precise number of men killed and wounded. The figures cited here are from Herwig, *The First World War*, 446. Whalen notes 2.3 million dead and 4.3 million wounded in his study. Whalen, *Bitter Wounds*, 40, 55–6.

10 Richard Bessel cites a figure of 2.7 million permanently disabled men, but does not distinguish between amputees and other forms of disability. Richard Bessel, *Germany After the First World War* (Oxford: Oxford University Press, 1993), 275.

11 See injury table in Whalen, *Bitter Wounds*, 55–6.

12 Michael Howard, *The Franco-Prussian War: The German Invasion of France* (New York: Collier Books, 1969), 453. Of course it should also be noted that the Franco-Prussian War lasted just five short months.

13 Boris Urlanis, *Bilanz der Kriege* (Berlin: VEB Deutscher Verlag der Wissenschaften, 1965), 94.

14 The number of disabled amputees even exceeded those left in the wake of the U.S. Civil War (1861–1865). According to Figg and Farrell-Beck although some

60,000 soldiers underwent amputation surgery, only 45,000 survived the procedure. Laurann Figg and Jane Farrell-Beck, 'Amputation in the Civil War: Physical and Social Dimensions', *Journal of the History of Medicine and Allied Sciences*, Vol. 48: 454–75. Figures cited on p. 454.

15 For a demographic analysis and statistics on war-time death rates according to age, as well as region and marital status, see Bessel, *Germany after the First World War*, 9–10; especially the table on p. 9.

16 For more on the shift in battle strategy see Roger Chickering, *Imperial Germany and the Great War* (New York: Cambridge University Press, 1998), 66–71; Herwig, *The First World War*, 181–99; Gilbert, *The First World War*, 230–57.

17 Gerald Feldman, *Army, Industry and Labor in Germany, 1914–1918* (Providence: Berg, 1992), 301.

18 Feldman, *Army, Industry, Labor*, 117. For more on this see also Friedrich Aereboe, *Der Einfluss des Krieges auf die landwirtschaftliche Produktion* [Carnegie Endowment for International Peace. Division of Economics and History] (New Haven: Yale University Press, 1927).

19 See W. Hoffmann, et al., *Die deutschen Ärzte im Weltkriege; ihre Leistungen und Erfahrungen* (Berlin: E.S. Mittler und Sohn, 1920) and Konrad Lau, et al., 'Die Organisationen für die Versorgung des Heeres', in *Der grosse Krieg, 1914–1918: Volume 9: Die Organisationen der Kriegsführung* (Leipzig: Barth, 1923). Chapter 6 entitled 'Feldsanitätswesen' (pp. 401–539) can be found in Part 2, Vol. 9 in this multi-volume work.

20 See for example Hermann Cron, *Imperial German Army 1914–18: Organization, Structure, Orders of Battle* (Solihull: Helion & Co, 2002), or D.B. Nash, *Imperial German Army Handbook 1914–1918* (London: Ian Allan, 1980).

21 See for example Hugo Natt, *Zwischen Schützengraben und Skalpell: Kriegstagebuch eines Arztes, 1914–1918*, edited by Heinrich Hesse and Bernhard Natt (Gutenberg: Computas Druck Satz & Verlag, 2010) and Horst Naujoks, ed. *Äskulap in Kurland und Wolhynien, 1914–1919: Feldpostbriefe und Tagebuchseiten von Hans Naujoks, kgl.preuss. Feldunterarzt* [Archiv der Zeitzeugen], 20 (Münster: Monsenstein und Vannerdat OHG, 2012).

22 Christian Kliche, *Die Stellung der deutschen Militärärzte im Ersten Weltkrieg* (Dissertation: FU-Berlin, March 20, 1968). Regarding *Der Spiegel*'s list of medical dissertations of dubious sounding merit, see 'Haken ohne Wert', *Der Spiegel*, Vol. 29 (1969), 60. Ten years later, another student in the medical faculty wrote a somewhat longer dissertation on the politics of German doctors during the First World War, but this too received little scholarly attention – although one wonders if this was because its focus was on exposing the political leanings of so-called 'apolitical' medical personnel and not their actual medical war-time experiences. See Godwin Jeschal, *Politik und Wissenshaft deutscher Ärzte im Ersten Weltkrieg* [Würzburger medizinhistorische Forschungen, 13] (Hannover: Horst Wellm Verlag, 1977).

23 Here for example, in addition to Whalen, *Bitter Wounds*, see James M. Diehl, *The*

Thanks of the Fatherland: German Veterans after the Second World War (Chapel Hill: University of North Carolina Press, 1993), introduction and chapter 1; and Bessel, *Germany after the First World War.*

24 Here for example see James M. Diehl, *Paramilitary Politics in Weimar Germany* (Bloomington: Indiana University Press, 1977); James M. Diehl, 'The Organization of German Veterans, 1917–1919', *Archiv für Sozialgeschichte,* Vol. 11 (1971): 141–84; and most recently Deborah Cohen, *The War Come Home: Disabled Veterans in Britain and Germany, 1914–1939* (Berkeley: University of California Press, 2001).

25 See Whalen, *Bitter Wounds.*

26 See Cohen, *The War Come Home.*

27 Stephen R. Ward, ed. *The War Generation: Veterans of the First World War* (Port Washington, N.Y.: Kennikat Press, 1975). I consider Klaus Theweleit's two-volume study on the misogynist and proto-fascist yearnings of the *Freikorps* to fall into this category as well. See Klaus Theweleit, *Male Fantasies,* 2 vols. Trans. by Stephen Conway (Minneapolis: University of Minnesota Press, 1985–1989).

28 See for example Paul Lerner, *Hysterical Men: War, Psychiatry, and the Politics of Trauma in Germany, 1890–1930* (Ithaca: Cornell University Press, 2003); and Jason Crouthamel, *The Great War and German Memory: Society, Politics, and Psychological Trauma* (Exeter: University of Exeter Press, 2009); Marc Micale and Paul Lerner, *Traumatic Pasts: History, Psychiatry, and Trauma in the Modern Age, 1870–1930* [Cambridge Studies in the History of Medicine] (Cambridge: Cambridge University Press, 2001); Eric J. Leed, *No Man's Land: Combat and Identity in World War I* (Cambridge: Cambridge University Press, 1979); Ben Shephard, *A War of Nerves: Soldiers and Psychiatrists in the Twentieth Century* (Cambridge: Harvard University Press, 2001).

29 See Wolfgang U. Eckart and Christoph Gradmann, eds, *Die Medizin und der Erste Weltkrieg* (Pfaffenweiler: Centaurus, 1996); Roger Cooter, Mark Harrison, and Steve Sturdy, eds, *War, Medicine, and Modernity* (Stroud: Sutton, 1998); Roger Cooter, Mark Harrison, and Steve Sturdy, eds, *Medicine and Modern Warfare* (Atlanta: Rodopi, 1999).

30 See for instance the essays in Eckart and Gradmann, *Die Medizin und der Erste Weltkrieg,* as well as those in Cooter, et al., *War, Medicine, and Modernity.*

31 Susanne Michl, *Im dienste des 'Volkskörpers': deutsche und französische Ärzte im Ersten Weltkrieg* (Göttingen: Vandenhoeck & Ruprecht, 2007).

32 See Hans-Georg Hofer, Cay-Rüdiger Prüll, and Wolfgang U. Eckart, eds, *War, Trauma, and Medicine in Germany and Central Europe (1914–1939)* [Neuere Medizin und Wissenschaftsgeschichte, 26] (Freiburg: Centaurus Verlag, 2011).

33 Daniela Claudia Angetter, *Dem Tod geweiht und doch gerettet: Die Sanitätsversorgung am Isonzo und in den Dolomiten 1915–1918* [Beiträge zur Neueren Geschichte Österreichs, 3]. (Frankfurt: Peter Lang, 1995). Angetter's published dissertation offers a nice overview of the organisation of Austrian military medicine on the southwest front, the impact of chemical weapons on

their medical practices, medicine in the Habsburg navy, and the contributions of private and philanthropic organisations to soldier care during the war. She also offers a very brief, but interesting, comparison of parallel services developed for soldiers in Italy. Although interesting, however, her study reveals nothing about developments in the German Army or Germany at this time. Angetter has also considered the development of military medicine in in the longue duree of Austrian medical history – including a brief section on the Great War. See Daniela Angetter, *Krieg als Vater der Medizin: Kriege und ihre Auswirkungen auf den medizinischen Fortschritt anhand der 2000-jährigen Geschichte Österreichs* (Wien: Österreichischer Kunst- und Kulturverlag, 2004). Brigitte Biwald has also published on Austrian military medical care during the war. However, despite linguistic and educational similarities between German and Austrian doctors, their war-time experiences were in completely separate national, military, and administrative contexts and should for those reasons not be considered identical. For more on Austria, see the two-volume dissertation from Brigitte Biwald, *Von Helden und Krüppeln: Das Österreichisch-Ungarische Militärsanitätswesen im Ersten Weltkrieg* (ÖBV & hpt Verlag: Vienna, 2002).

34 Leo van Bergen, *Before My Helpless Sight: Suffering, Dying, and Military Medicine on the Western Front, 1914–1918* (Burlington, VT: Ashgate, 2009).

35 See for instance the essays in Roger Cooter, Mark Harrison, and Steve Sturdy, eds, *Medicine and Modern Warfare* (Atlanta: Rodopi, 1999).

36 See Roger Cooter, 'Medicine and the Goodness of War', *Canadian Bulletin of Medical History/Bulletin canadien d'histoire de la médecine,* Vol. 7, No. 2: 147–59. For more on the centrality of this thesis, see Roger Cooter, 'War and Modern Medicine', pp. 1536–73 in W.F. Bynum and R. Porter, eds, *Companion Encyclopedia of the History of Medicine* (1993), especially pp. 1541–6.

37 In addition to the previously cited articles and essay collections, see also Derek Linton, 'The Obscure Object of Knowledge: German Military Medicine Confronts Gas Gangrene during World War I', *Bulletin of the History of Medicine,* Vol. 74 (2000): 291–316; William H. Schneider, 'Blood Transfusion between the Wars', *Journal of the History of Medicine and Allied Sciences,* Vol. 58, No. 2 (2003): 187–224.

38 See Mark Harrison, 'Medicine and the Management of Modern Warfare', *History of Science,* Vol. 34 (1996): 379–410.

39 Mark Harrison, *The Medical War: British Military Medicine in the First World War* (Oxford: Oxford University Press, 2010) and Mark Harrison, *Medicine and Victory: British Military Medicine in the Second World War* (Oxford: Oxford University Press, 2004).

40 Wolfgang U. Eckart and Alexander Neumann, *Medizin im Zweiten Weltkrieg: militärmedizinische Praxis und medizinische Wissenschaft im 'Totalen Krieg'* [Krieg in der Geschichte, Vol. 30] (Paderborn: Schöningh, 2006).

41 Seth Koven, 'Remembering and Dismemberment: Crippled Children, Wounded Soldiers, and the Great War in Britain', *American Historical Review,* Vol. 99 (1994):

1167–202; Joanna Bourke, *Dismembering the Male: Men's Bodies, Britain, and the Great War.* (Chicago: University of Chicago Press, 1996).

42 Jeffrey S. Reznick, *Healing the Nation: Soldiers, Caregivers and British Identity During World War I* (Manchester: Manchester University Press, 2005).

43 Sabine Kienitz, *Beschädigte Helden: Kriegsinvalidität und Körperbilder 1914–1923* [Krieg in der Geschichte, 41] (Paderborn: Schöningh, 2008).

44 See for instance Ana Carden-Coyne, *Reconstructing the Body: Classicism, Modernism, and the First World War* (Oxford: Oxford University Press, 2009).

45 See Marina Larsson, *Shattered Anzacs: Living with the Scars of War* (Seattle: University of Washington Press, 2009).

46 See Julie Anderson, *War, Disability, and Rehabilitation in Britain: 'Soul of a Nation'.* (Manchester: Manchester University Press, 2011) and Beth Linker, *War's Waste: Rehabilitation in World War I America* (Chicago: University of Chicago Press, 2011).

47 For casualty statistics, see Whalen, *Bitter Wounds*, 39–40, 55–6; Urlanis, *Bilanz der Kriege*; Cohen, *The War Come Home*, 4. For arguments on how the German experience was different, in addition to Michl, *Im dienste des Volkskörpers* and the essays in Hofer, et al., *War, Trauma, and Medicine in Germany,* see also Cay-Rüdiger Prüll, 'Pathology at War' pp. 131–62 in Cooter, et al., eds, *Medicine and the Management of Modern Warfare* (Amsterdam: Rodopi, 1999).

48 A useful and brief overview of the origins of medical specialisation can be found in George Weisz, *Divide and Conquer: A Comparative History of Medical Specialization* (New York: Oxford University Press, 2006), xi–xxx.

49 Michael Geyer, 'The Militarization of Europe, 1914–1945', p. 79 in John R. Gillis (ed.), *The Militarization of the Western World* (New Brunswick: Rutgers University Press, 1989).

50 Geyer, 'The Militarization of Europe', 80.

51 For a good introduction to the concept of medicalisation see Peter Conrad, *The Medicalization of Society: On the Transformation of Human Conditions into Treatable Disorders* (Baltimore: Johns Hopkins University Press, 2007).

52 In Roger Cooter's definitive work on the history of orthopaedics in Great Britain, he argues that the Great War was more of a caesura, than a watershed in the medical field's development. In his study which examined the field's development in Great Britain within its broader social, economic, and political contexts, Cooter argues that the two world wars were not as instrumental to its success as has been argued. For more on the development of orthopaedics in Britain and the United States, see Roger Cooter, *Surgery and Society in Peace and War: Orthopaedics and the Organization of Modern Medicine, 1880–1948* (London: Macmillan, 1993). For more on how the professional development of orthopaedics in Germany contrasted with the British case see chapter 1 of this book. See also, Heather Perry, 'The Thanks of the Fatherland? WWI and the Orthopaedic Revolution in Disability Care', in Hofer, Prüll, and Eckart, eds, *War, Trauma, and Medicine in Germany and Central Europe.*

1

HEALING THE WAR-DISABLED: THE RE-ORIENTATION OF GERMAN ORTHOPAEDICS

> Its goal is to place modern orthopaedic techniques of splint-setting and fracture bandaging, treatments for joint fractures, physical therapy, and the fitting of new prostheses, etc in the service of the military. (Dr Fritz Lange, *War Orthopaedics*, 1915)[1]

> The war opened up whole new areas of specialty for orthopaedics. The treatment of gunshot fractures, their traction, methods of transport, their subsequent straightening, were all challenges which placed high demands on orthopaedic techniques. ... And thus during the storm of war a new science was born – War Orthopaedics. This science blurred the sharp division between orthopaedics and surgery and therefore these boundaries had to be re-configured once again. (Dr Fritz Lange, *The Handbook of Orthopaedics*, 1922)[2]

In August 1914 the Munich orthopaedist Fritz Lange was dispatched to Cambrai in the north of France to work in a Bavarian Army field hospital. On his railway journey, he was waylaid unexpectedly in Zweibrücken, where local doctors pleaded with him to treat the wounded soldiers who had been recently left there. These men's injuries were so severe that their unit's medical officers had decided that transporting them any further was too risky; thus, when the field hospital was forced to move on, these men had been left behind. Moving them might have either worsened their wounds or spread infection throughout the patient ranks. None of the town's available doctors had been trained in surgery, and before Lange's arrival, it had seemed likely that these men would die. After securing the necessary military permissions for a temporary delay, Lange headed to the nearby hospital to treat these wounded heroes of the nation.[3]

He was shocked at what he found. Woefully unprepared, Zweibrücken authorities had placed the wounded soldiers in a scantily furnished schoolhouse which they had converted into a makeshift casualty station. Still in their dirty uniforms and blood-soaked field dressings, the men lay on straw pallets on the floor. The stench of gangrene hung in the stale air. With no beds, operating tables, surgical instruments, or hospital facilities, Lange was forced to tend more than a hundred men over the next couple of weeks. Like other civilian doctors who left for the field with no idea what to expect, he had had the foresight to bring some medical equipment with him from his clinic in Munich. Still, with few supplies or resources, Lange was compelled to operate on over a hundred bullet wounds and shattered limbs, improvising procedures to accommodate the filthy and inadequate conditions that both he and his patients faced.[4]

In the weeks that followed, Lange realised that the techniques he and other doctors used at home did not transfer well into the war environment. The traction bandages originally designed to attach to sturdy hospital bed frames were useless on field stretchers, as were the soft plaster casts preferred by surgeons at the time. Ultimately deciding that the situation called for him to 'break all the rules', Lange devised new splints which used the men's own bodies for stability, and he made his casts from plaster-of-paris, a material generally rejected by his colleagues. He also discovered that plaster-of-paris could be used to make temporary 'walking casts' for the men, so they might move about on their own – necessary now that gurneys, trolleys, and extra hands were not there to assist the wounded in getting around. A week later, Lange found himself improvising medical instruments as well, even bending silver table forks into surgical retractors because his military supplies had still not arrived. In the end, much to his own surprise, every man he treated survived and, satisfied with their health, by late September 1914 Lange continued on to Cambrai.[5]

Years later, Lange admitted that in the early days of August 1914 he had been uncertain about the role of orthopaedists in the Great War, but that by the end of the year their mission had become much clearer to him.[6] Through his experiences first in Zweibrücken and then later in Cambrai, Lange had begun to realise that the emerging medical specialty of orthopaedics would be central to the healing of Germany's severely injured soldiers – that its expertise would be crucial in the physical rehabilitation of the disabled. The horrific nature of the soldiers' wounds, the poor bandaging carried out by medics, and the unhygienic conditions of the battlefields combined with the long train or wagon journeys to medical facilities had all signalled to him that the skills of orthopaedists would be invaluable in this war. But, at the same time, Lange could see that if he and his colleagues were to be successful in their efforts, they would need to revise many of their techniques. The wounds of this war were markedly different from the injuries orthopaedists had typically faced in peacetime, while the makeshift environments in which he and others were forced to treat the men were not conducive to many established procedures. Orthopaedists, he concluded, would have to re-think their approach to healing injured bodies if they were to be of use to the nation at war.[7]

This chapter examines the impact of the First World War on orthopaedic medicine in Germany and argues that the war-time experiences of doctors in the battlefields and behind the lines inspired them to transform their profession. More specifically, it traces how the high incidence of severe injury among German soldiers prompted the nation's orthopaedists to re-direct their energies toward the treatment and rehabilitation of trauma victims – a move which helped them not only to carve out a new sphere of medical expertise for themselves, but also to establish unprecedented influence over the social and economic policies of the war-time empire. By proving that their healing talents were indispensable to the nation at war, German orthopaedists gained what had eluded them in peacetime – state-sanctioned recognition as a medical specialty. For German orthopaedists, the First World War ushered in a professional revolution.[8]

Orthopaedics and 'cripple-care' in Germany before the war

Before the First World War orthopaedics was a marginal field within both academic medicine and the larger constellation of 'cripple welfare' [*Krüppelfürsorge*] in Germany. Although the art of orthopaedics had been practised since ancient times, by the early twentieth century, the area had not yet achieved status as an independent specialty within German medicine. This lack of recognition can be attributed to several important historical factors: existing divisions among orthopaedic practitioners, the absence of an organised system of disability care, and the national system of social insurance. In the years before the war, orthopaedists in Germany were struggling with specialisation.

The term 'orthopaedics' was coined by Nicolas Andry in 1741 and as the Greek roots of the word imply, straightening the malformed bones of children was the historical root of the discipline.[9] Since the days of Hippocrates medical practitioners had been concerned with the treatment of physical abnormalities even though they did not often understand the cause of these so-called 'birth defects'. These conditions included both genetic and developmental malformations of the musculo-skeletal system, but in either case they were conditions generally recognised as children's ailments because of their manifestation at birth or in early childhood. Orthopaedic disorders encompassed such specific conditions as scoliosis (spinal curvature), kyphosis (hunchback), clubfeet, and knock knees. Eventually they grew to include even those impairments of the locomotor system that were acquired, such as infantile paralysis (polio), stiffened limbs, or arthritic joints.

Over time, both lay healers and university-trained doctors developed therapies for treating these conditions, concentrating primarily on non-invasive procedures such as the stretching or splinting of body parts. Such 'conservative' procedures aimed to straighten misshapen bones by re-directing their growth without cutting into the body. Before the eighteenth century, this kind of 'bloodless surgery' was preferred over invasive surgical procedures, which were generally unsuccessful and likely to result in infection and death.[10]

With the rise of pathological anatomy, medical knowledge about the body increased dramatically. Recognising the difference between tendons, ligaments, nerves, and muscles – as well as how they worked – helped physicians better understand the physiological causes behind many orthopaedic conditions. By the eighteenth century, more daring surgeons began experimenting with invasive procedures for clubfoot or stiffened joints. Still, before the discovery of anti-sepsis and anaesthesia, open surgery remained painful, and risky for both patients and surgeons. Because there was no clear understanding of germ theory, those patients who caught post-operative infections were likely to die. Surgeons meanwhile tended to avoid risky, invasive procedures because failures damaged their professional reputations. Patient deaths also had a negative impact on surgeons' careers. More to the point, however, because few Germans could afford these treatments – conservative or surgical – orthopaedics as a specialty remained an impractical career choice for many doctors.

In spite of the low demand for their services, by the nineteenth century orthopaedics had become a more common practise among some doctors who specialised in more lucrative fields. Paediatricians offered orthopaedic treatments to bourgeois families who could afford their services. Similarly surgeons treated wealthier clients, while charging heavy fees in exchange for the professional risk they took in performing such procedures.[11] Additionally, in response to growing social concerns about the fate of 'crippled children', religious, voluntary, and communal organisations began founding and supporting 'cripple homes' – residential institutions which offered these children a combination of physical care, guardianship, and education. Doctors wishing to concentrate on orthopaedic treatments might thus find employment in these philanthropic spaces. However, their compensation was low and these institutes often housed not just the physically disabled, but also the developmentally challenged and mentally ill. For poor families, this kind of assistance was a welcome solution to providing for children for whom they were unable to care themselves. However, in the nineteenth century, many bourgeois families balked at the stigmatisation such public confinement would give their children. In the nineteenth century, Krüppelfürsorge was not a viable career for most German orthopaedists and these residential institutes for disabled children became largely associated with poor relief, not medical treatment.[12]

By the last third of the nineteenth century, however, all of these conditions began to change. Germ theory and the sanitation revolution were having a radical impact on surgery. With the introduction of early anaesthetics such as chloroform and ether, surgeons were able to operate on sedated patients whose still bodies allowed them time to perfect invasive procedures that had been impossible to perform on conscious ones. The discovery of anti-sepsis increased dramatically the patient survival rate from these surgeries, because for the first time post-operative infection might be prevented, even if it could still not be healed. Orthopaedic surgery improved and invasive procedures became both more common and less expensive. Surgeons began to specialise in the field.[13]

In 1891, the surgeon Albert Hoffa (1859–1907) published a textbook of the specialty which outlined the practices of orthopaedic surgery and instructed students in their operation. In the *Textbook of Orthopaedic Surgery* [*Das Lehrbuch der orthopädischen Chirurgie*], Hoffa included not just the corrective techniques of invasive surgical intervention but also the conservative therapies of 'bloodless surgery'. Although the manual clearly described how surgeons might intervene in cases of club foot, scoliosis, muscle atrophy, and congenital disabilities, the book still presented orthopaedics as a subfield of surgery, not an independent specialty. Indeed, in the book's introduction, Hoffa struggled to balance the development of the field with its subservience to surgery, voicing his wish that the text itself might serve as proof that orthopaedics was working hard to be a 'worthy daughter to her mother, General Surgery'.[14]

Orthopaedics might thus have remained simply a sub-field of surgery, an area within the larger discipline and not one worthy of medical specialisation – except that in Germany, orthopaedic surgeons were slowly becoming marginalised within their own profession. The advancements in anaesthesia and anti-sepsis had not simply contributed to the evolution of invasive orthopaedic procedures; they had opened entirely new surgical fields. By 1901 surgeons were more interested in perfecting procedures which focused on the body cavity – the stomach, lungs, and other internal organs. Corrective surgery for growth deformities ceased to pique professional interest and many authorities considered the 'bloodless surgery' of conservative orthopaedists to be hardly worth their consideration. By 1900 less than one-seventh of the eighty papers presented at the annual conference of the *German Association of Surgeons* were orthopaedics-related. In response to their own marginalisation at professional conferences, in1901 those German physicians who self-identified as 'orthopaedic surgeons' founded their own professional society, *The German Society for Orthopaedic Surgery* [*Deutsche Gesellschaft für Orthopädische Chirurgie*, DGOC] but in the end this did little to increase their professional profile or secure their position among fellow surgeons. Nor did it change the fact that their services were still costly and beyond the financial reach of most Germans.[15]

The industrial revolution and its medical consequences only furthered the marginalisation of orthopaedic surgeons in German medicine and society.[16] The rapid industrialisation and urbanisation of nineteenth-century Germany significantly impacted medical development. The mechanisation of production in factories increased the incidence and degree of accidents among workers, as labourers were caught up in the swift industrial machinery of the modern age. Hospitals moved away from serving (or housing) terminal patients and began to include acute trauma care as part of their services.[17] Moreover, industrial accidents were not confined to workers in the factories. Modern urban transportation, such as railways, streetcars, and automobiles, brought new varieties of trauma, which required acute medical care, as well. Pedestrians, passengers, and drivers in these rapidly travelling vehicles were frequent victims of accidents in fin-de-siècle cities.[18]

In response to growing social unrest among the population, and pragmatic concerns about national health, the German government passed a series of ground-breaking social insurance laws in the 1880s. Accident, sickness, and invalidity insurance provided for the welfare of injured citizens; however, an intricate web of bureaucracy became necessary for the adjudication and award of these claims. Medical doctors came to play a significant role within this system as both healers and evaluators of injury, and thus national insurance created new areas of employment for the nation's physicians. However, because orthopaedic surgeons concentrated on correcting congenital and growth abnormalities and not traumatic injury, a new medical field emerged to specialise in this new area. Traumatologists, doctors who practised so-called 'accident surgery' [*Unfall-chirurgie*], were trained in the trauma centres of hospitals where they treated the victims of these sudden, industrial accidents of modern society. Thus, whereas Roger Cooter has argued that in Great Britain the development of orthopaedic medicine benefited directly from industrialisation, the rise of work-place accidents, and the railway system, in Germany the emergence of these phenomena benefitted the growth of other health fields and medical disciplines in the nineteenth century. By the early twentieth century, it was Germany's traumatologists – and not orthopaedists – who had emerged as specialists in accident care.[19]

Moreover, Worker Insurance Medicine [*Arbeiter-Versicherungsmedizin*] evolved as a medical field dedicated to treating and evaluating the victims of workplace accidents. Worker Insurance Doctors, specialists trained in this area, were especially crucial in determining how and to what extent a worker had been injured. This was important because the German insurance system was designed to encourage worker recovery, not to award lifelong pensions. Moreover, those injured on the job were entitled to different compensation than those whose injuries were the result of leisure activity. Those workers who could be returned to full-time work in any capacity were expected to do so, even if it meant a change of vocation. In fact pensions were calculated in order to encourage their recipients to resume work. Sickness pensions were temporary and terminated once the doctor determined that a worker could be returned to work, while accident pensions were calculated low enough such that a return to the workplace was necessary for most recipients. Only those injured workers who were designated by doctors as permanently 'crippled' by their accidents and unable to work at all received invalidity pensions. Thus Worker Insurance Doctors were trained in healing injuries as well as determining the residual work capacity of the injured body. They were not, however, trained in rehabilitative treatments.[20]

Physical rehabilitation was a therapy regimen not generally encouraged under the German insurance laws. Medical treatment under the system was designed to return injured labourers to the workforce quickly, but not required to heal them completely. Thus patients were healed enough to enable them to return to work, but not necessarily to their former job or work capacity. Instead of full physical recovery, insurance programmes focused on occupational therapy – therapeutic regimens designed to increase the labour power, not the full recovery of injured workers. This re-training of the injured body primarily took place in medico-mechanical institutes, where gymnasts and physiotherapists might use lay therapies to re-educate weakened muscles or stiffened joints. Accident pensions were used to make up the income labourers lost when their injuries prevented them from either earning their previous wages or returning to their jobs.[21]

Thus while the passage of health insurance legislation did foster an increase in doctors and surgeons who specialised in accident and disability medicine, there was little space in this medical constellation for orthopaedists, who focused primarily on congenital not acquired disability. Moreover, children who were born with disabilities or who developed them in early childhood were not covered under this insurance system. Their care and treatment continued to be costly and for those whose families could not afford private treatment, institutions and homes remained their only option for medical care. At the same time, the ongoing industrialisation of Germany only increased the incidence of growth malformations in the nation's children, as squalid living conditions and undernourishment promoted rickets, tuberculosis, and bone infections (*osteomyelitis*) among the urban youth.[22] By the dawn of the twentieth century, the sphere of German orthopaedists' work had expanded far beyond the 'straightening of children's bones' and included the foot ailments of adults, the joint problems of arthritics, and the consequences of malnutrition and disease among the urban proletariat.[23] Yet at the same time, as a profession, they were largely still associated with poor relief and private patients. In the years before the war, German orthopaedists started to realise that they constituted a distinct discipline – one which required more state support if they were to achieve specialty status.

Early attempts at specialisation

The growing conviction that orthopaedics was a distinct field of expertise manifested itself in a campaign to gain recognition from the German imperial state as an autonomous discipline within the medical community. In a movement led by a handful of prominent representatives, most importantly Konrad Biesalski and Fritz Lange, German orthopaedists began to systematically carve out their practical proficiencies while also defining a specific patient population. In addition to outlining the parameters of their field, German orthopaedists founded their own journals, published their own specialised textbooks, formed professional organisations, and began to demand clinical space in hospitals, as well as their own teaching chairs in university medical schools. As Claudia Huerkamp has pointed out in her study of doctors in nineteenth-century Prussia, these kinds of organisational manoeuvres were crucial markers of professionalisation. They signalled the break between university-educated doctors and lay healers and were significant steps toward 'establishing themselves as experts with extensive professional autonomy based on specialised scientific training', the crucial markers of professionalisation.[24] When the empire's orthopaedists claimed exclusive access to specific patients, called for acknowledgement of their expertise in certain ailments, and demanded separate clinics, they were establishing themselves as a professional specialty. In the face of increasing marginalisation, they determined to demonstrate their importance to both the state and the public.

In 1906 Dr Konrad Biesalski, a Berlin paediatrician specialising in the care and treatment of disabled children, began to define a distinct patient population for Germany's orthopaedists. In order to identify those citizens needing their specialised services, as well as to publicly underscore the ever-widening reach of disability throughout the nation, he conducted the first empire-wide census of Germany's disabled population. Called the 'Cripple Census' [*Krüppelzählung*], this attempt to quantify and describe disabled Germans within the empire was intended to outline the scope of orthopaedics. By surveying the incidence of disability across Germany, Biesalski aimed to present the Imperial government with a comprehensive report of the current work facing orthopaedists, and to underscore the vast public need for their services.[25] According to the statistics which Biesalski gathered, in 1906 there were over 100,000 disabled children – that is, youth under the age of fifteen. Of these, some 50,000 were in need of institutional placement, for which there were roughly 4000 spaces available in homes throughout the empire.[26] Biesalski's census did not measure the number of disabled adults, or offer a total of the empire's disabled citizens (adults and children). This is partly because his goal in 1906 was to collect information to support his call for increasing the financial and institutional support for the nation's needy children.[27] In the years before the war, Biesalski, like many of his fellow orthopaedists, still considered his primary medical responsibility to be toward disabled *children*. Still, the Cripple Census did call public attention to the need to devote more resources to orthopaedic care in order to prevent an epidemic of crippledness [*Krüppeltum*] throughout the Empire.

Biesalski used the figures from the Cripple Census to call for the creation of more residential homes and institutions for the disabled. One of his first responses to this information was to found an institute in Berlin for treating disabled children. In 1906 he opened the doors to his *Krüppel-Heil- und Erziehungsanstalt für Berlin-Brandenburg* with the idea that his small centre would offer disabled children more than simply a home, but would in fact provide them with treatment and experimental healing therapies. His five-room apartment in southern Berlin provided space for up to eight children and here he used both surgery and physical therapy in treating his young patients. Over the next eight years, he expanded his undertaking as he gained both public attention and private financial support, so that after moving operations once in 1907, he was able to open his own free-standing institution. On April 20, 1914, a few months before the war broke out, Biesalski officially inaugurated the 'Oskar-Helene-Home for the Healing and Education of Invalided Youth' in Berlin.[28] Biesalski was not the only orthopaedist to found a private institute for disabled children at the time, and these pre-war years marked the founding of several such establishments around the German Empire in response to the growing need for orthopaedic treatment centres. New homes or charity institutes were founded in Munich, Wolfshagen (Posen), Brandenburg, Cologne, Zwickau, and Braunschweig among others.[29]

In addition to highlighting the growing need for their expertise, in the early years of the twentieth century German orthopaedists were breaking away from their 'parent disciplines' and founding new, specialised professional groups in order to increase their public profile. The German Association for Cripple-Care [*Deutsche Vereinigung für Krüppelfürsorge*, DVK] was formed in 1909 as a direct consequence of the Cripple Census taken three years earlier. The goal of the association was to link the various care-giving institutions, schools, and associations which attended to disabled Germans. It was a broadly oriented organisation whose membership included many non-medical personnel such as social workers, lay healers, government bureaucrats, and charity groups, but which was guided primarily by orthopaedists. Formally established on April 14, 1909, the organisation took as its highest priority the standardisation of care and the centralisation of information regarding the treatments and remedies for the disabled in Germany. As the organisation's first president, Dr Eduard Dietrich, medical advisor to the Prussian Ministry of Spiritual, Educational, and Health Affairs, declared in his inaugural address,

> Everywhere concern has been wakened, now the task is to maintain this interest and to continually reinforce it. The executive committee believes that this can best be accomplished through the creation of a German-wide organisation which will pull together and coordinate all factors of Cripple Care. Its main purpose will be to liberally propagate information – both verbal and written, hold conferences, and manage the press.[30]

For these reasons the DVK also founded its own journal whose first issue came out just before the organisation's formal establishment. The *Zeitschrift für Krüppelfürsorge* [*Journal of Cripple Care*] was an interdisciplinary journal.[31] Its mission was to unify and standardise information about disability care and treatment within the otherwise decentralised German Empire. In addition to printing articles for both lay and professional care-givers on all aspects of the discipline, it offered its readers short notices dealing with medical, teaching, and economic news, government bulletins, case studies of rehabilitated patients, and updated lists of welfare offices across the empire.[32] Moreover, in an effort to ensure the widest possible publicity for these newly developed treatments, in 1910 the DVK began holding biannual conferences in cities across the empire, which not only facilitated the intellectual exchange of ideas and experiences among doctors, but – by inviting members of the popular press – helped to keep orthopaedists and their achievements in the public eye.[33]

At roughly the same time the German Society for Orthopaedic Surgery changed its name to the German Orthopaedic Society [*Deutsche Orthopädische*

Gesellschaft, DOG]. Although at first glance this name change may seem only semantic, the shift from calling themselves 'orthopaedic surgeons' to 'orthopaedists' reflected the physicians' effort to distinguish themselves and their healing specialty as a medical field *independent* of surgery – and not simply a subset within that 'parent field'.[34] Moreover, just as orthopaedists were beginning to distance themselves from surgeons in their professional associations in the first decade of the twentieth century, so too did they begin laying the educational framework for maintaining the occupational standards they were in the process of establishing – a move clearly evident with the publication of the first modern orthopaedic textbook in Germany.

In 1914 the Munich orthopaedist, Fritz Lange (1864–1952), published the first edition of his *Textbook for Orthopaedics* [*Lehrbuch der Orthopädie*].[35] In many ways, Lange was a natural choice for drafting the groundbreaking text which formally declared the separation of orthopaedics from surgery. An orthopaedist of international recognition, he had trained in Jena, Munich, and Vienna before accepting a position in 1908 at the University of Munich as the first full professor [*Professor ordinarius*] of orthopaedics in Germany.[36] In addition to teaching, however, he maintained an active research agenda and, as part of a personal mission to advance orthopaedic treatment among the needy, in 1913 he opened the first public, state-funded orthopaedic clinic in Germany.[37] His technique for tendon transplantation was known throughout the world as the 'Lange method', and he had published extensively in the fields of paediatric orthopaedics, flat feet, paralysis, and tuberculosis. Lange was a path-breaker in the field and his ideas and suggestions carried much weight among his readers – both at home and abroad.[38]

In drafting the first textbook for the specialty, Lange had two goals: to establish the independence of modern orthopaedics from surgery and to clearly delineate the various fields of expertise within the discipline. He positioned his book as the successor to Hoffa's earlier manuals on orthopaedic surgery, while simultaneously underscoring the new parameters of the discipline. 'There is no doubt that the field of orthopaedics has greatly expanded in the past eight years', he wrote, before nodding to the advancements made in treating polio, infantile cerebral paralysis, rheumatoid arthritis, and joint dislocation.[39] Indeed, he added, the expertise of orthopaedists had evolved so much that the field's name now stood in question, and he proceeded to argue that the previously used appellations for their discipline no longer adequately identified the scope of their work. In explaining his point, he elaborated that the term *Extremitätenchirurgie* [surgery of extremities] was inaccurate because it could only designate surgery on limbs or the outermost parts of the body and failed to include spinal malformations, which were still a main focus of orthopaedics. He pointed out that specialists in other countries – indeed other areas of Germany – still understood orthopaedics as the field of 'paediatric surgery'. However, this was also an inadequate term for the field, as it left out the treatment of flatfoot and rheumatism in adults. As he considered an earlier descriptive for their work, 'the treatment of deformities', Lange noted that many contemporary orthopaedists were now treating certain nervous disorders with orthopaedic techniques, and that in these cases their patients did not suffer a *physical* deformity of any kind.[40]

Lange also emphasised that is was especially important to distance orthopaedics from traumatology – the 'accident surgery' [*Unfallchirurgie*] practised primarily on acute injuries and infections. Acknowledging that trauma cases required quick surgical responses, he argued that 'orthopaedic afflictions' required rather the slow, patient, dexterous hand of a surgeon who was not responding to the time pressures associated with most accident victims. Moreover, he pointed out, these same orthopaedic cases were often given too little attention by traumatologists, who were more focused on other procedures. The new orthopaedics was not to focus on emergency surgery, but rather the overall functioning and healing of the human locomotor system.[41] For Lange, the 'modern orthopaedics' marked not just a significant break with the past, but a clear demarcation from accident and emergency surgery.

In addition, Lange argued that the 'modern orthopaedist' should be concerned not simply with surgical procedures, but also with the entire repertoire of post-operative patient treatments for the disabled. He meant that when orthopaedists took on the healing of a disabled patient, it was irresponsible to leave their follow-up care in the hands of the simple bandagist, or physical therapist.[42] Modern orthopaedists needed to be trained and competent in all stages of care for the severely injured patient, and the new textbook reflected this principle. Furthermore, the ideas presented in the volume were not the intellectual fruit or opinion of one man, as was Hoffa's series of textbooks, but more importantly, the result of an ongoing intellectual exchange among orthopaedic specialists from across the discipline. Lange's manual culled the knowledge and experience of his colleagues from Hamburg to Vienna, Breslau, and Würzburg, to present this first comprehensive text of the discipline, which he touted as 'derived of the practice, for the practice'.[43]

The new textbook was far-reaching in its scope. At 790 pages, Lange's volume was shorter than Hoffa's final manual, but was divided into fifteen chapters (as opposed to Hoffa's which had just five). Each of the chapters was written by an area specialist. Altogether they covered general orthopaedics, growth malformations, chronic bone infections, congenital bone dislocation, orthopaedic treatments for nerve disorders, torticollis (wryneck), spinal deformities, spondylitis (inflammation of the vertebrae), and malformations of the arms, legs, and feet. Although many of these areas had received mention in Hoffa's book, in Lange's book they received more detailed discussion and specialised therapeutic instruction.[44]

By early 1914 the specialisation efforts of German orthopaedists were in full swing. They had founded professional organisations devoted to spreading information about the field – both at the lay and specialist levels. National and international conferences had been established to further the intellectual exchange of ideas. New publications, including a German-language professional journal and the first specialist teaching manual, showcased the wide variety of treatments evolving within the new orthopaedics. Yet despite this groundswell of professional activity, on the eve of the war orthopaedics had still not achieved formal recognition as a medical specialty. Few universities required instruction in the field as part of their medical curriculum and the subject remained excluded from examination in the state's medical boards. Thus, those students who studied orthopaedics did so voluntarily, and in addition to their required course load. The only university with a full professor's chair and dedicated clinic was the one in Munich, headed by Lange himself. Only the universities in Berlin, Vienna, Leipzig, and Freiburg offered any sort of orthopaedic clinical instruction, and even these institutions had to rely on one Associate Professor or non-specialist services.[45] Without the steady access to patients which university clinics would have guaranteed, or the inclusion of orthopaedics in the core curriculum of medical education, the field could not establish itself or continue its development. The Great War – and the casualties it brought with it – compelled the German state to recognise the importance of orthopaedics.

War orthopaedics: the impact of war on the discipline

When the German Empire declared war on August 4, 1914, the orthopaedic response was swift. In step with their compatriots, orthopaedists pledged to place their talents in the service of the nation. Many, like Lange, were immediately posted to field and evacuation hospitals at the front. Others, like Biesalski, spent the war years at home, organising care and resources for the wounded warriors who returned from battle. Whether at home or in the field, this rush to support the Empire was inspired by deep patriotism; however, the orthopaedic community also saw in this war-time service the opportunity to prove the usefulness of their nascent specialty. In demonstrating how their expertise might heal the disabled soldier, Germany's orthopaedists recognised the chance to emerge from under the professional shadow of surgery and child medicine.

By mid August Biesalski had begun coordinating many of the nation's orthopaedic and disability resources for the war effort. At the behest of the German Empress Augusta Viktoria, he sent out a call to the nation's private orthopaedists and charity institutions urging them to inventory their resources, and to place them in the service of the wounded. With the support of the Empress, Biesalski was able to bring many of the existing homes for disabled children under his direct supervision.[46] By January 1915, Germany's 'cripple care' community had placed fifty-four clinics, recuperative institutions, and healing centres in the service of the nation's wounded soldiers.[47] Orthopaedists who remained at home pledged to care for the wounded.

Orthopaedists who were sent to the field were unprepared for what they found there. The challenges of the Great War – the harsh environmental conditions, the destructive capacity of modern weapons of mass destruction, and the limited mobility of trench warfare – prompted orthopaedists to revise many of their practices. Lange's own experiences in Zweibrücken revealed that in the first month of the war not only were orthopaedists treating soldiers in unsanitary, makeshift facilities, but were also working with limited supplies and instruments. Despite these conditions, however, Lange improvised treatments and saved these men's lives. He took the lessons learned at Zweibrücken with him to Cambrai where he continued experimenting with how to treat shattered bones, severed limbs, and other wounds of war. Throughout these early months of the war, he meticulously recorded his successes and failures in treating the wounded with the aim of compiling a set of treatment guidelines for military medical personnel.

In 1915 Lange published a field manual for army doctors entitled *War Orthopaedics* [*Kriegs-Orthopädie*]. In it, he detailed the ways in which 'modern orthopaedics' could respond to the war-time situation. Lange outlined techniques for setting splints, bandaging compound fractures, prepping the wounded for transport, making use of physical therapy, and fitting amputees for prostheses – techniques which he had developed during his experiences in Zweibrücken and Cambrai. His goal was to educate military medical personnel – whether orthopaedic specialists or not – to place these specialty innovations in the service of the nation's wounded. This service was crucial, Lange emphasised, because orthopaedics was all that stood between the German Empire and the 'threatening crippledom' of war.[48] The war demanded the skills of all doctors, he argued, 'especially orthopaedists, who, thanks to their technical expertise, can make themselves particularly useful to our wounded'.[49]

The proposition – that orthopaedists were particularly well-equipped to respond to the trauma and injuries of war – probably surprised many contemporary doctors, especially coming as it did from the pen of Fritz Lange.

Just a year earlier in the *Textbook for Orthopaedics,* he had argued against the usefulness of orthopaedics to trauma medicine.[50] Yet Lange now argued that *all* German doctors should learn the rudiments of orthopaedics in order to tend the war-wounded. During the first few months of war, he had clearly started reconsidering the relationship between orthopaedics and trauma – no doubt due to his own experiences.

In the introduction to *War Orthopaedics,* Lange argued that the place of orthopaedics in war had shifted recently in significant ways. Whereas the expertise of the specialty had been marginal in earlier wars, it was now central. This shift, he explained, was occurring for two reasons. First, he pointed out that the 'old orthopaedics' – with its primitive techniques and materials – had offered its patients and practitioners limited results. Second, and more importantly, there had been little demand for orthopaedic treatment, because there had been *so few survivors* with severe injuries. Lange used the example of the Franco-Prussian War (1870–1871) in which the mortality rate among amputees and the severely injured had been between 80 and 90 per cent. Most German soldiers from that war had died from their severe wounds, making follow-up orthopaedic treatment unnecessary. The current war-time situation was different, he insisted, because not only were proportionately fewer amputations being performed, but the mortality rate among those operated upon had fallen to just 3 per cent. For Lange, this was significant in two ways. First, it indicated that physicians were now able to treat many injuries conservatively, without resorting to surgical amputation. Secondly, the survival rate among surgery patients had increased dramatically. Here he noted that in Zweibrücken where he faced 100 patients suffering from severe bullet wounds, in only one of these instances was he compelled to remove the injured soldier's limb. More significantly, though, ensuring the long-term recovery of these men required specialised initial preventive care so that follow-up treatment would be successful. Orthopaedics, he underscored, was indispensable to medical officers and workers in the nation's field hospitals.[51]

Orthopaedists were also useful, Lange continued, because of their expertise in the long-term care of the physically disabled. He pointed out that because this war would produce a far greater number of disabled veterans [*Kriegskrüppel*] than previous wars, orthopaedists would be in demand for years to come. Their familiarity with paralysis, nervous disorders, tendon transplantations, and limb reconstruction therefore made them vital to the after-care and reconstruction of the wounded. 'The war has brought us a huge number of wounded who desperately require orthopaedic treatment', Lange wrote. 'How great this number is, we still don't know; but one thing is certain:

it is much greater than any doctor – including the orthopaedists – had ever suspected before the war.'[52]

Yet, claimed Lange, the low professional status of orthopaedists before the war now placed German military medicine in a disastrous situation. The nation suffered from a dearth of these trained specialists. Because orthopaedics had not been recognised as an autonomous medical specialty before the war, the field had lacked the teaching and research resources that other medical fields received. There was no *Staatsexam* for orthopaedics, that is, no medical-board qualifying examination. Without the pressure of such an exam, few students took classes in the field and thus many contemporary doctors in Germany had little familiarity with the subject.[53]

Moreover, Lange continued to his readers, the instruction of those students who had expressed interest in the specialty had been hampered by their lack of access to patients. Historically orthopaedic cases had been housed in institutional homes or private medical clinics – spaces to which medical students had no access. To make matters worse, the few students that did exist now found themselves stripped of the doctors who could be teaching future specialists, as most practising orthopaedists had been called up.[54] As the numbers of wounded soldiers far outstripped the numbers of qualified specialists, Lange had concluded that the only solution was through remedial education. The best solution was to train all field-hospital doctors and medics in the specialty as soon as possible. Only with their help would it be possible to prevent the 'threatening crippledness' that countless wounded now faced.[55] Thus the purpose in writing *War Orthopaedics* was to 'place modern orthopaedic techniques of splint-setting and fracture bandaging, treatments for joint fractures, physical therapy and the fitting of new prostheses, etc in the service of the military.'[56] To Lange the fate of Germany's disabled – indeed the fate of the army itself – lay in the hands of the nation's orthopaedists.

Demonstrating the discipline's usefulness to the nation's disabled, as well as its armed forces, both continued and modified Lange's quest for specialty recognition. He argued not only that the field was exceptional among other medical fields, but also that the specialty's unique skills and training were of particular value to a nation at war. *War Orthopaedics,* thus, was more than just an orthopaedic how-to manual for general practitioners who found themselves at the front. Lange was aware that military authorities, not just doctors, would be reading his manual. Its publication marked an attempt to carve out the centrality of orthopaedic expertise to the long-term care and welfare of the nation's disabled soldiers while ensuring that the German state became aware of this.

War Orthopaedics provides a rare glimpse of medical innovation in the chaos of conflict (as opposed to the more typical recollections and memoirs of military doctors published after a war). The manual had six chapters: transporting the wounded; treating bullet-wound fractures; post-operative care for bullet wounds; treating bone dislocations; injury-related paralysis; and artificial limbs. While many therapies were geared toward treating war-related injuries, others focused on adapting orthopaedic procedures to war-time conditions. For instance, instructions on transporting the wounded included new methods for immobilising the injured, so further bodily damage might be prevented. Physical therapy was introduced as a way of retraining a body part that was stiffened by weakened or reconstructed tendons. Orthotics and other orthopaedic inserts were discussed as ways to treat or compensate for injured limbs. While few of these procedures were new, they were re-fashioned for field and triage conditions.[57] In fact, some of the healing methods were so new that Lange admitted to his readers that some were still undergoing perfection.[58]

Fritz Lange was not the only one to improvise in the face of mounting war-time casualties. Orthopaedists throughout Germany published innumerable articles, pamphlets, and books detailing their war-time innovations. In leading medical journals, they recounted the various ways in which they were responding to the challenge of healing soldiers and their successes in 'reclaiming' the bodies of the wounded. Whether at home or in France, orthopaedists were on the frontlines of soldier care, and they used their experiences to carve out this new sphere of expertise for themselves.[59]

The 1915 treatise from Dr Adolf Silberstein was a case in point. Based upon a talk he had given in early March that year to a local doctors' association, his essay *War Invalid Care and Welfare* [*Kriegsinvalidenfürsorge*] related many current features of the emergent care for the nation's war wounded, while detailing ways to improve and centralise the larger efforts. Drawing on his experiences as the Chief Medical Officer of the Bavarian Royal Orthopaedic Reserve Lazarette (hospital) in Nuremberg, Silberstein emphasised the importance of early orthopaedic intervention in the healing of the wounded. Like Lange, he argued that the rehabilitation of the wounded was better guided by a specialist in long-term care than the surgeon who only saw the patient as an 'interesting surgical case to perform' and then 'sew up and discard'.[60] He noted that intensive occupational therapy [*Arbeitstherapie*], as practised by orthopaedists, was important not just for exercising maimed limbs, but also for its 'psychic' healing effects. Keeping disabled soldiers employed at 'real work' in the blacksmith, saddlery, and cabinet-making 'orthopaedic workshops' while they underwent other treatments proved that the wounded could be made fit for work again. Moreover, he assured his readers, disabled soldiers soon came to 'cherish the blessing [*Segen*] of work' and looked forward to their return to civilian life. In the hopes of influencing government policy, he argued that every military lazarette should be assigned at least one orthopaedist and should construct its own orthopaedic workshop, so that military and medical officials could more accurately assess and treat every wounded soldier.[61]

In Münster, Dr Hermann Paal, the Surgeon General [*Landesarzt*] for the province of Westphalia, also argued that orthopaedists were best suited to lead the rehabilitation of the nation's injured soldiers. In a speech to a local doctors' association in late September 1915, he too emphasised the role of orthopaedics in the emerging area of 'war-disabled care' [*Kriegsbeschädigtenfürsorge*], and regretted the lack of attention to this specialty in medical schools before the war. He also underlined the importance of orthopaedic treatments such as occupational and physical therapy. He noted that wood-working and metal-working studios were particularly beneficial to the rehabilitation of the wounded, but that field and garden work was also medically productive. In the Bethel Institute in Bielefeld, he observed, over thirty different workshops re-educated the bodies and minds of the wounded – all under the watchful eye of an orthopaedist.[62] Dr Max Böhm, leader of the orthopaedic lazarette for the XX. Army Corps in Allenstein, worked with one-armed soldiers in the fields of East Prussia, and published extensively on the ways to rehabilitate amputees for farm labour.[63]

From the outset of the war, discussions among Germany's orthopaedists centred on how they might best respond to the acute wounds of the soldier while also keeping an eye to his future. In doing so, they tied the centrality of their expertise to the long-term recovery of the nation's wounded servicemen. However, this portrayal of orthopaedics as crucial to trauma care was a firm departure from pre-war conceptions of the discipline – both among orthopaedists themselves and the wider medical and lay communities. Thus in addition to educating their professional brethren regarding the benefits of orthopaedics war-time medicine, orthopaedists focused on re-educating the public.

Reinventing orthopaedics: treating the wounded, treating the nation

Although most orthopaedic articles were aimed at a medical or military audience, Lange and others spread the message among the general population as well. As early German military victories gave way to stalemates on the western front, many Germans feared the spectre of endless streams of returning casualties. As Lange and other orthopaedists triaged soldiers at the front, doctors who remained at home faced the task of convincing their compatriots that orthopaedics could not just save the lives of the nation's wounded warriors, but perhaps their futures too. For a population caught in the early stages of 'total war', the notion that this previously marginal discipline promised the salvation of the empire was welcome.

By January 1915 some 30,000 German soldiers had returned from the front brutally injured in some way. It was now clear that the war which was expected to be over by Christmas had no end in sight. In response to growing apprehension among the nation's citizens regarding the fate of the wounded, the German government opened a medical exhibit in the halls of the *Reichstag*. The *Exhibit for Wounded- and Sick-Care* educated Germans about medical treatments being organised for injured soldiers, highlighting the recent advancements in orthopaedics and related fields. At the opening ceremony, Biesalski gave a speech entitled 'The Ethical and Moral Meaning of War-Disabled Care and its Organisation within National War Relief', in which he outlined ways that the new, modern orthopaedics was responding to the needs of the soldier.[64]

Biesalski confessed that despite years of experience treating disabled children, he had quickly realised that the task of healing soldiers – disabled adults – required more than simply applying the therapies used for one patient population to another. This was due not only to the lack of national 'cripple care' medical standards but also to the variety of treatments and healing professionals engaged in this care in Germany. The random, decentralised disability care, which had sufficed for Germans before the war, would be a disastrous system for treating returning soldiers. In touring the institutions and universities throughout Germany, he had taken notes and suggested improvements to each clinic he visited. In trying to consolidate and centralise the nation's resources, he enriched both his own knowledge and that of others, while also spreading ideas for new treatments.[65]

Biesalski concluded that there were three ways in which orthopaedic expertise was of particular use in the treatment of the war wounded: preventive therapy, surgery, and medico-mechanical therapy. 'Preventive therapy', he explained, employed early intervention and treatment to prevent permanent disability [*Krüppeltum*], and to promote healthy healing of the wound. One successful variety of preventive therapy was the 'plaster technique', which relied on hard casts, metal braces, and slings and weights to immobilise and strengthen the injured body part. The 'plaster technique' was, according to Biesalski, a difficult treatment regimen to learn, but it could be used with great success by those who truly mastered it.[66]

Invasive surgery was the second way in which orthopaedists' skills could benefit the severely injured soldier. Advances in surgery and the introduction of reliable anti-sepsis made it possible to re-open wounds after partial healing

– something unthinkable in the time of Germany's previous war. For instance, Biesalski exclaimed,

> you can take someone who has become paralysed on one entire side of his body, because he was shot in the head, and much later, remove the bullet from his brain or drain the abscess; then you'll see to your great joy and surprise, how the previously limp side of the body slowly begins to move.[67]

He also explained how damaged nerves and tendons could be replaced with ones from another part of the injured's body, that soft tissue could be inserted into stiffened joints to promote easier movement, and how poorly mended fractures could be surgically reset to heal properly.[68]

Finally, noted Biesalski, orthopaedists could offer the injured soldier the healing wonders of 'medico-mechanical therapy'. This therapy denoted a wide variety of external physical treatments, which used specially constructed equipment to rejuvenate the sick or injured body through external manipulation. Biesalski explained that hot air, diathermy, electric shock, and even heat lamps could revive weakened nerves and limbs, while external weight could strengthen atrophied muscles. Knowing precisely how to reanimate the injured body with these modern devices had become a core skill of the modern orthopaedist – who, unlike lay competitors, was medically trained in the use of these machines.[69]

The optimism and confidence which Biesalski exuded in his 1915 lecture was put to the test over the next few years as the number and severity of casualties rose exponentially. What began as a response to war became a crucible for the emergent specialty of orthopaedics. In responding to the new challenges of total war, orthopaedists developed techniques for treating the wounded, reinventing and expanding the scope of their field along the way.

Conclusion

When the First World War broke out, German orthopaedists were still struggling to define their discipline as a modern medical specialty. Until 1914, there had been little patient demand for orthopaedists. In the years before the war, most disability services – public and private – had concerned themselves with the welfare of poor, congenitally disabled children. Privately run 'cripple homes', supported by religious or charity groups, took on the responsibility of caring for the indigent disabled – offering them some basic medical attention, primary education, and a home when their families could not. Paediatricians and surgeons however, developed orthopaedic treatments for wealthier Germans who could afford their private services. Some orthopaedists, such as Konrad Biesalski and Fritz Lange, interpreted the medical care and treatment of the nation's disabled children as crucial to national public health, and opened clinics for the less fortunate. As Klaus-Dieter Thomann has persuasively argued, German orthopaedists struggled in the pre-war years to wrest the care of disabled children away from confessional groups and religious societies which simply institutionalised them, in order to offer them medical treatment which might improve their bodies.[70]

Disabled adults, on the other hand, were more generally allocated pensions under the German national insurance system. However accident and invalidity insurance was designed more to defuse a volatile working class than to promote a healthy citizenry. Invalidity pensions offered enough financial assistance to support its recipients, but it was only dispensed to those injured workers who were completely incapable of any work. Accident insurance, however, was orchestrated such that total physical recovery of the injured worker was rarely necessary. Medical treatment that sufficed to return the injured to any paid work was considered sufficient to most Germans. It was easy for middle-class Germans to blame workplace accidents on recalcitrant workers, while employers were able to quickly replace lost workers from a large pool of labour. Given the already marginalised status of orthopaedics within the medical community, they were accorded little regard within the complex, bureaucratic apparatus of the German Empire's national insurance system. With few patients and limited financial incentive, the physical rehabilitation of disabled adults was not a priority before the war, and their long-term care was most often the responsibility of the state, their families, and sometimes work or fraternal aid societies.

In addition to its low profile in German society, orthopaedics had not yet earned the academic recognition enjoyed by other modern medical disciplines. Historically orthopaedics had straddled paediatrics and surgery, and in Germany it had not formally been recognised as a specialty. Before the war, only one university had a professorship in the area and few others offered courses in the field; it was considered too insignificant. Without teachers or classes, of course, few universities had felt the need to build orthopaedic clinics in their teaching hospitals. Without clinics – and the healthcare that such facilities provided those who could not afford the services of private physicians – orthopaedists did not have steady access to a patient population, a situation which is generally necessary to promote research and encourage innovations. Finally, because orthopaedics was not a designated medical specialty, subject to examination [*Prüfungsfach*], Germany's various state governments did not include the subject in their professional board exams [*Staatsexamen*]. The cumulative effect of these conditions was that there existed little academic or professional incentive to study the field – and thus it attracted few students.[71] In 1914 orthopaedics remained at the margins of German medicine.

The First World War profoundly changed this situation. The heavy casualties among the empire's young, fit, male population inspired innovation and expansion within the ranks of Germany's orthopaedists. Medical journals specialising in surgery, disability care, and orthopaedics brimmed with information about how to use orthopaedics in the treatment and rehabilitation of Germany's wounded soldiers. Orthopaedists positioned their expertise as crucial to military medicine so that first responders might prevent widespread disability within the ranks. At the same time, they argued that modern orthopaedics had an important social role in restoring an empire being 'crippled by war'. By emphasising how their specialist knowledge and skills could restore and rehabilitate the injured body of the German soldier, orthopaedists argued that their work was of national importance. Over the course of the next four years, they used these same arguments to extend their medical authority into other areas of military organisation, disability medicine, and social welfare for the war-disabled.

Notes

1 Fritz Lange and J. Trumpp, *Kriegs-Orthopädie* [Taschenbuch des Feldarztes, Vol. III] (Munich: J.F. Lehmann Verlag, 1915), iii.
2 Fritz Lange, ed. *Lehrbuch der Orthopädie*. 2nd ed. (Jena: Gustav Fischer, 1922), v.
3 Fritz Lange, *Ein Leben für die Orthopädie: Erinnerungen von Fritz Lange* (Stuttgart: Ferdinand Enke, 1959), 117–18.
4 Lange, *Ein Leben für die Orthopädie*, 119–22.
5 Lange, *Ein Leben für die Orthopädie*, 117–18.
6 Lange, *Ein Leben für die Orthopädie*, 116.
7 Lange, *Ein Leben für die Orthopädie*, 119–22.
8 For a contemporary perspective on these changes, see the introduction to Fritz Lange's *Lehrbuch der Orthopaedie* (1922).
9 The term 'orthopaedia' in fact combines the two Greek roots: *orthos* 'to straighten' with *paideia* 'the training of children': *Webster's New World Dictionary*, 3rd college ed (Cleveland: Webster's New World, 1988), 956–7. Aspects of the discipline can be traced back to ancient Greece, India and Egypt. In fact, Hippocrates was said to have practised the art of straightening the spine and clubbed foot. For a pre-war account of the history of orthopaedics, see Albert Hoffa, *Lehrbuch der orthopädischen Chirurgie*, 5th ed. (Stuttgart: Ferdinand Enke, 1905), 1–9.
10 Lange, *Lehrbuch der Orthopädie*, 2nd ed. (1922), 1–2.
11 Here the example of Adolf Lorenz is a good one.

12 Klaus-Dieter Thomann, *Das behinderte Kind: 'Krüppelfürsorge' und Orthopädie in Deutschland 1886–1920* (Stuttgart: Gustav Fischer, 1995), 8–28; 175–8, 192.

13 Lange, *Lehrbuch der Orthopädie*, 2nd ed. (1922), 4. D. Wessinghage, 'Die Gesellschaften deutscher Orthopäden in den ersten 20 Jahren', *Der Orthopäde*, Vol. 30, No. 10 (2001), 675–84.

14 See the various textbooks for orthopaedic surgery by Hoffa, including *Lehrbuch der orthopädischen Chirurgie* and *Lehrbuch der Fracturen und Luxationen für Aerzte und Studierende*, 2nd ed. (Würzburg: Stahel, 1891).

15 Wessinghage, 'Die Gesellschaften deutscher Orthopäden', 675–8.

16 Arnim Braun, *Oscar Vulpius: Leben und Werk: Ein Wegbereiter der Orthopädie und orthopädischen Chirurgie in Heidelberg* (Heidelberg: Guderjahn, 1997), 24–5.

17 For more on the changing nature of hospitals and acute care see Johanna Bleker, 'To Benefit the Poor and Advance Medical Science: Hospitals and Hospital Care in Germany, 1820–1870', pp. 17–33 in Manfred Berg and Geoffrey Cocks, eds, *Medicine and Modernity: Public Health and Medical Care in Nineteenth- and Twentieth-Century Germany* (Washington, D.C.: German Historical Institute, 1997).

18 For more on the potential dangers of urbanisation and industrialisation and the concomitant rise in hospital acute care, see Guenter B. Risse, *Mending Bodies, Saving Souls: A History of Hospitals* (New York: Oxford University Press, 1999), especially 467–70. For more on the increased incidence of accidents following the rise of urban transportation, see Anton Rosenthal, 'The Arrival of the Electric Streetcar and the Conflict over Progress in Early 20th-Century Montevideo', *Journal of Latin American Studies*, Vol. 27, No. 2 (1995), 319–42; Viviana A. Zelizer, *Pricing the Priceless Child: The Changing Social Value of Children* (Princeton: Princeton University Press: 1994); and Nathan D. Wood, 'Becoming Metropolitan: Cracow's Popular Press and the Representation of Modern Urban Life, 1900–1915' (Dissertation: Indiana University, 2004), especially his chapter, 'Planes, Trams, and Automobiles: The Dangers and Allure of Modern Technology'. I thank Nathan for sharing his expertise in the history of urbanisation and modern transport and technology with me.

19 For more on the history and evolution of accident surgery, see Franz Povacz, *Geschichte der Unfallchirurgie* (Heidelberg: Springer, 2007). For more on the growing importance and specialisation of orthopaedics in Great Britain, see Cooter, *Surgery and Society in Peace and War*.

20 For more on the evolution of Worker Insurance Medicine and its role within the larger constellation of German social insurance, including sickness, accident, and invalidity insurance, see F. Gumprecht and G. Pfarrius, *Lehrbuch der Arbeiter-Versicherungsmedizin* (Leipzig: Barth, 1913).

21 Gumprecht and Pfarrius, *Lehrbuch der Arbeiter-Versicherungsmedizin*, xix–xxi. For more on the lack of state interest and support for physical rehabilitation, see Greg Eghigian, *Making Security Social: Disability, Insurance, and the Birth of the Social Entitlement State in Germany* (Ann Arbor: University of Michigan Press, 2000), 132–5.

22 Thomann, *Das behinderte Kind*, 21–5, especially 23. Rickets is a disease of the skeletal system, generally found in children, which results from the absence of vitamin D, and is characterised by a softening of the bone. Tuberculosis is a bacterial infection characterised by the forming of tubercles, or small, rounded nodules, on various tissues of the body. Osteomyelitis is a bacterial infection of the bone marrow or bone itself.

23 Hoffa, *Lehrbuch der orthopädischen Chirurgie*, preface.

24 The nineteenth century witnessed the emergence of a variety of professionalisation movements including not just German medicine, but also other 'free' (service-for-fee) professions such as law, engineering, and chemistry. In addition to these 'service-for-fee' professions, other occupational groups such as teachers and clergy were also establishing their professional standards and credentials. For more on professionalisation see Charles E. McClelland, *The German Experience of Professionalization: Modern Learned Professions and their Organizations from the Early Nineteenth Century to the Hitler Era* (New York: Cambridge University Press, 1991). For a discussion which concentrates on the professionalisation of medicine specifically see McClelland, *German Experience of Professionalization*, 73–87; and Claudia Huerkamp, 'The Making of the Modern Medical Profession, 1800–1914: Prussian Doctors in the Nineteenth Century', pp. 66–84 in Geoffrey Cocks and Konrad H. Jarausch, eds, *German Professions, 1800–1950* (New York: Oxford University Press, 1990), especially 66–7.

25 Thomann, *Das behinderte Kind*, 121–59.

26 Membership flyer of the 'Deutsche Vereinigung für Krüppelfürsorge' [DVK] (ca. 1924–1926), BArch R86/1272. See also, Thomann, *Das behinderte Kind*, 137–41.

27 Thomann, *Das behinderte Kind*, 137–41. See Thomann also for a discussion of the history of children's cripple-care more specifically and its relation to orthopaedic medicine.

28 Thomann, *Das behinderte Kind*, 215–17. Biesalski initially opened a small clinic under his own auspices in May of 1906 which could house ten children. At the same time he began raising funds for a larger home with an attached clinic which was eventually named the 'Oskar-Helene-Heim für Heilung und Erziehung gebrechlicher Kinder', in honour of its benefactor, the industrialist Oskar Pintsch. Although the first children moved in on April 20, 1914, the official dedication ceremony held in the company of the German Empress Augusta Victoria was not held until May 27, 1914. See 'Historie des Oskar-Helene-Heims' in *Oskar-Helene-Heim: 80 Jahre Feier* (1994). Pamphlet given to the author June 1998, personal collection.

29 For instance, Dr Fritz Lange founded the first public, state orthopaedic clinic in Munich (Bavaria) in 1910 and its doors opened December 1913 – again, just before the war. For more on Lange see his memoirs, *Ein Leben für die Orthopädie*, 92; and also 'Lange, Fritz' in *Wer is Wer?* (Lübeck: Schmidt-Rönhild, 1950–), 231. For a list of homes for the disabled in Germany in 1909, see Konrad

Biesalksi, *Umfang und Art des jugendlichen Krüppeltums und der Krüppelfürsorge in Deutschland* (Leipzig: Voss, 1909), 146–51.

30 Eduard Dietrich, 'Eröffnungsansprache zur konstituierenden Versammlung', *Zeitschrift für Krüppelfürsorge* 1909/1910, Vol. 2, No. 1: 7–8. Dietrich and Biesalski had known each other since university where they had both been members of the same student corps (fraternity) and studied medicine together. The growth of the DVK was certainly not hurt by the two men's long-standing friendship.

31 BArch R86/1272. Membership flyer (ca. 1924–1926), 2: 'Werde- und Wirkungsgang der Deutschen Vereinigung für Krüppelfürsorge e.V.'

32 BArch R86/1272. Membership flyer (ca. 1924–1926). 2: 'Werde- und Wirkungsgang der Deutschen Vereinigung für Krüppelfürsorge e.V.' See also Thomann, *Das behinderte Kind*, 214.

33 Thomann, *Das behinderte Kind*, 219–21.

34 H.W. Neumann, '100 Jahre Orthopädie in Deutschland', *Zeitschrift für Orthopädie und ihre Grenzgebiete*, Vol. 139, No.5 (2001): 373–4.

35 Fritz Lange, *Lehrbuch der Orthopädie*(Jena: Gustav Fischer, 1914). Although Lange was the principal editor and author of the textbook, the list of contributing authors included Dr von Aberle (Vienna), Dr Bade (Hannover), Dr von Baeyer (Munich), Prof. Dr Konrad Biesalski (Berlin), Sanitätsrat Dr Gaugele (Zwickau), Prof. Dr Ludloff (Breslau), Dr Preiser (Hamburg), Prof. Dr J. Riedinger (Würzburg), Dr L. Rosenfeld (Nürnberg), and Prof. Dr Spitzy (Vienna). *Lehrbuch der Orthopädie* (1914), titlepage.

36 In 1903 Lange was named 'Professor extraordinarius' at the University of Munich. In 1908 he was promoted to 'Professor ordinarius' – the German equivalent of 'full Professor' and chair of the subject.

37 Schön Klinik Redaktionsteam [Editorial Team], 'Von der Wiege der Orthopädie zum Multispezialitätenzentrum: Die Anfänge. Wie alles began'. Schön Klink, www.schoen-kliniken.de/ptp/kkh/okm/klinik/profil/geschichte/ (accessed November 8, 2013).

38 For more on Lange's position in the first chair of orthopaedics and leading role in Germany, see Doris Schwarzmann-Schafhauser, *Orthopädie im Wandel: Die Herausbildung von Disziplin und Berufsstand in Bund und Kaiserreich(1815–1914)* (Stuttgart: Franz Steiner, 2004), 182–6. See also Fritz Lange and Hans Spitzy, eds, *Chirurgie und Orthopädie im Kindesalter* (Leipzig: Vogel, 1910). For more on Lange's high regard in the international medical community, see the editorial written in honour of Lange's 1910 address to the American Orthopaedic Association, Robert W. Lovett, 'Editorial', *J Bone Joint Surg Am.* 1910; s 2–7: 556–7.

39 Lange, *Lehrbuch der Orthopädie* (1914), v.

40 Lange, *Lehrbuch der Orthopädie* (1914), v–vi.

41 Lange, *Lehrbuch der Orthopädie* (1914), v–vi.

42 Lange, *Lehrbuch der Orthopädie* (1914), vi.

43 Lange, *Lehrbuch der Orthopädie* (1914), vi–vii.

44 Compare Lange, *Lehrbuch* (1914), ix–xvii and Hoffa, *Lehrbuch* (1905), ix–xiv.

45 Hans-Heinz Eulner, *Die Entwicklung der medizinischen Spezialfächer an den Universitäten des deutschen Sprachgebiete*(Stuttgart: Ferdinand Enke, 1970), 394.

46 On August 13, 1914 the empress sent a letter to the president of the DVK – Biesalski's old school friend, Eduard Dietrich – encouraging them to not only carry on their work, but also simultaneously to expand their efforts in two directions. First, she requested that the existing homes not only continue to take in disabled children, but that they broaden their scope of their care by taking in those children whose at-home, full-time care kept their mothers from important war-time work. Second, she requested that the rehabilitative institutions and workshops of the disability community prepare themselves for taking on the duties of healing and re-training the severely wounded. Given that the empress herself had little expert knowledge of orthopaedic care but that she had attended the opening of Biesalski's Berlin clinic in 1906, it is not implausible that Biesalski himself might have enlisted the empress's aid in his project of centralising the 'cripple care' resources under his own authority by suggesting that she author such a letter. Konrad Biesalski, 'Die ethische und wirtschaftliche Bedeutung der Kriegskrüppelfürsorge und ihre Organisation im Zusammenhang mit der gesamten Kriegshilfe' [Vortrag im Rahmen der Ausstellung für Verwundeten- und Krankenfürsorge im Sitzungssaale des Reichstags gehalten am 13. Januar 1915] (Leipzig: Leopold Voss Verlag, 1915), 4–5. See also Edward T. Devine, *Disabled Soldiers and Sailors: Pensions and Training* [Preliminary Economic Studies of the War, 12] (New York: Oxford University Press, 1919), 288–9.

47 Biesalski, 'Die ethische und wirtschaftliche Bedeutung', 4.

48 Lange and Trumpp, *Kriegs-Orthopädie*, iii.

49 Lange und Trumpp, *Kriegs-Orthopädie*, 8.

50 Lange, *Lehrbuch der Orthopädie* (1914), v.

51 Lange und Trumpp, *Kriegs-Orthopädie*, 7–8. Lange does not offer much statistical evidence to support this argument, but rather relies more on anecdotal support. Moreover, it should be emphasised that while the absolute number of amputation surgeries performed in WWI was much higher than that of the Wars of Unification, Lange was arguing that the incidence of amputation was statistically lower than in previous wars due to the new alternative responses to war trauma.

52 Lange und Trumpp, *Kriegs-Orthopädie*, i.

53 Both McClelland and Huerkamp discuss the importance of the state certifying boards (Staatsexam) as a measure of professional proficiency among individual doctors, as well as a marker of disciplinary autonomy and professionalisation among medical specialisms. See Huerkamp, 'The Making of the Modern Medical Profession', 67–70; and McClelland, *The German Experience of Professionalization*, 55, 119.

54 Lange und Trumpp, *Kriegs-Orthopädie*, 8.

55 Lange und Trumpp, *Kriegs-Orthopädie*, iii–iv, 8.

56 Lange und Trumpp, *Kriegs-Orthopädie*, iii.

57 Lange und Trumpp, *Kriegs-Orthopädie*, 156–82.
58 Lange und Trumpp, *Kriegs-Orthopädie*, iv.
59 The hundreds of articles written about this subject are too numerous to cite here; however, a look in any medical journal during the war years bears out this assertion. For a useful contemporary summary of articles in the field, see for instance, Prof. Dr A. Koehler, *Die Kriegschirurgie des Jahres 1917*, [*Veröffentlichungen aus dem Gebiete des Militär-Sanitätswesens*, No. 76] (Berlin: August Hirschwald, 1921), especially pp. 124–30. Copy in BA-MA PHD 6/163/12.
60 Adolf Silberstein, *Kriegsinvalidenfürsorge* [Würzburger Abhandlungen aus dem Gesamtgebiet der praktischen Medizin, 15] (Würzburg: Curt Kabitzsch, 1915): 119–30; remarks about surgeons' disregard for patients on p. 122–3.
61 Silberstein, *Kriegsinvalidenfürsorge*, 119–30.
62 [Hermann] Paal, *Kriegsbeschädigten-Fürsorge und Ärzte* (Münster: Universitätsbuchdruckerei Johannes Bredt, 1915). This is a reprint of a speech he held on 16 September 1915.
63 Max Böhm, 'Ueber den Armersatz bei Landwirten', *Münchener medizinische Wochenschrift*, January 22, 1918, Vol. 65: 99–100.
64 Biesalski, 'Die ethische und wirtschaftliche Bedeutung', 4. Biesalski cites the figure of 30,000 wounded in this speech.
65 Biesalski, 'Die ethische und wirtschaftliche Bedeutung', 5. See also, Konrad Biesalski, 'Praktische Vorschläge für die Kriegskrüppelfürsorge', Sonderabdruck aus der *Zeitschrift für Krüppelfürsorge* (Leipzig, Leopold Voss Verlag, 1915).
66 Biesalski, 'Die ethische und wirtschaftliche Bedeutung', 6–7.
67 Biesalski, 'Die ethische und wirtschaftliche Bedeutung', 7.
68 Biesalski, 'Die ethische und wirtschaftliche Bedeutung', 7. When referring to Germany's last war, Biesalski means the Franco-Prussian War.
69 Biesalski, 'Die ethische und wirtschaftliche Bedeutung', 7–8. These therapies are discussed further in chapter 3.
70 For a detailed discussion of this see Thomann, *Das behinderte Kind*.
71 Lange and Trumpp, *Kriegs-Orthopädie*, v.

2

RE-ARMING THE DISABLED: WWI AND THE REVOLUTION IN ARTIFICIAL LIMBS

> 'I wanted to become head forester once.'
> 'So you may still', I assure him. 'There are splendid artificial limbs now; you'd hardly know there was anything missing. They are fixed on to the muscles. You can move the fingers and work and even write with an artificial hand. And besides, they will always be making improvements.' (Erich M. Remarque, *All Quiet on the Western Front*, 1929)[1]

All Quiet on the Western Front is still considered by many to be 'the greatest war novel of all time'.[2] But in 1929, the year it was published, this book was largely perceived as the voice of a lost generation – a generation still reeling from the trauma of the Great War. The novel tells the story of a young student, Paul, who experiences the horrors of battle in the trenches, and ultimately realises the pointlessness of war. As he watches his comrades die or become severely wounded he begins to question the values and ideals of the society he is defending.

Erich Maria Remarque was himself a wounded German veteran of the Great War and he drew upon his own experiences when writing this story. His status as an ex-serviceman is what lent the novel such credibility, and earned its author both the ire and adoration of readers around the world. Remarque's descriptions of Paul's life in the trenches, of the growing distance between Paul and his family at home, and of the mocking attitude of his comrades toward the European rulers whose decisions had resulted in such carnage, struck a familiar chord with millions. Thus, while *All Quiet on the Western Front* was not a true story, the themes, events, and conversations portrayed in the book reflected a reality that many Germans in 1929 could recognise. When Paul tells his wounded friend Franz that the new artificial limbs will not only hide his disfigurement, but will restore his body, he is not just trying to cheer him up. Paul is voicing a sentiment that Remarque and his contemporaries knew to be true: the Great War had revolutionised prosthetic limbs in Germany.

Although the medical goals of German orthopaedists shifted during the First World War, they were still limited by pre-war technology. They quickly realised that if they were going to restore the bodies of the nation's disabled soldiers, they were going to need more than the artificial limbs which had been available before the war. Those prostheses had been designed for either cosmetic appearance or simple gestures, neither of which would help send the permanently injured man back to work. Imbued with a sense of their new wartime mission, orthopaedists developed a wide variety of new artificial limbs – arms, hands, and legs capable of heavy work. No longer satisfied with simply hiding the disfigurement or facilitating the routine gestures of daily life, they enlisted the help of industrial scientists, mechanical engineers, and efficiency experts in designing these new prostheses. Over the course of the war, orthopaedists revolutionised the design and manufacture of artificial limbs, not simply healing the severely injured body, but ultimately restoring it.[3]

This chapter examines the revolution in German prosthetic technology. It examines artificial limbs before the war, and offers an analysis of why those devices were considered inadequate for sending the wounded back to work. Next the chapter analyses the impulses which drove the development of wartime prostheses. Then, through a series of close readings of particular artificial limbs, it demonstrates how embodied notions of class guided the corporeal re-creation of disabled soldiers. Because German artificial limb development concentrated so heavily on the creation of prosthetic arms, rather than legs, this chapter reflects that imbalance in its discussion. However, it also sheds light on why human arms were in some ways more difficult to replace than legs. Finally, the chapter highlights the ways in which orthopaedists argued that their specialised knowledge should earn them primacy of place in directing these developments.[4]

Artificial limbs before the First World War

Orthopaedists did not invent the first artificial limbs, nor were prosthetic devices unknown in Germany before the First World War. Ersatz limbs for missing body parts can be traced back to the third century B.C.E. Pliny the Elder told the story of the Roman soldier, Marcus Sergius, who, during the Second Punic Wars (218–201 B.C.E.), lost his right hand in combat, was fitted with an iron artificial one and thus returned to battle.[5] Artisans in the Middle Ages expended much skill and energy in crafting ingenious but expensive replacements for lost body parts. Several stunning medieval iron arms survive to the present day – the products of ironsmiths more generally remembered for their weapon making.

The arm of the medieval Germanic knight, Götz von Berlichingen is one familiar to many through the work of Goethe. According to the arm's lore, the knight designed the arm himself after having his right hand shot off by a musket during the 1504 siege of Landshut, but the arm itself was forged by a weapons-smith in Olnhausen. The intricate mechanics of the hand included knuckles, which allowed the fingers to bend into the shape of a fist or tightened grip, and clasp objects either by pushing the limb's fingertips against a surface or with the wearer's healthy hand. Expensive and unwieldy – even for a knight – artificial limbs such as these were intended more to display the advances of artisanal craftsmanship than for use in daily life. Indeed there is no evidence that Berlichingen ever wore the now famous arm that bears his name. The pristine condition in which at least one of these limbs has survived today has led some to speculate that it was delivered straight to the glass display case and never used.[6] The important point is that the intention behind these designs was to fashion an artificial limb which could hide the bodily disfigurement of its wearer, either by resembling a glove or piece of battle armour. Over the next 300 years artificial limbs mimicked this 'passive' design. Whether made of wood, metal, leather, or a combination of these materials, the artificial arms and hands resembled the human body, but could hardly operate in the same way. Stiff, and bendable only at artificial joints, these arms depended upon the intervention of the healthy hand for movement, if they moved at all.

By the nineteenth century, artificial limb manufacturers were designing 'voluntary arms' – arms which might be manipulated with the remaining muscle of the residual limb. These designs relied on muscle adduction and abduction to open and close the artificial hand, without the aid of the healthy one. Most designs employed a cord, which was attached to the artificial thumb and ran alongside the length of the prosthesis under the wearer's clothing. This cord was then attached to a strap which wrapped around the wearer's torso or rump. Lifting the residual limb would open the fake hand by tugging the thumb cord taut. Similar tension in the other direction might pull the hand shut. However, because of their delicate construction, weak springs, and pulleys, these limbs could hold only the lightest of objects.[7] Moreover, their expense put them out of the reach of many.[8] Indeed, they were more likely to be used to showcase advances in design, than to be actually worn or used by amputees, and perhaps might better be understood as prosthetic examples of the fascination that enlightenment scientists had with automata in the eighteenth and nineteenth centuries.[9] In spite of their technological advances, they were not *practical, useful* arms.

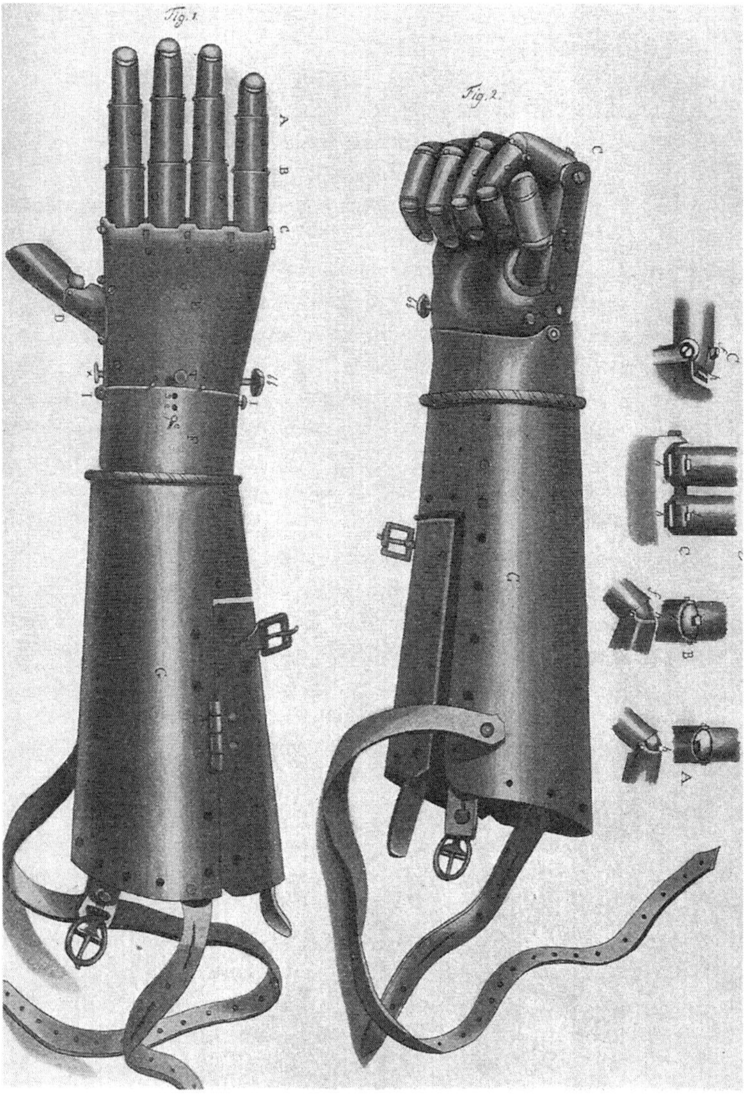

1 The iron artificial limb of the medieval knight Götz von Berlichingen, made in 1509.

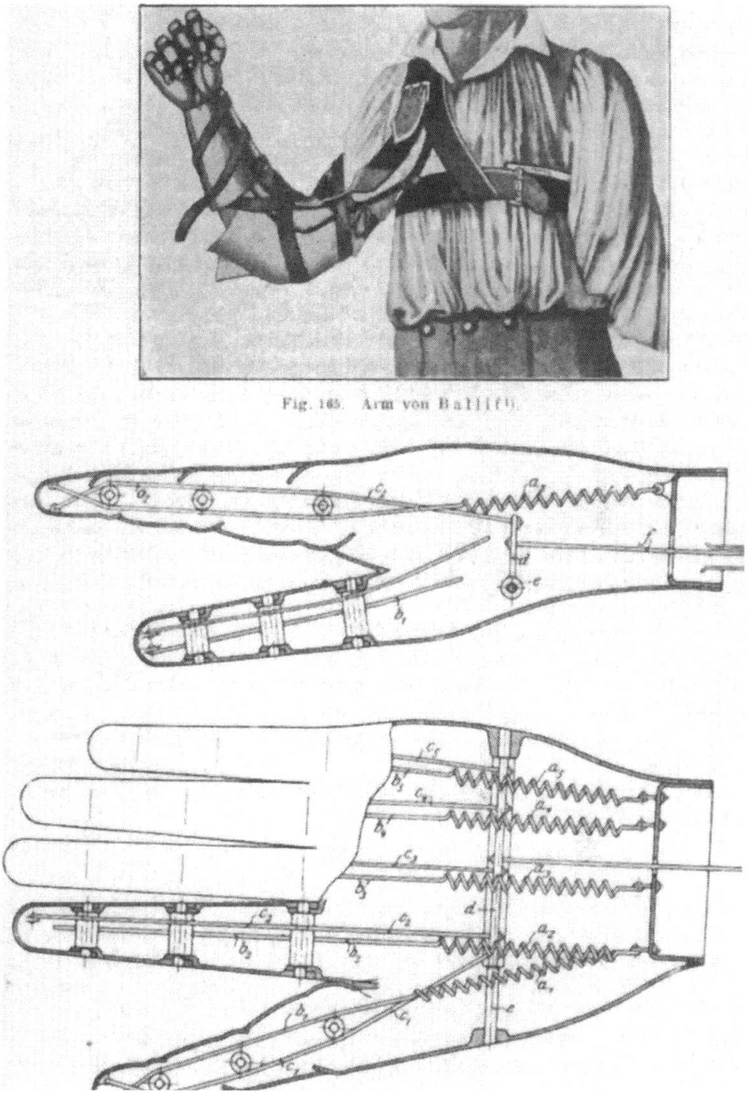

2 This artificial arm by the Frenchman Ballif was the first to employ cords for operating the prosthesis.

By the dawn of the twentieth century, designers were concentrating on cosmetic prostheses that might best reproduce the fine mechanics of the human body, and resemble it as much as possible, as well.[10] Expensive and intricately designed arms replicated the movements of the human hand better than the earlier attempts. There was just one drawback to these arms – their lack of strength. The fine mechanics and multiple parts made them ultimately too fragile for arduous work.[11] These arms were intended for social engagements, or the polite society one encountered at church or on Sunday afternoon strolls. In these instances hiding the disfigurement was of paramount importance, and it is from these circumstances that the ubiquitous slang terms used by doctors and laypersons for this kind of artificial arm – *Sonntagsarm* (Sunday-arm), *Schönheitsarm* (beauty arm), and *Schmuckarm* (decorative arm) – derived their meanings.

They were also far too expensive for most disabled Germans. Although the national insurance implemented in the 1880s provided for accident care, such as pensions and medical treatment, the responsibility for these fell to the injured worker's employer liability insurance [*Berufsgenossenschaft*]. Just as the standards for 'medical recovery' were set by the Worker Accident Doctors – doctors whose jobs and salaries were at the discretion of the firms who employed them – so too were the standards developed for the prosthetics given to accident victims. Not surprisingly, Accident Insurance Doctors did not recommend such expensive limbs to their patients. Rather they assigned them basic work claws and peg legs, cheap limbs which cost employers much less than Sunday Arms.[12]

The *Arbeitsklau* – the so-called 'work-claw' – was a crude claw-like apparatus. It was a sleeve covering the amputated stump with a long, narrow cylindrical rod affixed to its end and to which could be fastened either a hook or pincer. One of the earliest work-claws was the model from Grillpeau and Le Fort developed in 1867 and depicted in Figure 3.[13] Though simple in its design, clearly an arm such as this one with a small cup or receptacle on its end allowed its wearer to hold or steady, however precariously, a tool or other work implement. Exchanging the holding receptacle for the hook (E), offered the wearer another use for the 'arm', such as carrying an object. Though these devices offered little cosmetic value to amputees, they did return some function to the wearer. At the outbreak of war two familiar models were the Nyrop and the Rosset Claws.[14]

The Nyrop Claw basically resembled a pincer with three tines. Two of these were next to each other, often curved at the end, forming a double-pronged hook. The third was placed opposite these two, as an opposable 'thumb', and could be opened and closed, resting securely between the two upper tines

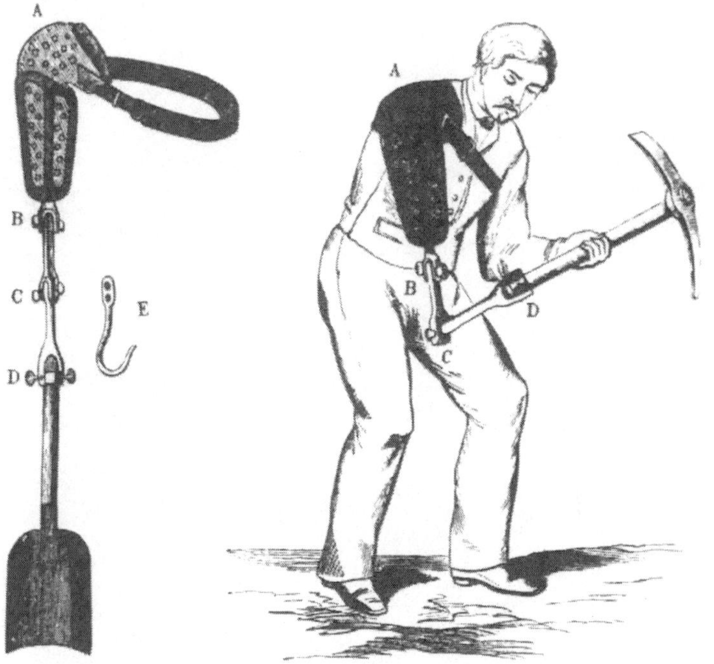

3 An example of a basic Arbeitsklau [work-claw] by Grillpeau and Le Fort.

when locked into place. The claw had to be manually opened, closed, and locked or unlocked by the healthy hand; and, though it in no way resembled a human arm or hand, it was useful for carrying items with handles. So useful, in fact, that it served as the model for all subsequent work-claws. The Rosset Claw, developed by a doctor in Freiburg of the same name, was an improvement on the Nyrop Claw in that the 'thumb'-piece could be swivelled for more variance in grip as demonstrated in Figure 4. And, although prosthetic devices such as these could not perform all the tasks of the human hand, the Nyrop and Rosset Claws offered their wearers more function than any other contemporary prosthetic apparatus available to amputees – though of course, a cosmetic one was better able to mask the disability by completely replicating the appearance, even if not usefulness, of the human arm.[15]

By the outbreak of war, there was no single German, or even European, prosthesis that could reproduce the appearance, strength, agility, and movements of the human arm; nor even a highly functional one capable of any real

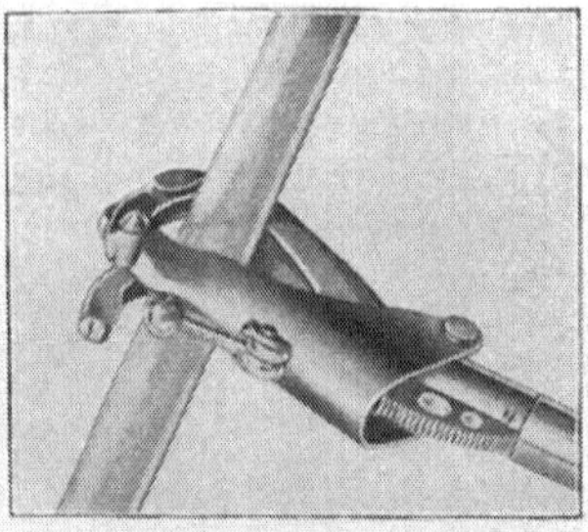
Fig. 429.

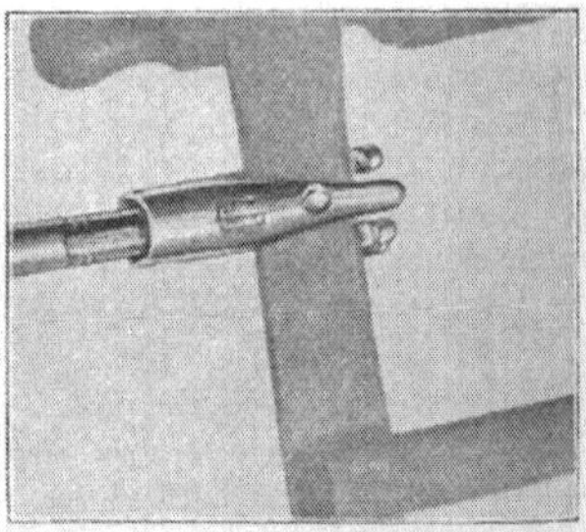
Fig. 430.

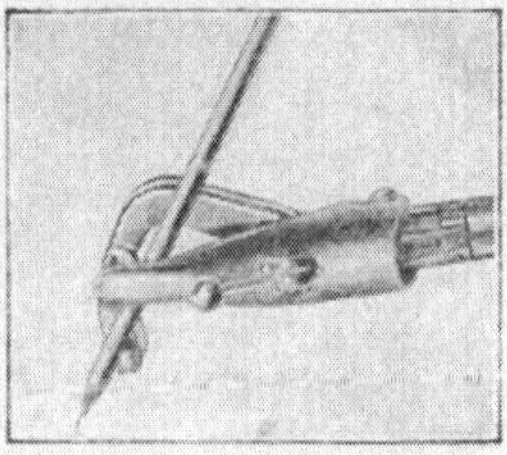
Fig. 431.

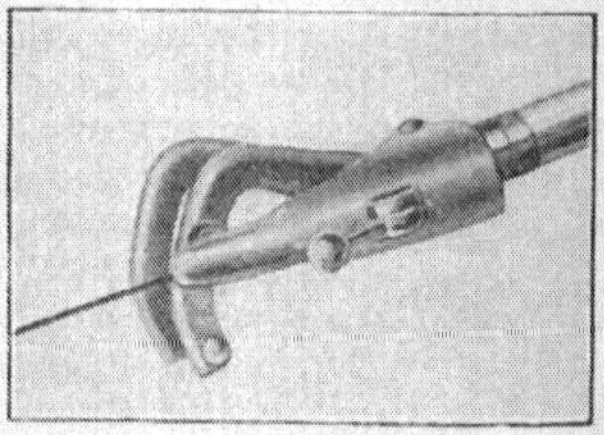
Fig. 432.

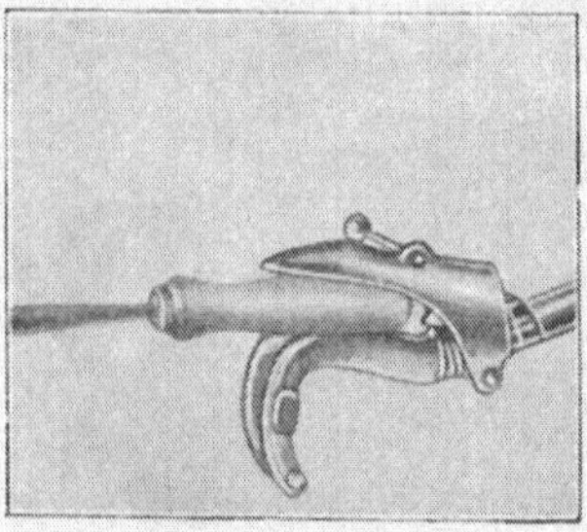
Fig. 433.

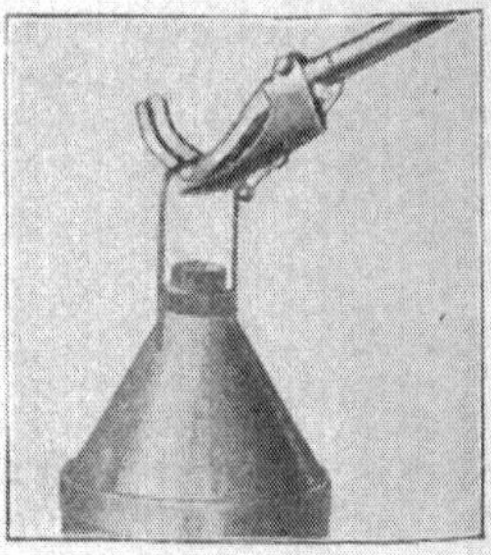
Fig. 434.

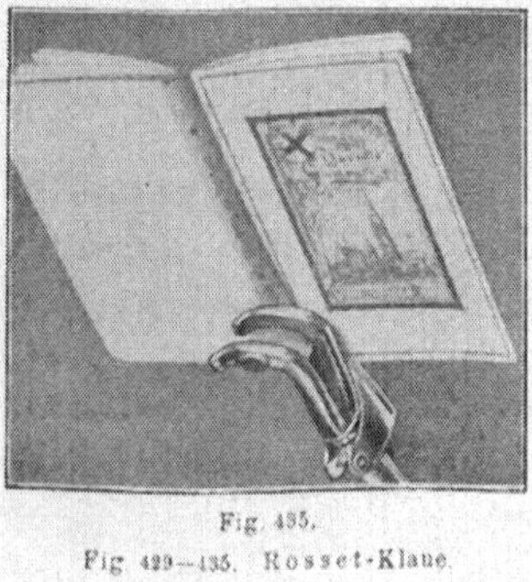
Fig. 435.

Fig. 429—435. Rosset-Klaue.

4 These images of the Rosset Claw depict the various grips it offered wearers.

work. The arm closest to meeting either of these qualities was the American-made Carnes Arm – a marvel of design and function. The limb was remarkable in a number of ways: in its simplification of movements, its compromise in hand design, and in its easy manufacturability. Carnes had combined the opening and closing of the hand in one gesture, so rather than having to rely on various awkward back-and-forth movements of the wearer's torso or rump, the hand could be opened or closed with a simple jerk of the amputated limb's shoulder. Carnes had also re-centred the source of the arm's movement, not only making the limb's construction less complicated, but also making the arm's harness smaller and less dependent upon the wearer's body. The design itself was a compromise between hands with individually movable fingers and fixed ones. The hand was crafted with its four fingers affixed to each other, but they were designed such that they could bend as a whole at the knuckles. Thus although the hand's fingers could not move separately, they did form a cup or hook when bent. Finally, through the application of American taylorised principles of design and construction, Carnes produced these arms quickly. Unlike the masterworks of German artisan production, the Carnes Arm was made of discrete, interchangeable parts.[16] However this arm had to be imported, and with the trade blockade in place during the war, this was a prosthesis which like many American goods became even more costly and unattainable in Germany.[17]

Germany's orthopaedists were in unanimous agreement that this prosthetic selection left the medical community woefully unprepared for the masses of disabled soldiers generated in the war.[18] These devices, though remarkable in mechanical design or resemblance to the human body, left much to be desired in terms of functioning capacity. When the trainloads of wounded began returning from the front, Germany's orthopaedists quickly realised that if they were going to make good on their pledge to return the thousands of Germany's war-disabled to the workforce, the supply of arms – both in number and design – would be insufficient.

Revolutionising the artificial body: the impact of war on prosthetic limb design

Orthopaedists found that sending the wounded back to work required a significant change in designing artificial limbs and a redefinition of 'usefulness' in prosthetic design. Pre-war Sunday-Arms would be inappropriate to assign to the multitude of Germany's war-disabled because they were essentially 'useless' in the workplace. As Biesalski noted in his 1915 *War Cripple Welfare*:

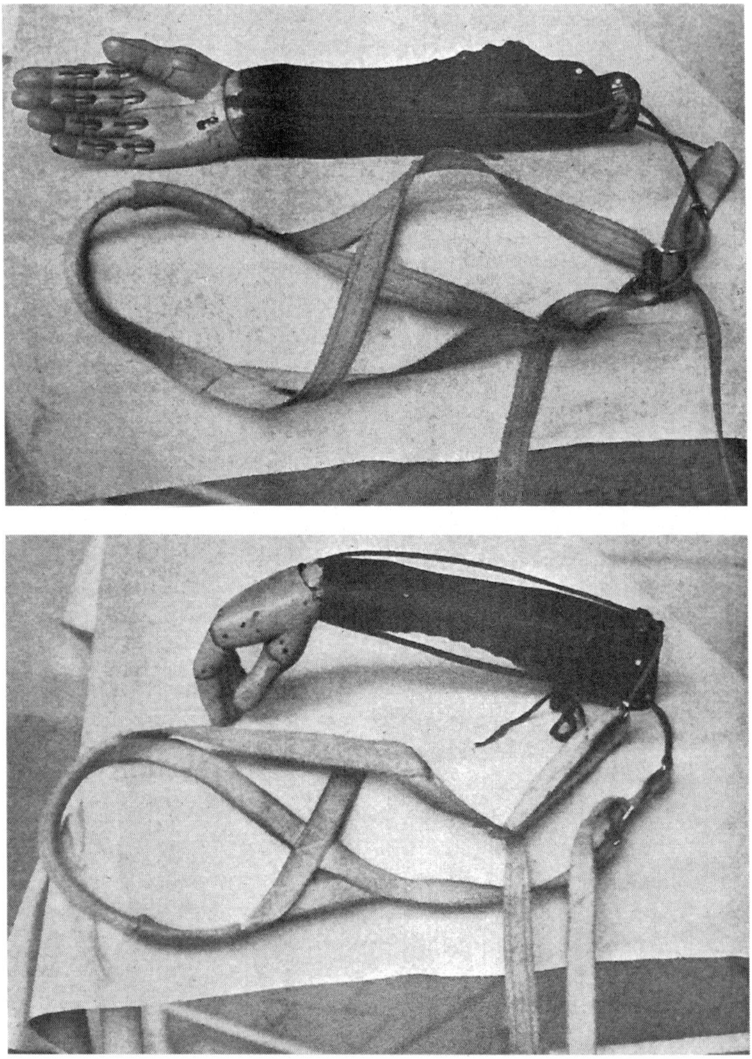

5 The American-made Carnes Arm.

An artificial arm with a hand is, as all lay-people must be told, essentially useful for nothing more than to hide the disfigurement. That is, it should be worn during strolls and used for simple movements: eating, holding a piece of paper, while writing and reading, etc. For any kind of *important function,* it has little value.[19]

Lange, too, described them as having a 'hand which due to the inexpedient movement of the outer three fingers was practically useless – even for simply holding or carrying an object'.[20]

However, even those pre-war prostheses designed to return some functioning capacity to the disabled's body proved insufficient as well. The orthopaedist Adolf Silberstein noted how the new rehabilitation demands necessitated new artificial limb designs as well. Before the war, he reminded his colleagues, no one had seriously expected an amputee to return to his profession – with or without a prosthetic limb. Certainly no one had expected the disabled to earn a full-time living with these devices. Under the accident insurance system, workers who had lost an arm or a leg were usually granted pensions of between 60 and 70 per cent of their pre-injury income, thus any work to which they returned was generally much less demanding; they were not returned to their original positions. Although he noted that some experimental subjects had demonstrated great dexterity with specially constructed limbs, even these amputees had been employed in orthopaedic workshops. That is, they remained in the rehabilitation institute; none had ever faced job competition on an open market.[21]

In order to return the nation's disabled soldiers to their pre-war lives, orthopaedists had to re-think the design and function of artificial limbs. They needed prostheses which would enable an amputee to perform to the same capacity, endurance level, and skill that their able-bodied competitors could. New guidelines in the designing of artificial limbs would have to be followed so the wounded could resume being 'productive members of human society'.[22] Hermann Gocht, a Berlin orthopaedist who began focusing on limb design during the war, noted that the disabled themselves often 'erroneously' emphasised the importance of the artificial limb's capacity to hide the disfigurement. He pointed out, however, that in the design of artificial limbs,

> It is the restoration of function, that is the ability to work again and the ability to accomplish something, which is of the greatest importance. Moreover, this is not simply with respect to the limbs of the severely injured and his will to work, but also for the general public, for the entire nation, and for the state [*für die Allgemeinheit, für das ganze Volk, für den Staat*].[23]

Restoring a soldier's ability to work, rather than his physical appearance, became the primary goal of prosthetic design during the war. Thus function eclipsed cosmetic value as it became increasingly apparent that the construction of a human-looking artificial arm capable of 'productive work' remained impossible. In explaining design goals for the new prostheses, one doctor remarked, 'The human hand – whether it be performing high-culture or serving the wage-labourer – remains at present irreplaceable. It is especially impossible to fulfil demands that a prosthesis take into consideration both appearance and work ability.'[24] Orthopaedists could not combine a practical, useful arm with a cosmetic one, so they dispensed with attempts to hide the disability. They focused on replacing the functional capacity of the hand and not its appearance. Function began to dictate form in the design of prostheses. This principle had significant consequences not only for the development of artificial limbs, but also for the role of the disabled body in the German wartime economy.

In re-designing substitutes for lost body parts, orthopaedists turned to the theories and practices of *Arbeitswissenschaft,* or the 'science of work'. With the rise of industrial capitalism, so-called 'human engineers' emerged to study the physical motions of the body at work. They analysed the speed, angles, thrusts, power, and especially energy deployed by workers' bodies at their jobs. These human engineers conceptualised the human body much like a piece of industrial machinery which could be finely tuned and trained. Their studies were designed with the goal of harmonising the physical movements of the human body with the increasing mechanisation of work under industrial capitalism. By streamlining the corporeal activity of a worker, German scientists of work aimed to eliminate wasted motion and increase worker productivity.[25]

German orthopaedists adopted a similar set of principles. Rather than leave the development and construction of prosthetic devices to craftsmen in workshops, as their predecessors had done, modern orthopaedists worked directly with engineers, motion photographers, mechanics, and surgeons to craft new designs which could better replicate the functions of the body. Until the early twentieth century, most designs for artificial limbs had been either developed or especially contracted by amputees. The process was costly, so the nobility or other well-to-do members of society were the catalysts for their design. These limbs were then crafted by skilled artisans or metal-smiths.[26] However, modern orthopaedists had concluded that in order to provide capable, productive artificial limbs to their patients, they would have to abandon the practice of leaving their development to either the amputee himself or to the hit-or-miss skill of the artisan who chanced to receive the contract for its construction. The isolated, ad hoc design and manufacture had not created the sturdy, capable arms that orthopaedists now required, nor had it resulted in manufacturers outside of a small community. Positioning themselves now as experts in the repair and rehabilitation of the body, orthopaedists decided to become more active in their design.[27]

Thus orthopaedists joined forces with engineers and scientists of work, and began analysing the motion patterns of the human body in the workplace.

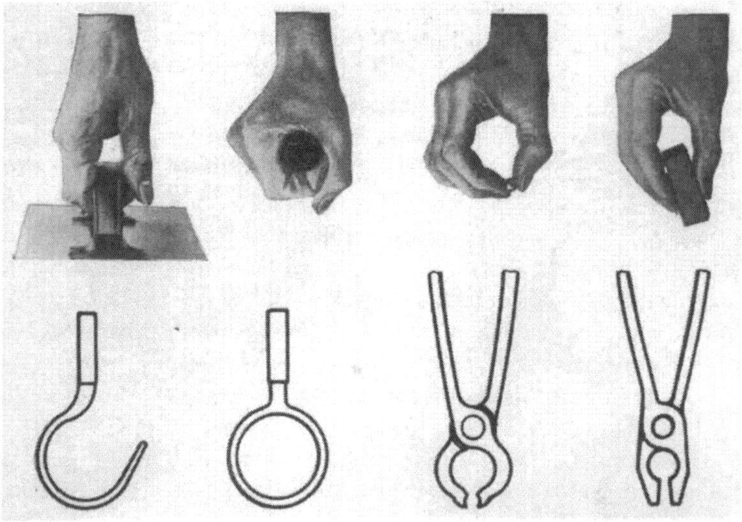

6 Image of the different hand grips which war-time prosthesis designers attempted to replicate.

In studying what one orthopaedist called the 'statics and mechanics of the human body' (what today we might refer to as ergonomics or kinesiology) they examined the human form at rest and in motion, minutely detailing the actions and strength necessary in the body's movements.[28] Engineers helped them to determine which were the most common positions, grips, and formations of the human hand – whether at work or rest. These included grips which resembled hooks, rings, pliers, and wrenches as seen in Figure 6.[29] They then collaborated to craft limbs which replicated these shapes.[30] By analysing the body-in-motion as a series of discrete movements, doctors determined which functions a worker had 'lost' along with his arm or leg. They then focused on creating a corresponding 'work-arm' [*Arbeitsarm*] which was capable of performing these functions.

Although orthopaedists also developed new artificial legs, the creation of specialised 'work-legs' was less of a concern. The majority of professions did not require the trained and dexterous use of the leg in the performance of work. Most productive labour was performed by the human hand. As one orthopaedist noted in early 1915, the basic principles for creating artificial legs and arms were similar. The only significant difference was that 'solving the problem of the artificial hand was much more complicated, due to the fact that arms and hands have to fulfil far more functions than do legs'.[31]

Although specialised legs were not necessary for performing skilled labour, they were important for stabilising the body and providing humans with basic transportation. Whether walking or riding a bicycle, the nation's disabled veterans needed to be mobile if they were going to return to work. Thus, while the productive economy of the German labour force did not require work-legs as much as work-arms, there was still a demand for sturdy lower-limb prostheses. For instance, industrial workers who used their feet for pushing pedals or regulating speed of machinery needed artificial feet that might be easily and accurately manoeuvred. Some workers performed their labour while standing, particularly agricultural workers and service personnel, and their limbs needed to be manoeuvrable as well. Consequently, though orthopaedists spent less time and attention on the design of prosthetic legs, there was a need for reliable, sturdy artificial limbs beyond the typical pre-war peg-leg – a need which they sought to meet.[32]

Once this new direction in artificial limb design had been articulated, Germans across the empire took this mission to design new body parts for the disabled seriously. Orthopaedists, surgeons, engineers, scientists – even craftsmen – drafted hundreds of plans and designs for artificial limbs – all of which needed to be tested and evaluated.[33] According to one report there was a 'flood of inventions – especially of work-prostheses, because the old artificial limbs, which had focused on more cosmetic goals, were not so well-oriented for practical work'.[34]

The German military itself soon recognised the significance of the improvements being made in prosthetic design. In order to evaluate these inventions, in 1915 the War Ministry erected the Centre for Artificial Limb Testing [*Prüfstelle für Ersatzglieder*] in Berlin. This institute was charged with the careful testing of each new device created during the war. During the war, countless recovering amputees were used as test subjects for determining the suitability of these limbs for the industrialised workplace.[35] To gather these devices, the War Ministry sent questionnaires to the Medical Offices in each Army Corps asking for information about the prostheses they were using in their reserve hospitals – including detailed descriptions of their designs and manufacture, and even images. The Ministry also requested samples of these artificial limbs be sent to Berlin for evaluation and inclusion in a permanent public exhibit on new developments in prosthetic technology.[36]

As the numbers of these inventions increased, the War Ministry established branches of the office to help alleviate the pressure on the Berlin headquarters and speed up the process.[37] Take for example the Dresden branch of the Prüfstelle für Ersatzglieder. As part of their mission statement, they included the 'Erlangung von Unterlagen über Neuerscheinungen und Abgabe von

Gutachten' of various new prosthetic devices. Once having ordered and tested the various new prosthetic designs available, they would send these evaluations and recommendations to the various disabled war veterans' organisations. The Dresden office took especial pride in having established the particular usefulness of the Webereiansätze Koselak, that is, Koselak's 'weaver's hand' which according to their tests enabled an amputee to achieve an output rate of 90 per cent of that of a healthy, able-bodied worker. Using these methods of ergonomics and kinesiology, orthopaedists and engineers tested efficiency and measured the productivity of these new prosthetic creations.[38] They also offered construction advice to engineers and mechanics who were inventing new devices, drawing on their own experiences and the experiences of the office's test subjects.[39]

In addition to evaluating the new artificial limbs, orthopaedists conducted scientific studies of the movements of the human body – both whole, able bodies and disabled ones outfitted with prostheses. They studied the motions of the foot as it stepped, tapped, or powered pedals. Using film, x-ray images, and specially built obstacles, they studied the gait of an able-bodied person and then compared it to that of one wearing a particular leg prosthetic.[40] One orthopaedic study made use of the new technology of slow-motion photography, a technique used by German and other European scientists of work in their analyses of the human body as well.[41]

At first, designs for new artificial limbs concentrated on designing 'universal prostheses', artificial arms which could fulfil all the functions of the human arm and which could be indiscriminately distributed to the wounded. Once the Prüfstelle für Ersatzglieder in Berlin had distilled the functions of the human hand into four essential grips, these shapes became the baseline requirements for an artificial hand. The Centre determined that the four necessary hand formations were: the 'pincer-grip', which facilitated picking up an object between the tips of the thumb and fingers; the 'fist-closure', which implied closing the hand like a fist around an object to grip it; the 'ring-closure', which was most useful for closing the hand around an object; and the 'clamp-grip', which held an object, such as a pencil, between the thumb and the fingers (Figure 6).[42] The hope was to design a single arm that would fulfil all these functions and that could be distributed to all war amputees. However, soon orthopaedists confronted the fact that different occupations put divergent demands upon the human body. Certain kinds of work relied on specialised body movements and thus necessitated more specialised arms. For these reasons, prosthetic design eventually broke down along vocational lines. Design – and more importantly, distribution to individual disabled soldiers – became linked to the pre-war (or pre-injury) occupation of the maimed soldier. The project of rebuilding the disabled's body thus became linked to re-building class structure in war-time Germany.[43]

In 1915, the German Association of Engineers [*Verein deutscher Ingenieure*] published guidelines establishing the basic requirements of a prosthetic arm appropriate for artisans, skilled workers and other labourers. Acknowledging the importance of orthopaedic treatment and care, the association had drawn upon the principles of orthopaedic rehabilitation in formulating these goals.[44] The guidelines mandated that:

1. the arm should only function as a work arm, not as a cosmetic arm;
2. the arm should be such that it is worn over the clothing and can be easily and without help put on by the wearer;
3. the power source should come from an uninjured part of the body, preferably the shoulder;
4. the arm stump should not serve to carry the tool holder or be cramped by the prosthetic sleeve;
5. the stump's potential for movement should be maximised;
6. to keep production expenses low, the same arm should be able to be used by both left- and right-handed amputees;
7. it should be able to be used by amputees from all occupations;
8. it should be simple enough for the wearer to be able to keep it clean and in good working order; and
9. it must be resilient and reliable enough for all necessary uses;[45]

One good example of the attempt to create a standard or 'universal' work-arm was the Work-Arm for War-Injured Craftsmen, Workers, and Farmers [*Arbeitsarm für kriegsbeschädigte Handwerker, Arbeiter und Landwirte*] developed by the Siemens-Schuckert-Werke in Nürnberg.[46] This device was a tool-holder with interchangeable working implements. It consisted of a leather harness which could be strapped around the wearer and a metal shoulder-ring which fitted snugly on the residual limb of the amputee. From the shoulder-ring extended two metal rods, which formed the upper arm of the prosthesis. At the end of this 'arm' was a metal joint into which any number of specially designed working 'hands' could be inserted and fastened (Figure 7). These 'hands' ranged in form and shape from simple tools, such as a hammer, to cutlery with elongated handles, and specially designed inserts whose free ends could be fitted and attached to corresponding industrial machinery while the wearer was 'at work'. This arm was suitable for nearly any amputee, regardless of his profession, needing only to be outfitted with the particular inserts necessary for completing his job. Figure 8 illustrates many of the 'hands' available

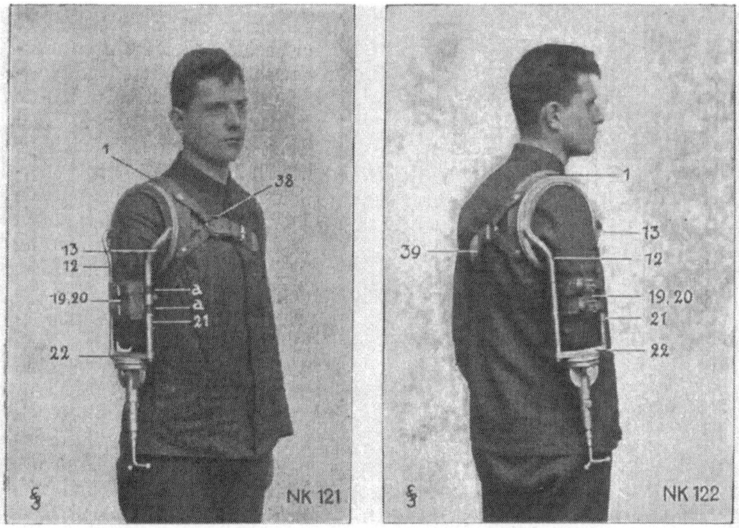

7 Siemens-Schuckert Universal Arm.

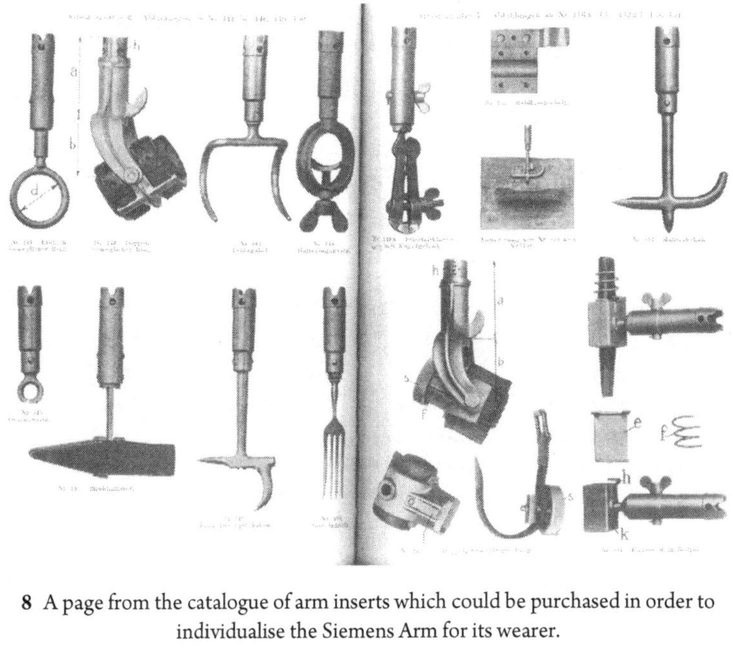

8 A page from the catalogue of arm inserts which could be purchased in order to individualise the Siemens Arm for its wearer.

with the arm. This prosthetic work-arm essentially attached a tool to its wearer, replacing the human arm with a simple instrument of work.

The Siemens Universal Work Arm had many advantages to recommend it. Its design maximised the remaining strength of the residual limb. Its easy assembly and disassembly made it possible for amputees to clean and maintain it themselves without much, if any, assistance.[47] Siemens had also designed over fifty-eight ready-made hand-inserts that could be purchased (separately, of course) and used for outfitting the disabled to return him to work.[48] And, while the arm had not been tested in every working-class profession, the firm noted that workers in heavy industry and farming were able to regain anywhere from half to two thirds of their labouring capacity with its use. Further studies suggested that the arm would be useful in other professions as well.[49] For all appearances, the Siemens Arm appears to have met each of the criteria required in the engineering society's guidelines.

The Siemens Arm also appeared to make good on its promise of universal application. The arm and its many hand-inserts were compatible with many occupations, whether carpenter, farmer, draughtsman, locksmith, lathe-turner, cabinet-maker, tinsmith, or other categories of manual labour.[50] One advertising catalogue noted that a cabinet-maker [*Tischler*] would need to buy a 'head-prop' (#134: Kopfstütze für Bohrleier) for drilling, but also a 'holder' (#106: Greifer für Bohrleier) which could only be used in conjunction with 'guide-discs' (#107: Führungsplatten).[51] In addition, the attachment joint conformed to a standard hand attachment size as regulated by the artificial limb testing centre in Berlin.[52] Any hand-attachments and most work tools produced by other manufacturers could be used with the Siemens Arm. It was thus a universal tool-holder, as well as a universal 'arm'. In the artificial arm industry, 'hands' became standardised and interchangeable, much like the soldier-workers who eventually received them.[53]

The Siemens Arm was nevertheless a costly one. For instance, the three cabinet-making 'hands' mentioned above cost 19.90 Reichsmarks (RM).[54] However, a well-equipped *Tischler* needed up to twenty-four inserts. Together they totalled at least RM 200.00, not including the initial outlay for the arm itself, which amounted to RM 225.00.[55] So, although general arms might be universal, and more economical to produce, they were not inexpensive for their wearers. Nevertheless, orthopaedists endorsed them. Silberstein called the Siemens Arm revolutionary in its design. Noting that other designs focused too heavily on outward appearances, he claimed that for the working class, what was necessary was a machine, a device built by an engineer, not a doctor.[56] Silberstein argued, '[I]t is the first artificial arm which has been constructed exclusively as a work-tool. The uncompromising implementation of this idea – to create a machine and not an "arm" – led logically to considerable divergence from all previous systems.'[57]

The Siemens Arm was not the only new prosthesis which relied on interchangeable 'hands' to rebuild its wearer. The Jagenberg Arm and Rota Arm also relied on multiple hand inserts and were intended to send the disabled soldier back into workplace. The Jagenberg Arm, named after its designer, Emil Jagenberg, offered a variety of specialty inserts designed to be compatible with most machinery (Figure 9). The Rota Arm was even more universal. Developed by the engineer Felix Meyer, the Director of the Rota Works in Aachen, it was designed not only for heavy, industrial work, but also for 'lighter' office work or farming (Figure 10).[58]

The Siemens Arm, Jagenberg Arm, and Rota Arm physically attached these men to their work, binding their bodies to the machinery or tool in the effort to ensure efficient, smooth production. Ultimately not only were the hands themselves interchangeable, but so were the men who wore them. Perhaps a more utilitarian vision of the arm was as a tool itself which could attach any disabled body to any standard industrial equipment – whether a simple carpenter's plane or a piece of factory machinery. Many of these prosthetic 'hands' physically bound the disabled man to his work station. Attaching to the amputee on one end and to machinery on the other, the prosthesis literally blended the disabled man's body into his work. This quest for efficiency melted the boundary between man and machine. In these cases it was unclear whether the disabled man was working the machinery or the machinery was working the disabled man. As if to confirm Karl Marx's prediction that in the future the urban proletariat would become a mere 'appendage of the machine',[59] the disabled worker appeared as a kind of living appendage or *human prosthesis* to the technology of work he wore, as one sees when taking a closer look at Figures 9 and 10.

Whether or not an artificial limb which bound its wearer to factory equipment increased worker efficiency, the physical binding of the disabled man to his work could actually prove inefficient, even hazardous. Dr Ferdinand Sauerbruch, the noted German surgeon, pointed out two fundamental problems with an arm of this kind. First, he argued that the replacing or exchanging of the 'hands' required the constant use of the healthy hand, taking more time than some experts acknowledged. The able hand had to loosen the joint, remove the old tool, exchange it for the new tool, secure it in the joint, and finally tighten the closure. An arm of this kind was useless to the double-amputee who, without the benefit of an able hand, could not open and close the joint himself. Secondly, quickly manoeuvring the work arm was crucial when the worker was attached to motorised machinery. Sauerbruch reported

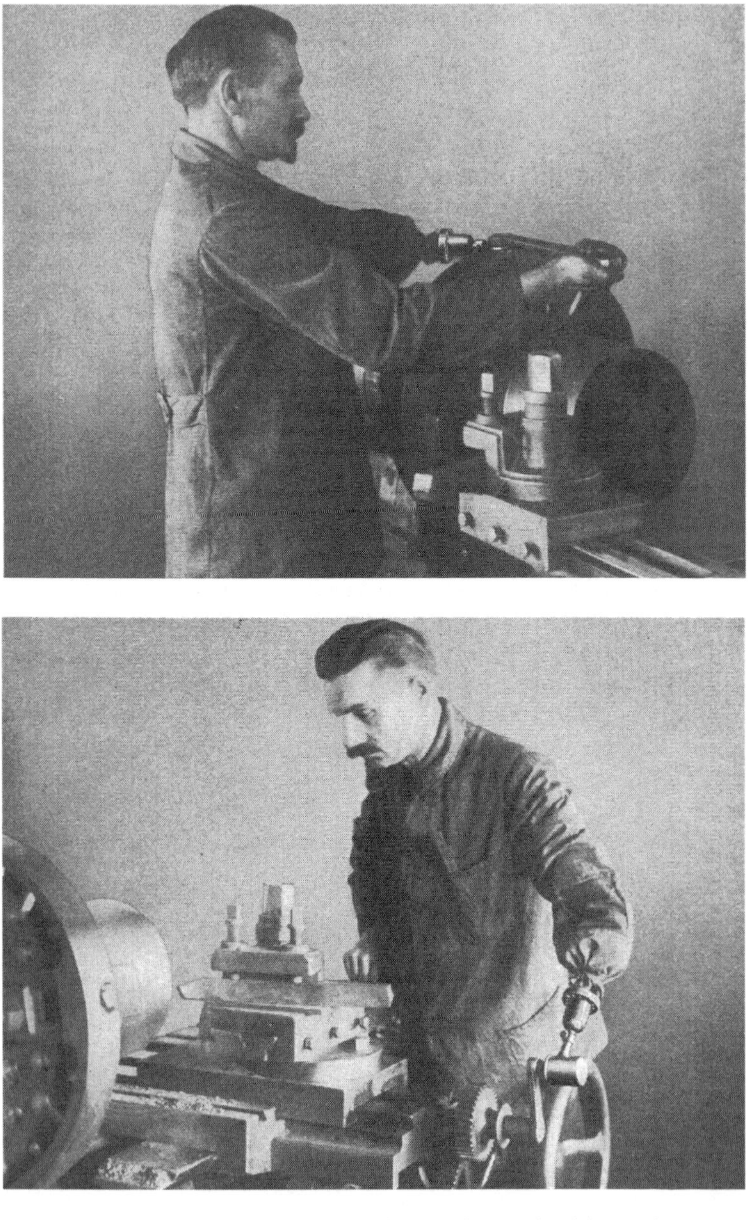

9 The Jagenberg Arm was conceived as a working tool and designed to be factory made.

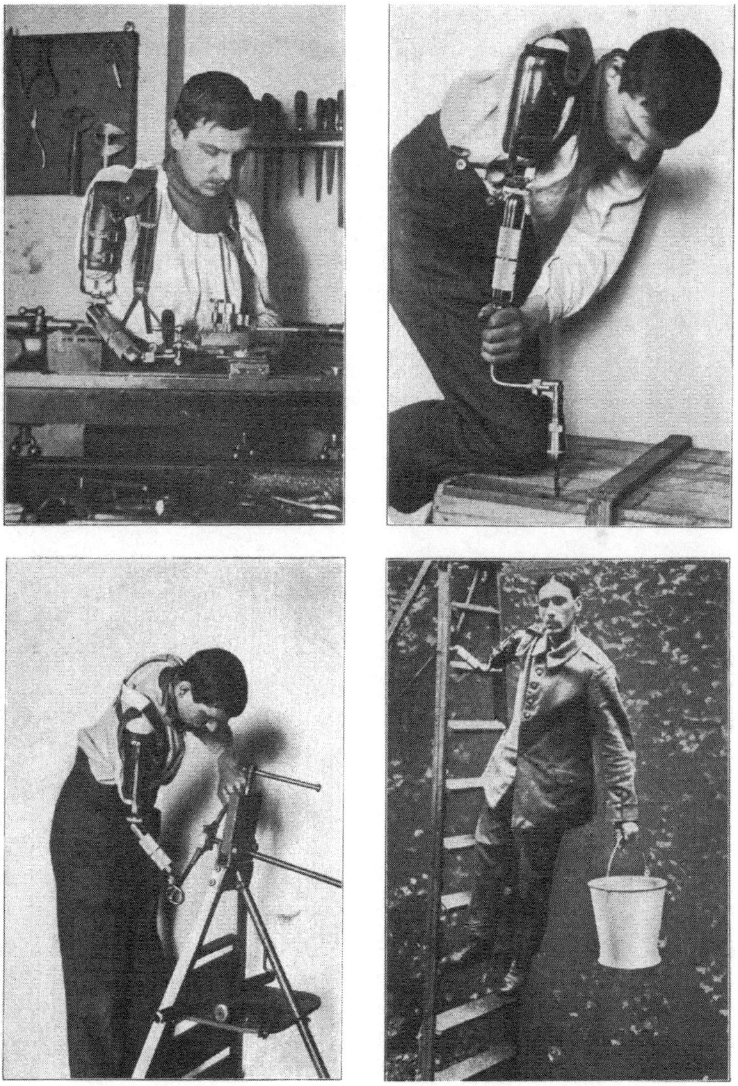

10 The Rota Arm pictured here was designed for light clerical work, as well as industrial and farming use.

observing the upper-arm stump of a disabled worker being ripped from his body when the prosthesis became caught in a factory machine.[60] An efficient and ergonomic design could thus not prevent all hazards in the workplace.

For some, the idea of a single, universal prosthesis was less popular, for as Dr Theodor Mietens, head doctor at the orthopaedic station in Kaiserslautern, remarked,

> In the question of the artificial arm it appears more and more self-evident that a universal appliance, as suitable in all ways as the natural human hand is, can neither be developed, nor does it need be. And, the decorative-arm and the work-arm do not permit themselves to be combined in one and the same tool.[61]

So, some doctors began designing arms for specific occupational groups, such as agricultural workers, workers in light or heavy industry, and for *Kopfarbeiter* (literally: 'head-workers'), such as clerks, teachers, and shop assistants, whose work relied more on mental faculties than manual dexterity. This step was necessary, as Dr Peter Janssen noted, 'because of the demands we must place on an artificial arm, which are completely different, depending on whether it has to do with the Kopfarbeiter, the industrial worker or the agricultural worker'.[62] Doctors realised that developing job-specific artificial limbs created more efficient workers, so they began to concentrate on the manufacture of trade-specific prostheses. This philosophy of construction – letting function dictate form – led orthopaedists and engineers to design artificial arms that were highly specialised and divided along class lines. By war's end, German medical professionals had created well over 2200 different artificial arms, legs, and other prosthetic devices.[63]

One of the more specialised arms was a prosthesis designed for a piano tuner. A soldier, a former piano technician [*Klaviertechniker*], came to the arm distribution centre in Kaiserslautern wanting a device which could return him to his work. The serviceman had already sketched out an idea, and Mietens turned it over to the manufacturing firm of Emil Huber, which turned out the apparatus shortly thereafter. When it was finished, the hand's fingers had been fashioned to make the distance between them equal to the spacing intervals between a quarter, fifth, and full octave on the piano. The third finger was raised above the level of the other fingers, so it would neither hit nor rest upon the interlaying piano keys. Although the finger and wrist joints of this hand were not moveable, it was possible to order other 'tuning hands' whose fingers were set at different intervals. Mietens especially praised this arm.[64]

Another specialised limb was the Letter Carrier's Hand. This was a leather arm with a carved wooden hand which, from a distance, resembled a natural human hand. However, upon further inspection, the inside of the wrist

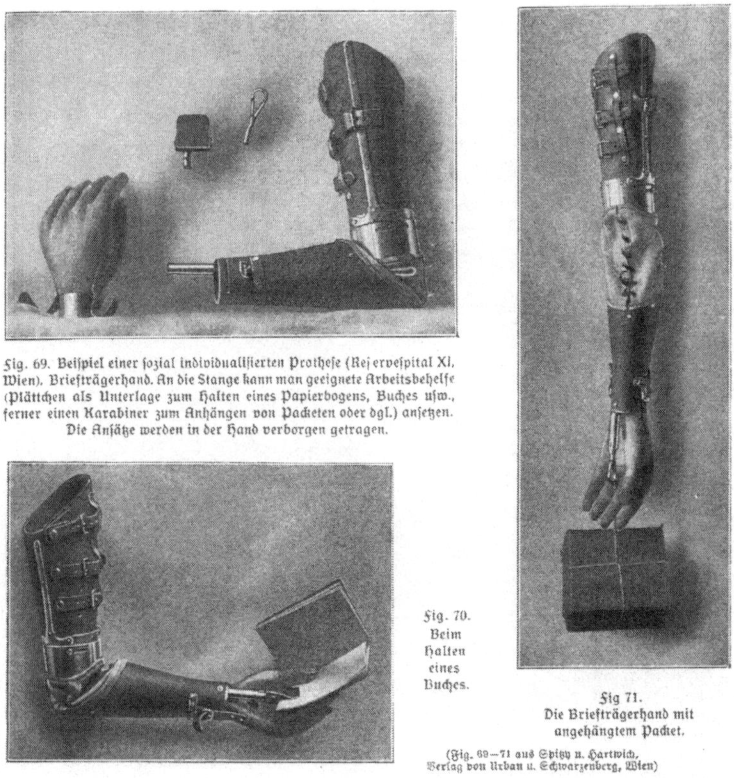

11 This Letter Carrier's Arm is an example of a custom or occupation-specific limb design.

included a small pipe into which several 'postal inserts' could be placed. These included a hook and a clamp, so the artificial hand might grasp the string of a package or bundle of letters with the inserts (Figure 11).[65]

Artificial arms and hands for farmers were also popular. The Keller Hand, a modern variation on the old-fashioned work-claw, was designed itself by a farmer, and considered ideal for agricultural work (Figure 12). This three-pronged metal claw was equipped with adjustable leather straps, which were threaded through a cylindrical opening at the base of the implement and belted around and through the tongs, allowing for the insertion or attachment of any number of farming tools to the work-hand.[66] The basics of this design proved so successful that it was quickly copied with additional variations.[67]

In another case, Hans von Baeyer, a Heidelberg orthopaedist working in

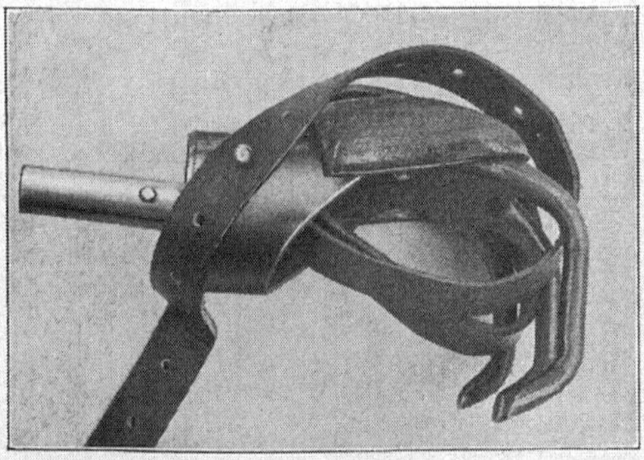

Abb. 12.

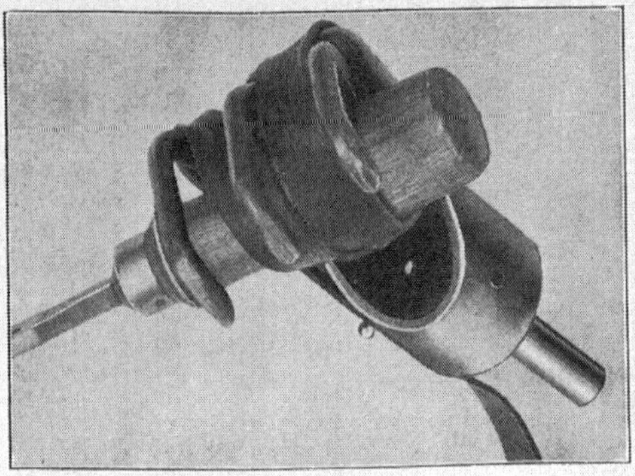

Abb. 13.

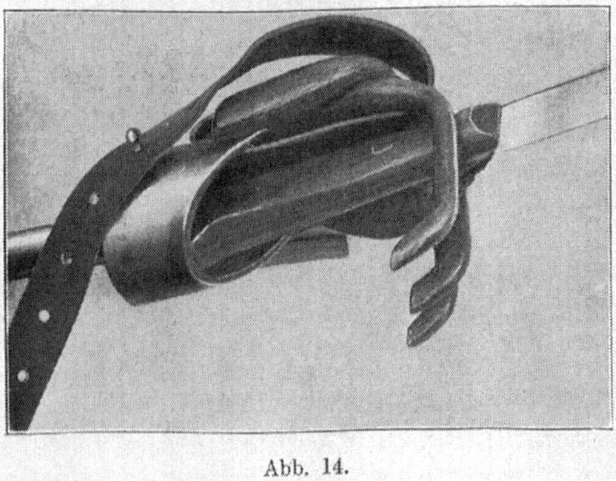

Abb. 14.

12 The Keller Hand was especially designed for farming and other agricultural work.

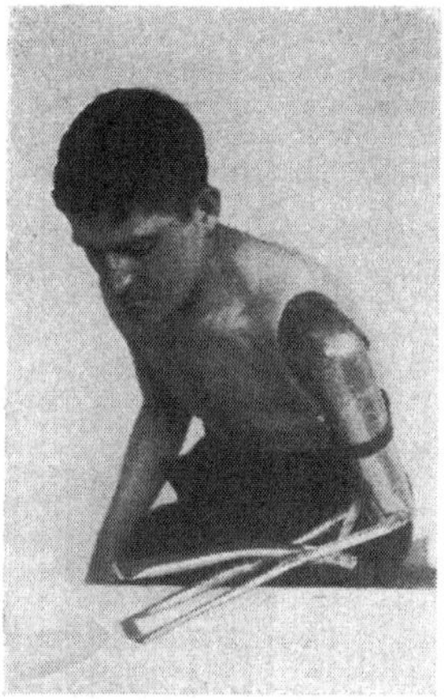
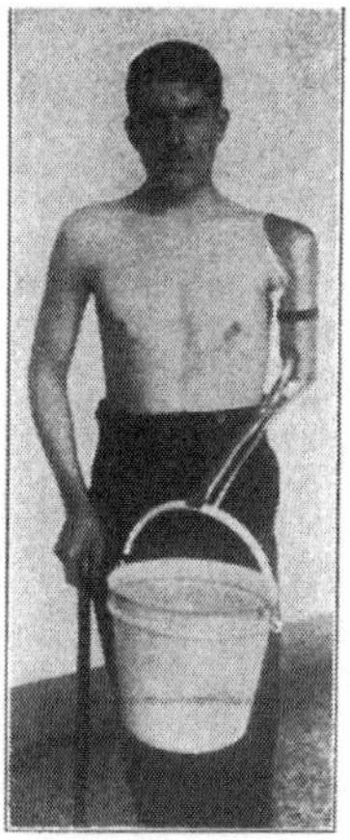
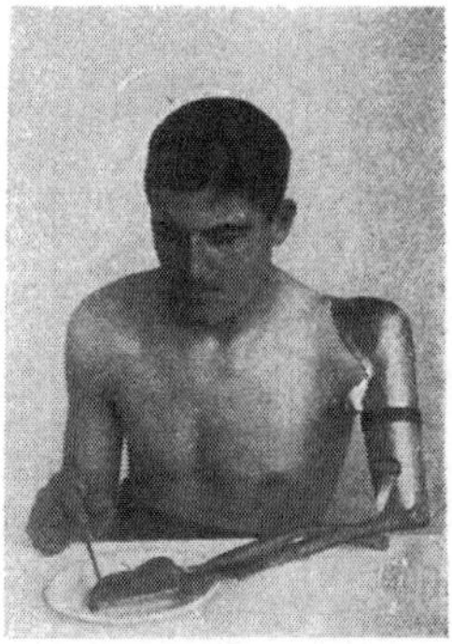

Fig. 97. 98. 99.
Armersatz bei Oberarmamputation mit Greifvorrichtung mittels Hebels nach von Baeyer-München.

13 Von Baeyer's device was lauded as cheap and easily reproduced, yet hardly offered much cosmetic value to its wearers.

one of the reserve hospitals in Trier, touted his personal design for a work-arm made of tin. Von Baeyer's arm resembled a giant pair of pliers, whose tongs were the length of a man's forearm (Figure 13). His primary goal was to create an arm which could be used independently of the able one. His construction allowed a man to open and close the 'branches' of the arm without help. The arm could be opened by pushing down on the 'elbow' joint, forcing open the clamp's tongs. Once open, the wearer could position the arm so that an object might be wedged between the stems of the clamp. Once positioned, the object's weight caused the arm's tongs to close together, thus forming a tight grip. Because the arm relied on the weight of the object it held, heavier objects created more secure grips.[68]

Baeyer emphasised the arm's practicality – it was cost-effective and easy to manufacture. He designed his arm from tin to help in alleviating the 'extraordinarily high' demand for prostheses, as well as to combat their increasing costs. In fact, prices for prosthesis increased as the war continued, not simply as a result of increased demand, but also as a result of the increasing scarcity of raw materials for manufacturing them. The leather typically used for fashioning the prosthetic 'sleeves' for residual limbs was becoming too costly. Therefore Baeyer's arm used sheets of .06mm thick tin, which was both inexpensive and malleable.[69] Although he viewed his arm as ideal, describing it as 'easily produced, cheap, cosmetically satisfactory, and able to be utilised without the help of a healthy arm', we have no records from users of the arm telling us if they agreed.[70]

The timely and inexpensive production of prostheses became increasingly important as the war continued. Economy found its way into descriptions of suitable and appropriate arm design. Mietens argued that a limb must 'have a good display of strength, freedom of movement, a simple construction, the use of which is easily learned, be easy to repair, and last, but not least, be cheap in price'.[71] Given the material demands of the war, this was a tall order; however, it was one with which other doctors agreed. Biesalski, too, supported the idea of inexpensive, factory-made arms, which could be taylorised for easy construction and repair. He argued that,

> Only then can prosthesis construction become so inexpensive that truly every disabled man could acquire that prosthesis which is absolutely suitable for him, just as the wide dissemination of the automobile, the bicycle, the electric light, etc. was first possible when the standard parts became factory-made, available cheaply and everywhere.[72]

Still, manufacturing companies could not keep up with the ever-increasing orders for artificial limbs. At the naval hospital in Hamburg, delivery of artificial arms lagged so far behind patient demand that doctors there developed their own models. Delays resulted in a long waiting periods for prosthetic limbs, creating increasing numbers of disabled sailors unable to begin their post-operative treatments and training. The long wait for appropriate prostheses posed a threat to the success of rehabilitation. Karl Nieny reported that while waiting for their limbs, '[t]here is no opportunity to keep them adequately busy and therefore they are losing quickly and in great quantity their desire to return to work, one which is most often impossible to re-instil'.[73]

For these reasons, Nieny and his colleagues at the Naval Lazarette had developed their own prosthetic arm, which they could factory-produce in Hamburg. Local production enabled the hospital to reduce the delivery time; it also saved money and facilitated quick repairs. The primary principle of development had been to 'create an instrument designed to replace the human arm in as many functional ways as possible, and most importantly in the performance of productive work'.[74] The Hamburg doctors concentrated on reproducing holding and grasping motions, so arms could act as clamps to hold tool handles, nails, and to steady machinery.[75] Nieny's arm included a specially designed stump sleeve, which enabled the shoulder joint to move back and forth, in addition to using a hinge joint at the elbow. This construction enabled more movement at the various joints, facilitating greater work capacity.[76] His model included several different 'hands', as well as a specially designed insert for farmers (see Figure 14).

Like most army hospitals, the Hamburg Naval Lazarette built a work-

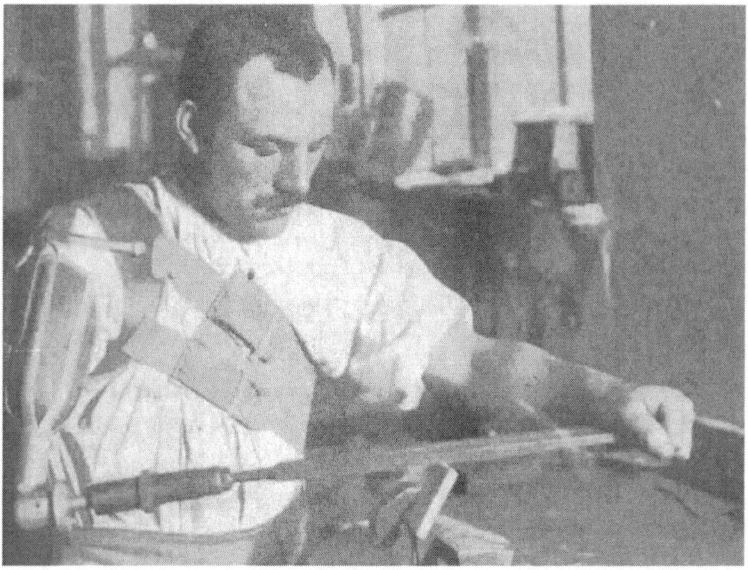

14 Nieny developed his arm to meet limb demands more quickly in the naval lazarette in Hamburg.

shop where the wounded men could practice the use of their arms. Here doctors were able to outfit and train the men in locksmithing, blacksmithing, and plumbing; cabinet-making, lathe-turning and other wood-working trades, some even as tailors, shoe-makers and harness-makers.[77] He regretted, however, that the majority of recovering sailors showed little interest in excelling in these exercises, preferring rather to relearn their penmanship and apply for positions in the government's postal or train administrations. Continued counselling and prompt limb delivery, Nieny was sure, would bring these men back in line. Wounded sailors from the 'educated professions', or those who were independent businessmen, showed far more enthusiasm for their pre-war work. In the final analysis, however, Nieny stated: 'given the importantance of rehabilitation for the national economy [*Volkswirtschaft*], there is no such thing as expending too much work or effort'; he urged his fellow orthopaedists to renew efforts at rehabilitation, despite the resistance of those more stubborn patients.[78]

Most of the arms were designed for the German Empire's manual workers – skilled, unskilled, artisanal, or agricultural. But not all Germany's war amputees required a modified tool-holder in order to resume their professions. The disabled Kopfarbeiter – or white-collar worker – was categorised and treated differently than injured manual labourers. In the main, they would return to work as civil servants, teachers, book keepers, office workers, or other non-manual vocations. Rationalising their motions was not necessary. This worker 'worked' with his mental faculties. Thus no 'teacher's arm' or 'civil servant's arm' was envisioned. Simple, cosmetic arms met the needs of the Kopfarbeiter. The physical work required in these professions consisted of holding papers, carrying light objects, or perhaps writing and filing. So disabled Kopfarbeiter received the so-called 'useless', but more anthropomorphic arms deemed inappropriate for disabled soldiers from the working classes.

Many orthopaedists ruled the Carnes Arm, or an artificial arm of similar construction, to be the ideal prosthesis for Kopfarbeiter (refer back to Figure 5, p. 54). Both Nieny[79] and Silberstein[80] recommended it for the 'intellectual professions'. In his lengthy analysis of the Carnes Arm, Dr Rudolf Ritter von Aberle noted its many advantages. The numerous levers and intricate gears enabled the wearer to perform more detail-oriented movements, which were beyond the scope of the more tool-like work prosthetics. These activities included tying a necktie, picking up coins from a flat surface, riding a bicycle, and taking banknotes out of a wallet. Men modelling the Carnes Arm were always depicted in civilian shirt and ties as in Figure 15.[81] According to von Aberle, an arm as delicate and finely crafted as the Carnes Arm could not withstand the heavy labour of the field and factory. Furthermore, he opined, its high price and costly repairs should reserve this arm for those patients in intellectual professions.[82] Paul Guradze, an orthopaedist from Wiesbaden, also identified the Carnes Arm as one strictly for Kopfarbeiter and intellectuals.[83] Engineers, too, argued that such a mechanically sophisticated arm was not appropriate for the working-class disabled. Not only was it impractical, but its high maintenance costs made it far more useful and valuable for the 'invalid intellectuals, especially for those in well-to-do circumstances'.[84] In short, the Carnes Arm was a middle-class arm.

It was not the only prosthesis available to Germany's middle class. Ferdinand Sauerbruch, who criticised the universal arms for industrial workers, had an invention of his own to promote – the Sauerbruch Arm. An accomplished surgeon of his day, Sauerbruch advocated arm designs which harnessed more directly the muscle power of the remaining stump of the amputee, updating the older vision of a 'voluntary arm'. He accomplished this via a surgical process he had developed especially for Germany's wounded soldiers, by creating a canal through the muscle of an amputee's residual limb. He then tunnelled through the tricep or bicep muscle, inserted an ivory rod through the remainder of the disabled soldier's natural arm, and harnessed that muscle for powering his device (see Figure 16). This was a new version of older model

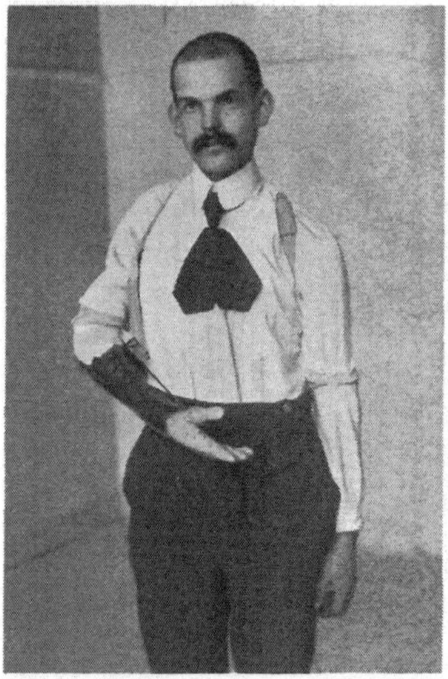

Fig. 222.

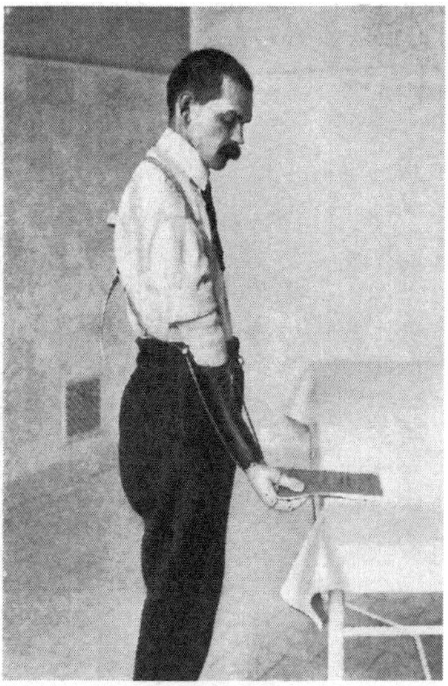

Fig. 223.

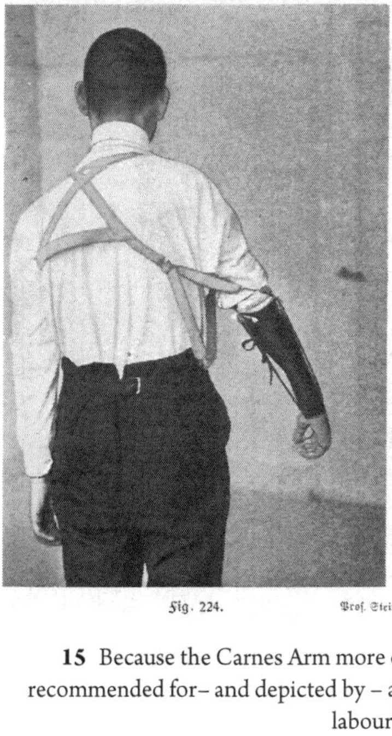

Fig. 224.

Prof. Steinthal, Stuttgart.

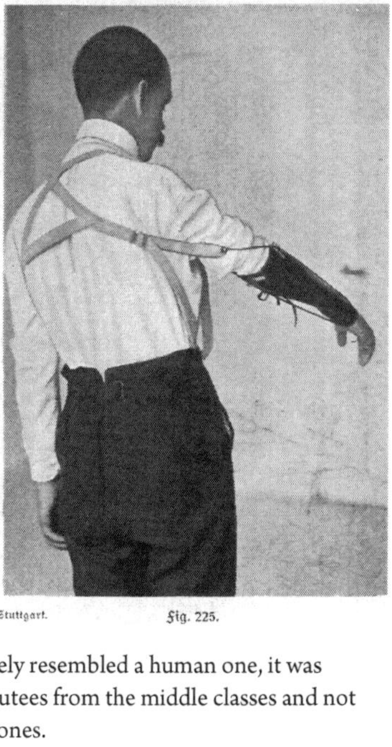

Fig. 225.

15 Because the Carnes Arm more closely resembled a human one, it was recommended for– and depicted by – amputees from the middle classes and not labouring ones.

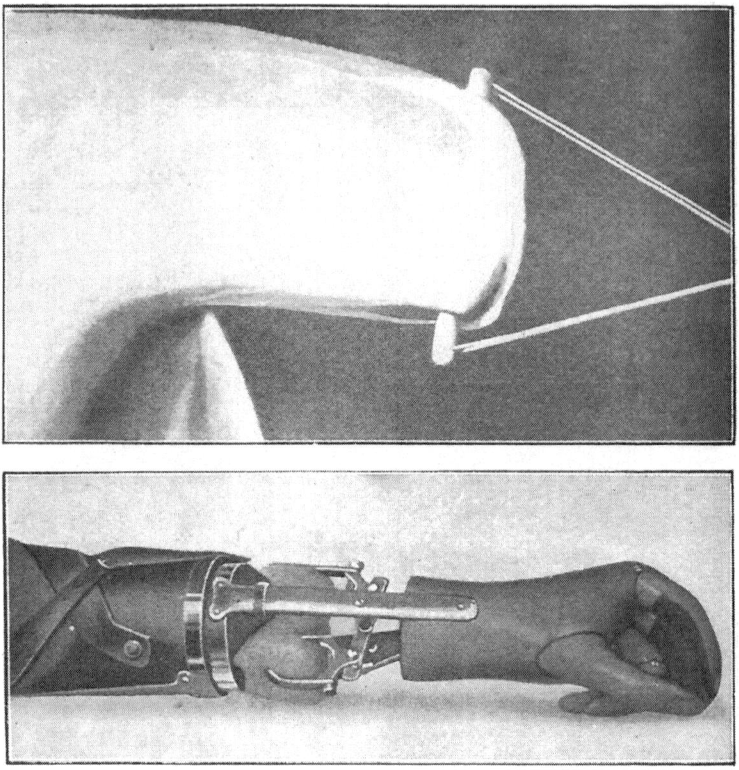

16 The Sauerbruch Arm was a prosthetic device operated by the remaining muscle in an amputee's stump.

'voluntary arms', in that it allowed the amputee to open and close the hand by attaching its mechanism to his physical body – provided of course, that he survived the surgery.[85]

As the war continued, not only were designs for limbs influenced by class and vocational differences, but the development of artificial arms became increasingly patriotic, as well. Orthopaedists sought to remove German doctors and patients from their dependency on foreign imports, emphasising the need to produce domestic limbs which did not stem from their belligerent foes. Max Cohn based his evaluation of the Carnes Arm, an American device, on personal experience – he wore it himself. At the 1916 emergency conference of the DOG, Cohn demonstrated the arm's usefulness in opening an umbrella and holding a pen. He then turned to the matter of its production.

'It is desirable that those with influence realise the importance of building this prosthesis here domestically in order to prevent a foreign firm – perhaps even an enemy one – from economically exploiting it after the war.'[86] Biesalski argued that German factories could design and manufacture an arm similar to the Carnes Arm at lower cost. He also noted, 'It can hardly lie within the taste of the German soldier to accept such a replacement arm, when the prosthesis possibly stems from the same source as the grenade which brought him down.'[87]

The U.S. entrance into the war in 1917 brought a more urgent push to develop German alternatives to the Carnes Arm. In May 1917, Lange himself introduced a new prosthesis to replace the American 'enemy' arm. The new Lange Hand was simple, sturdy, and inexpensive (see Figure 17). Weighing 200 grams, it was 300 grams lighter than the Carnes Arm and 'despite its light weight even hardier than any wooden hands produced yet'.[88] Lange concluded triumphantly, 'Therefore we now have every reason to rejoice that a German doctor has found the way to at least partly return to our amputees what the war has taken away from them.'[89]

Over the course of the war, the Imperial War Ministry was becoming increasingly interested in all these developments. In addition to gaining information on artificial limbs through the experiments at the Centre for Artificial Limb Testing in Berlin, military authorities sought to manage this information, too. Although medical knowledge and sanitation reports had been considered a matter of supreme military importance since the outset of the war, by 1917 the breakthroughs in prosthetic design became a matter of national security. In response to reports that the British government was becoming interested in the German advances in replacement limbs, the War Ministry imposed a ban on the publication or dissemination of any medical tract regarding developments in artificial limb or prosthetic technology.[90] The strategies designed for re-arming the disabled had become war-time state secrets.

Conclusion

By war's end, orthopaedists in Germany had established their authority in the design, distribution, and fitting of prosthetic devices. An area of rehabilitation technology which had been primarily the domain of artisans or engineers had become medicalised, that is, incorporated into the expert domain of medical professionals – the nation's orthopaedists. In the post-war years, they published a number of authoritative texts on artificial limb design, attributing the developments contained therein to their war experiences. In all of these, orthopaedists such as Gocht, Radike, and Schede linked the technical design

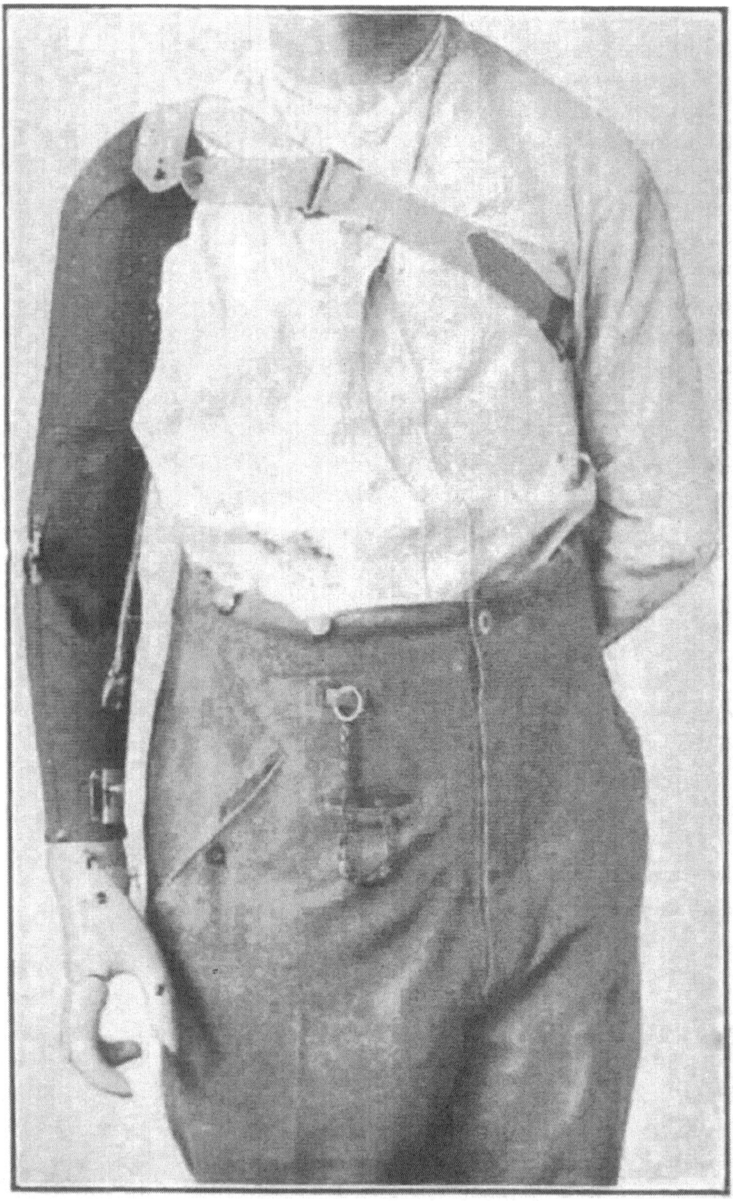

17 In response to U.S. entrance into the war, Lange developed this arm as a cheaper and more 'patriotic' replacement for the Carnes Arm.

of limbs to the medical goals of rehabilitation. They also focused on the importance of expert prosthetic fitting by orthopaedists, not bandagists, due to the demands of post-operative residual limb care and convalescent treatment.[91] In this aspect of their war-time development, Germany's orthopaedists ultimately differed substantially from those in Great Britain where, according to Cooter's analysis of their pre-professional 'adolescence', orthopaedists were 'lacking any persuasive scientific or technological foci for specialization'.[92]

Moreover, orthopaedists had established the importance of functional and not cosmetic designs in the manufacturing of artificial limbs. Herrmann Gocht maintained that the latter was tied more or less to the sensitivity of the disabled himself, who naturally considered hiding the disability to be of paramount importance. But medical experience, he argued, maintained that the limb's function was actually *more* crucial, not just for the severely injured soldier, but for society. As he noted, it was rather the ability of an artificial limb to offer the

> reproduction of function, that is the ability to be vocationally active again and to be able to perform valuable work, which is of greatest importance, and not just for the man whose limbs are damaged, but also for the general public, and for the entire nation [*ganze Volk*].[93]

During the war, orthopaedists were able to expand their medical authority into prosthetic design by linking technological goals with medical and social ones. Orthopaedists were not simply healing the nation's soldiers; they were sending them back to work and re-building a social order crumbling in the midst of war. Still, sending the disabled soldier back to work required more than simply 're-arming' his body. It included the development of an entire system of social and cultural reintegration, or *Wiedereingliederung*, a programme which orthopaedists were eager to lead.

Notes

1 Erich Maria Remarque, *All Quiet on the Western Front* [*Im Westen nichts neues*, 1929]. Trans. by A.W. Wheen (New York: Ballantine Books, 1982), 28.

2 See the multiple book reviewers' quotes printed in the frontmatter of the novel. Remarque, *All Quiet*, front matter.

3 Lange, *Lehrbuch* (1922), 553.

4 Other contemporary scholars have also analysed artificial limbs, while placing these studies in larger historical contexts. For an examination of the cultural and literary context of prosthetics in late eighteenth-century Germany, see Stefani Engelstein, 'Out on a Limb: Military Medicine, Heinrich von Kleist, and the Disarticulated Body', *German Studies Review*, Vol. 23, No.2: 225–44. For an anthropological analysis of the gendered nature of these technological reproductions and their

impact on interwar Germany, see Sabine Kienitz, 'Body Damage: War Disability and Constructions of Masculinity in Weimar Germany', pp. 181–203 in Karen Hagemann and Stefanie Schüler-Springorum, eds, *Home/front: The Military, War, and Gender in Twentieth-Century Germany* (Oxford: Berg, 2002). For a French perspective, see Roxanne Panchesi, 'Reconstructions: Prosthetics and the Rehabilitation of the Male Body in World War I France', *Differences*, Vol. 7, No. 3 (1995): 109–40.

5 R. Radike, 'Künstliche Arme und Hände', pp. 163–394 in Hermann Gocht, R. Radike, and F. Schede (eds), *Künstliche Glieder* [Deutsche Orthopädie, 2] (Stuttgart: Enke, 1920), 163. For a contemporary history of artificial limbs, see also H.H. Wetz, 'Zur Geschichte der Armprothetik', pp. 153–4 in *Geschichte operativer Verfahren an den Bewegungsorganen.* [Jahrbuch des Deutsches orthopaedisches Geschichts- und Forschungsmuseum, 2] (Darmstadt: Steinkopff, 2000).

6 Wetz, 'Zur Geschichte der Armprothetik', 156.

7 Radike, 'Künstliche Arme und Hände', 201; Wetz, 'Zur Geschichte der Armprothetik', 157.

8 Radike, 'Künstliche Arme und Hände', 205. Images of such arms by Eichler, Troschinski, and van Petersen can be found in Wetz, 'Zur Geschichte der Armprothetik'.

9 For an interesting discussion of the fascination that enlightenment natural philosophers had with automata and the technological reproduction of bodies in eighteenth-century Germany, see chapter 4 in Stefani Engelstein, *Anxious Anatomy: The Conception of the Human Form in Literary and Naturalist Discourse* (Albany, NY: SUNY Press, 2008).

10 Wetz, 'Zur Geschichte der Armprothetik', 163–5. The limits of space do not allow me to list each of the many and varied apparati that were developed in Europe at the time. However, Radike's chapter on artificial arms and hands does provide a good outline of the most well-known, and is recommended for further reading. See R. Radike, 'Künstliche Arme und Hände', 163–394.

11 Wetz, 'Zur Geschichte der Armprothetik', 157–60.

12 Gumprecht, Pfarrius, and Rigler, *Lehrbuch der Arbeiter-Versicherungsmedizin*, 103–5.

13 Wetz, 'Zur Geschichte der Armprothetik', 169–70.

14 Radike, 'Künstliche Arme und Hände', 242.

15 Radike, 'Künstliche Arme und Hände', 369–71.

16 Radike, 'Künstliche Arme und Hände', 215–23. See especially 215 for a description of the Carnes Arm's distinguishing characteristics.

17 For more on the war-time politics of the Carnes Arm and its impact on German artificial limb design, see the discussion at the end of this chapter, pp. 74–5.

18 Lange, *Lehrbuch*, 2nd ed. (1922), 553.

19 Konrad Biesalski, *Kriegskrüppelfürsorge: Ein Aufklärungswort zum Troste und zur Mahnung* (Leipzig: Leopold Voss Verlag, 1915), 12, emphasis mine.

20 Lange, *Lehrbuch der Orthopaedie.* 2nd ed. (1992), 553.

21 Adolf Silberstein, 'Bein- und Armersatz im Kgl. Orthopaedischen Reservelazarett zu Nuernberg', *Zeitschrift für orthopädische Chirurgie*, Vol. 37 (1917): 350–84, 361.
22 Silberstein, 'Bein- und Armersatz', 362–4.
23 Hermann Gocht in 'Bericht der ausserordentlichen Tagung der Deutschen Orthopädischen Gesellschaft', *Zeitschrift für orthopädische Chirurgie*, Vol. 37 (1916): 209–671; 215.
24 O. Witzel, 'Die Aufgaben und Wege fuer den Hand- und Armersatz der Kriegsbeschädigten', *Münchener medizinische Wochenschrift*, Vol. 44 (1915): 1491–2, 1491.
25 In Germany scientists emphasised the social utility of their discoveries – specifically the creation of more efficient workers, the reduction of fatigue (the debilitating 'mal de siècle'), and higher industrial productivity. Two good sources for further reading on this subject are: Matthew Hale's *Human Science and Social Order: Hugo Munsterberg and the Origins of Applied Psychology* (Philadelphia: Temple University Press, 1980) and especially Anson Rabinbach's *The Human Motor: Energy, Fatigue and the Origins of Modernity* (New York: Basic Books, 1990), 179–205.
26 Examples of these would be the arms of Ritter Götz von Berlichingen, Klingert's 'Marionette Arm' designed for an aristocratic soldier, and Count von Beaufort's prosthesis.
27 Radike, 'Künstliche Arme und Hände', 163–5.
28 Gocht, *Künstliche Glieder*, frontispiece.
29 G. Schlesinger, 'Die Mitarbeit des Ingenieurs bei der Durchbildung der Ersatzglieder', *Zeitschrift des Vereins deutscher Ingenieure* (1917): 737. Images of hand grips from Gocht, *Künstliche Glieder*, 30–2. See also Wetz, 'Zur Geschichte der Armprothetik', 169–70.
30 See for instance the chart of hand shapes and motions which Biesalski drew in explaining the usefulness of his Fischerklaue (Fischer claw). Next to each human hand in motion, Biesalski provided an image of the Fischer-claw performing the same task. These tasks included holding a nail, pulling a cord, holding a tool handle, and gripping a lever. In this way, Biesalski argued that his Fischer claw fulfilled all necessary motions, grips and abilities of the human hand at work. See Konrad Biesalski, 'Das neue Modell der aktiven Fischerhand und Arbeitsklaue', *Münchener medizinische Wochenschrift*, Vol. 65, No.39 (1918): 1078–9, 1078.
31 [Hans] von Baeyer, 'Prothesen aus Weissblech', *Münchener medizinische Wochenschrift*, Vol. 44 (1915): 1496–9; 1497.
32 For more on the importance of improving artificial legs and replacing the so-called 'peg leg', see Fritz Lange's discussion of artificial legs in Lange, 'Kriegs-Orthopädie', 157–73. For more on the development in artificial leg design, see the post-war summary in Lange, *Lehrbuch* 2nd ed. (1922), 543–52.
33 One of the more interesting, yet somewhat ridiculous, suggestions came from W. Castendyck in Mannheim. Castendyck suggested that artificial arms could be

improved by altering their construction so as to rely on the disabled's jaw muscles. Hoping to help out orthopaedists who were looking for other sources of energy for voluntary arms, he argued that the jaw muscle was the ideal source of control over arms. To that end, he sketched out a design for a clamp which resembled a metal clothes pin. This 'mouth clamp' could be attached to the shoulder and adjusted to mouth height. When the wearer wished to open his artificial hand, he could simply turn his face to the clamp, bite down on it, thus pulling on a cord and opening the hand's grip. Releasing the mouth clamp would then allow the hand to snap shut. Although Castendyck himself had not actually created or tested this system, he assured the journal's readers that he was available to consult if any engineer or scientist wished to follow up on his design. M. Castendyck, 'Ein Vorschlag zur Verbesserung der künstlichen Hand', *Zentralblatt für chirurgische und mechanische Orthopädie, Einschliesslich der gesamten Heilgymnastik und Massage*, Vol. 10 (1916) 137–9.

34 BArch R3901/8730. *Denkschrift über die Abbau und Auflösung der Heimatdank, Staats, und Lazarettwerkstätten*, 5.

35 BArch R3901/8730. *Denkschrift über die Abbau*, 5. For a contemporary account of this Centre, see the history of the development of medical technology at the Technical University of Berlin found on the web pages of that institute. FG Medizintechnik, 'Forschungsbereich Hilfsmittel zur Rehabilitation', Institut für Konstruktion, Mikro- und Medizintechnik, Technische Universität Berlin. www.medtech.tu-berlin.de/menue/forschung/schwerpunkte/hilfsmittelforschung/ (accessed November 8, 2013).

36 For more on the Prüfstelle see the correspondence between the Ministry of War in Berlin and the Medical Department of the Bavarian Army. BayHSta/Abt. IV, Stv GenKdo IAK SanA 308.

37 BArch R3901/8730. *Denkschrift über die Abbau*, 5

38 See BArch R3901/8730, 'Denkschrift über die Prüfstelle für Ersatzglieder, e.V. Dresden' January 4, 1921, 3–4.

39 BArch R3901/8730, 'Denkschrift über die Prüfstelle für Ersatzglieder', 4–5.

40 See for instance R. du Bois-Reymond, 'Physiologie des Armes und des Beins', pp. 69–104 in M. Borchardt et al., eds, *Ersatzglieder und Arbeitshilfen für Kriegsbeschädigte und Unfallverletzte* (Berlin, Springer: 1919).

41 BArch R3901/8730, 'Denkschrift über die Prüfstelle für Ersatzglieder', pp 5–6. The study referred to here is from this same document (Abb. 10–17). See Rabinbach, *The Human Motor* for more on the use of stop-motion photography in measuring and studying the body.

42 Steinthal, 'Wege und Ziele zum Problem der künstlichen Hand', *Bruns' Beiträge zur klinischen Chirurgie*, Vol. 106 (1917): 725–31; 726.

43 For more on this idea, see Heather R. Perry, 'Re-Arming the Disabled Veteran: Artificially Rebuilding State and Society in World War One Germany', pp. 75–101 in Katherine Ott et al. eds, *Artificial Parts, Practical Lives: Modern Histories of Prosthetics* (New York: New York University Press, 2002).

44 SHAD LVA III. Verein deutscher Ingenieure. Leitsätze über Fürsorge für Kriegsbeschädigte.
45 SHAD LVA III. Verein deutscher Ingenieure. Leitsätze über Fürsorge für Kriegsbeschädigte.
46 SHAD KA (P) 18188. *Mitteilungen über den Arbeitsarm der Siemens-Schuckertwerke Zweigniederlassung Nürnberg für kriegsbeschädigte Handwerker und Arbeiter und Landwirter*, A1–A2 (Nürnberg, 1918).
47 *Mitteilungen über den Arbeitsarm der Siemens-Schuckertwerke*, A5–A15.
48 *Mitteilungen über den Arbeitsarm der Siemens-Schuckertwerke*, B1–B26.
49 *Mitteilungen über den Arbeitsarm der Siemens-Schuckertwerke*, introduction.
50 'Anwendungsbeispiele'. *Mitteilungen über den Arbeitsarm der Siemens-Schuckertwerke*, C1–C2.
51 *Mitteilungen über den Arbeitsarm der Siemens-Schuckertwerke*, B5, B13.
52 *Mitteilungen über den Arbeitsarm der Siemens-Schuckertwerke*, B1.
53 The Centre for Artificial Limb Testing was the leader in standardising these medical technologies. See Boenick, 'Entwicklung der Medizintechnik'.
54 SHAD KA (P) 18188. *Preisliste 4 über den Siemens-Schuckert Arbeitsarm* (March 1918), 4–5.
55 *Preisliste 4 über den Siemens-Schuckert Arbeitsarm*, 4, 9. This does not include the price of two other pieces (*Stosslade, Greifklobe*) which were custom-made for each disabled Tischler and which therefore were priced upon order.
56 Silberstein, 'Bein- und Armersatz', 363–4.
57 Silberstein, 'Bein- und Armersatz', 382, quotation marks in original.
58 Felix Krais, ed., *Die Verwendungsmöglichkeiten der Kriegsbeschädigten in der Industrie, in Gewerbe, Handel, Handwerk, Landwirtschaft, und Staatsbetrieben* (Stuttgart: Krais Verlag, 1916), 62–4.
59 Karl Marx and Frederick Engels, *Manifesto of the Communist Party* (New York: International Publishers, 1948), 16.
60 Ferdinand Sauerbruch, 'Willkürlich bewegbare Arbeitsklauen', *Münchener medizinische Wochenschrift*, Vol. 10 (1918): 257–8, 257.
61 Theodor Mietens, 'Ein willkürlich beweglicher Arbeitsarm', *Feldärtzliche Beilage zur Münchener medizinische Wochenschrift*, No. 3 (1917): 100–3, 101.
62 *Kopfarbeiter* is a somewhat antiquated term not generally used today, but could be translated today as a 'white collar worker'. A discussion of both the term and its significance can be found later in this chapter. Peter Janssen, 'Was muss der Lazarettarzt von der Prothese wissen?', *Feldaerztliche Beilage zur Münchener medizinische Wochenschrift*, No. 12 (1917): 398–401, quote on p. 400.
63 A special volume of the German *Zeitschrift für orthopädische Chirurgie* was published in 1917 in an attempt to take stock of the state of German prosthetic design and offer a description of all the devices designed. At 828 pages and over 750 images, it still was not completely comprehensive. See 'Gesammelte Arbeiten über die Prothesenbau', *Zeitschrift für orthopädische Chirurgie*, Vol. 37 (Stuttgart: Ferdinand Enke, 1917). For another collection of limbs developed during the war

see M. Borchardt et al., *Ersatzglieder und Arbeitshilfen für Kriegsbeschädigte und Unfallverletzte* (Berlin, Springer: 1919). In this volume Konrad Hartmann claims that by the end of 1917, the Prüfstelle für Ersatzglieder had tested 2068 different limbs and other prosthetic devices. See Konrad Hartmann, 'Die Prüfstelle für Ersatzglieder', pp. 18–57 in Borchardt et al., *Ersatzglieder und Arbeitshilfen für Kriegsbeschädigte und Unfallverletzte*, 30.

64 Theodor Mietens, 'Eine künstliche Hand für einen Klaviertechniker', *Münchener medizinische Wochenschrift*, Vol. 67 (1920): 1055. Image also in this article.

65 Krais, *Verwendungsmöglichkeiten*, 53.

66 J. Riedinger, 'Zur Frage der Arbeitsarme', *Feldärztliche Beilage zur Münchener medizinische Wochenschrift*, No. 35 (1916): 1280–1, 1281.

67 These included agricultural hands from Lüer, Nieny (discussed below, pp.70–2), Schede, Berg, and Rosset. For more on these see Radike, 'Künstliche Arme und Hände', 359–63.

68 von Baeyer, 'Prothesen aus Weissblech', 1498–9.

69 von Baeyer, 'Prothesen aus Weissblech', 1496.

70 von Baeyer, 'Prothesen aus Weissblech', 1498.

71 Mietens, 'Ein willkürlich beweglicher Arbeitsarm', 101.

72 Konrad Biesalski, 'Ueber Prothesen bei Amputationen des Armes insbesondere des Oberarmes', *Münchener medizinische Wochenschrift*, Vol. 44 (1915): 1492–6; quote on 1496.

73 Karl Nieny, 'Die Behandlung und Ausrüstung der Amputierten im Marinelazarett Hamburg', *Zeitschrift für orthopädische Chirurgie*, Vol. 37 (1917): 302–22, 325.

74 Nieny, 'Die Behandlung und Ausrüstung', 318.

75 Nieny, 'Die Behandlung und Ausrüstung', 318–19.

76 Radike, 'Künstliche Arme und Hände', 174–5, 318–20.

77 Nieny, 'Die Behandlung und Ausrüstung', 328–9.

78 Nieny, 'Die Behandlung und Ausrüstung', 330–1.

79 Nieny, 'Die Behandlung und Ausrüstung', 327.

80 Silberstein, 'Bein- und Armersatz', 365.

81 Krais, *Verwendungsmöglichkeiten*, Appendix, Plate 31.

82 Rudolf Ritter von Aberle, 'Künstliche Gliedmassen für Kriegsverwundete', *Zeitschrift für orthopädische Chirurgie*, Vol. 35 (1916): 584–610, 601.

83 P. Guradze, 'Über Amputationsstumpf und Prothesen', *Zeitschrift für orthopädische Chirurgie*, Vol. 37 (1917): 83–93, 93.

84 Arthur Ehrenfest-Egger and Siegfried Neutra, 'Die Carnesarmprothese' Mitteilung des Vereins 'Die Technik für die Kriegsinvaliden' (1915) No. 2, as noted in *Zeitschrift für orthopädische Chirurgie*, Vol. 38 (1918): 695.

85 Lange, *Lehrbuch* 2nd ed. (1922), 561–2.

86 Max Cohn in 'Bericht der ausserordentlichen Tagung der Deutschen Orthopaedischen Gesellschaft', *Zeitschrift für orthopädische Chirurgie*, Vol. 37 (1916): 209–671; 264.

87 Biesalski, 'Ueber Prothesen bei Amputationen', 1494.

88 Fritz Lange, 'Eine neue Kunst-und Arbeitshand', *Feldaertzliche Beilage zur Münchener medizinische Wochenschrift*, No. 20 (1917): 661–4, 662.

89 Lange, 'Eine neue Kunst- und Arbeitshand', 664.

90 BayHStA/Abt. IV, Stv GenKdo I, AKSanAm 459. Directive from the Kriegsamt. Kriegsministerium. May 12, 1917 to all Deputy Corps Headquarters and all Sanitation Offices.

91 See for instance, Hermann Gocht, R. Radike, and F. Schede, eds, *Künstliche Glieder* [Deutsche Orthopädie, 2] 2nd ed. (Stuttgart: Ferdinand Enke Verlag, 1920), frontispiece.

92 Cooter, *Surgery and Society*, 5.

93 Gocht, *Künstliche Glieder*, 83.

3

REHABILITATION NATION: RE-MEMBERING THE DISABLED IN WAR-TIME GERMANY

> The war-disabled should not be left to their pensions alone, rather they must be brought to productive and profitable activities, in order that they may feel like useful, self-assured, and independent members of our industrious national body [*Glieder unseres arbeitsamen Volkskörpers*]. (Meissner daily newspaper, 1916)[1]

> Not until the war did orthopaedic practical therapy become the most obvious and self-evident treatment for injuries nor was it even applied in such wide scope before then. ('On the War Experiences of Orthopaedic Therapy', 1921)[2]

In March 1915 Dr Karl von Seydel, the Surgeon General of the Bavarian Army, recalled Fritz Lange from his post at the warfront. Citing recent innovations in the healing and rehabilitation of severely wounded men, von Seydel had decided to create Medical Advisory Boards, composed of orthopaedic specialists, who would be tasked with the oversight of the entire Bavarian Army's convalescent care facilities. Lange was being re-assigned to the home front as an advisor to the Medical Department of the Bavarian 1st Army Corps. As the casualties continued to mount, von Seydel had realised that a man like Fritz Lange was of far more value in Munich rehabilitating disabled soldiers than with the field hospitals at the front.[3] Just six months into the war, orthopaedists were being recognised as important figures in the healing of Germany's disabled servicemen.

This chapter examines the rehabilitation of the severely injured soldier. The orthopaedic mission to send the disabled back to work required more than simply healing their wounds; it meant re-inserting them back into the social and economic fabric of the German Empire. In order to accomplish this, the nation's orthopaedists had to create an entire network of structures designed for re-integrating the disabled soldier into the workforce. In doing so, men like Lange and Biesalski found themselves not just re-organising medical care and therapies for the wounded, but shaping disabled military and civilian welfare policies, as well. Thus as the war progressed, Germany's orthopaedists slowly expanded their influence beyond the hospital and into both military and private organisations. Over the course of the war, orthopaedists and their ideas became central to disability care and welfare.

This chapter begins with a brief description of rehabilitation in pre-war Germany and points out the limits that this system posed for the war-disabled. It then traces the path of the wounded soldier by first outlining his treatment under the military and then the civilian systems of medical care, while describing the ways in which new ideas of rehabilitation influenced their war-time reorganisation. Next follows a discussion of the specific restorative therapies used in the healing of the severely injured ex-serviceman. Then the chapter examines how the new project of medical rehabilitation influenced policies being developed for re-inserting the disabled veteran into the labour force. Called *Wiedereingliederung* by contemporaries, this social and cultural 're-membering' of the wounded soldier in the post-war German future was the long-term goal of the new rehabilitation.[4] Throughout, however, the chapter highlights how the social project of 're-membering' the individual soldier was fundamentally informed with underlying conservative goals of restoring a society caught in the social upheaval of war.

Medical rehabilitation before the war

Germany's orthopaedists did not invent the concept of physical rehabilitation during the First World War. Therapies for bodily restoration or 're-education' permeated nineteenth-century German society. Health spas, sanatoria, convalescent homes, and insurance infirmaries had evolved over the course of the century, offering a variety of treatments for different segments of the nation's population. In these institutions doctors, gymnastic instructors, and other medical personnel employed a variety of therapies for rejuvenating injured or debilitated bodies. These non-operative treatments were designed to strengthen muscles, stimulate nerves, or improve the overall constitution of a patient who had more often than not voluntarily undertaken such a 'cure'.

Among the repertoire of restorative procedures available in these institutions were gymnastics, medico-mechanical therapy, electric shock therapy, hydropathy, and massage. Therapeutic gymnastics [*Krankengymnastik*] was an organised system of bodily exercises initially created by the nineteenth-century Swede Peter Ling, who claimed to have cured his gout while fencing.[5] The precursor to modern physiotherapy, therapeutic gymnastics were designed to rejuvenate degenerating body parts. Gustaf Zander modified his compatriot's ideas through the invention of medico-mechanical therapy – a regimen which relied upon machines to exercise the body. By providing counter-balance to a patient's body with either a pendulum or weights, these therapeutic apparati allowed for the controlled, focused exercise of a specific area of the body. Others were designed to stretch or massage different body parts. Each of these treatments was designed to strengthen injured body parts through controlled supervised motions. Massage therapy, steam baths, sauna treatments, and electrical stimulation were also treatments used to rejuvenate the nervous and circulatory systems in order to encourage recovery.[6] All of these therapies were only to be administered by an expert, who in nineteenth-century Germany might be a physician with some orthopaedic training, but was more usually a gymnast, physical trainer, kinesiologist, or other lay practitioner who had undergone some training in the field.[7] However, as chapter 2 pointed out, orthopaedists spent the years before the war establishing their expertise as the university-trained medical professionals who should develop and lead, if not always personally administer, these therapies.

Despite the existence of these therapies, physical rehabilitation of the body was not always successful for a variety of reasons. Before the implementation of national insurance, treatments in health spas and residential health sanatoria were expensive luxuries that only wealthier Germans could afford. Bourgeois patients took these rest and nerve cures voluntarily as health vacations and were not there for serious medical treatment. Rarely were these Germans being restored to health for work. Disabled adults in 'cripple homes' might also have access to these treatments, but in group homes funded by charity, patients did not receive much individual or long-term attention. Largely conceived as poor relief, these institutions concentrated on housing, not treating their indigent residents.

The advent of social insurance increased national and state interest in physical rehabilitation. The focus on returning injured workers to the labour force prompted the founding of some new orthopaedic institutes for administering these therapies to workplace accident victims. However, these treatments focused on helping a patient reclaim the 'generic' use of an injured body part. In his discussion of these curative workshops, Greg Eghigian has concluded that despite the healing goals of these treatments, '[t]his did not mean that the therapy regimen was obliged to provide the disabled with the means to return to their former occupations or trades'.[8] They were also unpopular with workers, who tended to terminate their cures early or avoid them altogether.[9] Moreover, these types of treatments could offer very little to amputees who had no limbs to exercise or massage or to the blind who faced different challenges when being returned to work. For restoring the labour capacity of disabled soldiers, pre-war facilities and programmes for rehabilitating disabled adults were largely inadequate.

But the nation's orthopaedists had a second system of facilities at their disposal – those devoted to the care and welfare of disabled children. As chapter 1 pointed out, orthopaedists had concentrated primarily on the treatment of congenitally disabled youth. In the years before the war, many had developed of institutes for so-called 'crippled children'. Indeed, these had been the focus of Biesalski's 1906 Cripple Census, the results of which he had published in 1909 as *The Scope and Nature of Childhood Cripples and Cripple Welfare in Germany*.[10] As the casualties of the war mounted and the German military's internal system of soldier care proved inadequate, Germany's orthopaedists mobilised their resources to treat the nation's wounded.

Military care for wounded soldiers

In 1915 the care and treatment of disabled soldiers was formally split between military and civilian authorities. At a meeting that year of the DVK, it was established that the imperial government, under the auspices of the War Ministry, would be responsible for the treatment of the wounded soldier in so far as he could be restored to military service and for his service pension once released. However, once a soldier had been discharged from the armed forces, his medical care, social welfare, and rehabilitation fell to the civilian resources of the state or private organisations. Thus the treatment of disabled soldiers was divided into two distinct parts: military and civilian [*militärische Fürsorge* and *bürgerliche Fürsorge*]. To the military fell the immediate post-injury care of the wounded soldier, which might include field dressing, treatment in a stationary hospital behind the lines, emergency and/or amputation surgery, and general recovery at the home front before being well enough for discharge. Long-term convalescence, follow-up medical care, physical rehabilitation, and any other social welfare (besides the service pension) fell to the individual German states or to charitable organisations.[11]

The goal of the army's medical care was to keep the soldier fit for active duty, not take over his care in perpetuity. Thus the military care for the wounded soldier focused on restoring the soldier's health so that he could be made useful to the war effort [*kriegsverwendungsfähig*, kv]. Soldiers whose wounds could be healed within the army's medical organisation were sent back into the field as soon as they were declared fit. Even if his injuries made him incapable of further battle duty, however, he might still to be returned to useful service elsewhere within the army. Therefore soldiers might convalesce behind the lines and then be re-mobilised once declared fit for service in another capacity for the war effort. This might include being fit for base duty [*garnisonsverwendungsfähig*, gv] in the transportation or supply corps, or other work duty [*arbeitsverwendungsfähig*, av]. The army's medical care was therefore really designed to serve the needs of the military, not the individual soldier.[12]

Still, until a wounded soldier was discharged from military service, his physical care fell to the medical department [*Sanitätswesen*] of his Army Corps. Because the German army was not a single unified army, but rather a combination of state armies which centralised only during a time of war, there was no standard system of medical care for soldiers. The de-centralised nature of the peace-time armies resulted in the evolution of different approaches and standards of care within each of the empire's twenty-four Army Corps – most operating independently of one another.[13]

When the German Army mobilised in 1914, its medical services followed the military medical regulations established in 1907. Upon declaring war, the Surgeon General became known as the Chief Field Surgeon [*Chef des Feldsanitätswesens*] and was placed in charge of all medical matters in the theatre of operations: the field and the lines of communication [L of C].[14] The twenty-four Army Corps were organised into eight Army High Commands [Armeeoberkommando, AOK], each with its own Army medical officer [MO]. Each of the eight Army MOs had authority over the MO assigned to each Corps and L of C under his command. Each Army Corps included twelve field hospitals as well as MOs in charge of each division. Divisional units included MOs, hospital orderlies, and auxiliary stretcher bearers – in addition to the one or two medical companies assigned to each division. Medical-related orders followed the chain of command, although each Army MO and Corps MO had surgical and hygiene specialists to advise them.[15] The total strength of the Medical Department before the war was 2480 MOs and 5043 non-commissioned officers [NCOs].[16]

When a soldier was wounded in battle, he was first treated by his unit's MO who dressed his wounds enough so that he could be moved. Stretcher-bearers then carried him off the battlefield to where the ambulances were waiting. These might be either horse drawn or motorised, as both were being used by the German armies at this time. Ambulances transported the wounded soldier then to the casualty clearing station staffed by the medical company assigned to his division. Here he received first aid and might also undergo any emergency procedure or bandaging necessary to stabilise his condition for longer transportation. Here he might also receive something hot to drink – coffee, tea, cocoa, broth. Once he was declared 'transport ready', then the wounded soldier was transported to one of the nearby field hospitals attached to that army corps.[17]

The field hospital [*Feldlazarett*] was a mobile medical unit which could provide temporary medical aid to soldiers until these men could be removed to a stationary hospital. These were units of military doctors, administrators, sanitary officers, and orderlies assigned to each army corps. Field hospitals followed the corps divisions in wagons and busses carrying all the medical materials necessary for setting up a 400-bed infirmary – generally in whatever local town lay closest to the army's current battle location. Due to their transitory nature, field hospitals were makeshift facilities which often housed the wounded in shelled out buildings on hastily prepared straw pallets. The units carried iron operating tables with them and once quarters had been set up, they could erect an operating room for more serious operations.[18] It was to such a field hospital that Fritz Lange had been assigned when the war broke out. And it was for training medical personnel in these medical units that he had written *War Orthopaedics*.

Once a soldier had been treated at a field hospital, he was removed to a stationary hospital [*Etappenlazarett*]. Stationary hospitals were more permanent structures located in the army corps' communication areas [*Etappengebeit*] behind the battle lines. They were in easy supply distance from both the home front and the battlefield; thus they were also a middle space for transporting soldiers, doctors, medical supplies, food, and other materials between the army's headquarters and the battle areas. Stationary hospitals had to be prepared for hundreds of casualties as they would receive wounded soldiers transferred from all the field hospitals in the area. Soldiers not yet ready for transport would remain at the field hospital until the mobile unit needed to pack up and follow the troops. At this point, the stationary hospital would send forward a small unit to care for those soldiers who had been left behind until they could be brought back to the communications area.[19]

Due to their more permanent nature, stationary hospitals offered soldiers and doctors more resources. In addition to military medical personnel, one would find at these facilities volunteer nurses, Red Cross representatives, and more highly trained surgeons. Hygiene and contagion was of particular concern, and it was at these hospitals that contagious soldiers were quarantined in order to prevent the spread of disease to those at home or in the trenches. Given these concerns, stationary hospitals also had portable laundry facilities for maintaining hygiene. Soldiers might convalesce or wait to be transported by one of the hospital trains back to the home front if more complicated or longer-term treatment were deemed necessary.[20]

Soldiers who required more intensive or longer care than was available in the stationary hospitals were sent instead to a war hospital [*Kriegslazarett*], a larger medical facility which could offer more extensive services to the wounded and sick. War hospitals could handle not just intensive surgical cases, but included specialised departments for treating contagious disease, pulmonary conditions, eye disorders, dental problems, venereal disease, and could even offer patients access to x-ray machines.[21]

If the wounded soldier required medical treatment beyond what was available at the hospitals in the field or the communications areas, he was sent to his Army Corp's reserve hospital [*Reservelazarett*]. Reserve hospitals were located back at the home front and fell under the jurisdiction of the Deputy Medical Departments of each Army Corps district.[22] This was the final destination of the severely wounded serviceman. Here a soldier remained until he had fully recovered from surgery, illness, or broken limbs and returned to his unit in the field. In addition to their own military hospitals, the Deputy Medical Departments in each Corps district enlisted the help of local civilian institutions in the healing of the severely injured soldier during the war. Thus many reserve hospitals incorporated the facilities and personnel of nearby hospitals, university clinics, charity homes, and private institutes. When the infirmaries of private organisations such as fraternal aid societies or industrial concerns were enlisted into this system, they were generally referred to as auxiliary hospitals [*Vereinslazarette*].[23]

Given the structure of this war-time medical system within the Germany army, it should not be surprising that the care available to wounded soldiers varied according to local conditions and medical expertise. Field hospitals were dependent upon the facilities they could find while following the army. These could often be towns abandoned by residents, and whose buildings had been ravaged by artillery fire.[24] Medical personnel could range from expert surgeons to hastily trained MOs. Soldiers sent back to the home front for longer recovery might find themselves in either a larger, metropolitan area with plentiful facilities, such as Berlin or Munich, or they might end up in smaller towns with fewer resources. A 1919 study of soldier care in Germany noted that the 3rd Army Corps in Brandenburg-Prussia had perhaps the most developed system. With forty-three reserve hospitals of varying size it probably offered the widest scope of care to the wounded. Its largest affiliated institution, a recently constructed insane asylum near Görden, could offer 1000 beds and a 'curative workshop'. This kind of model system, however, could hardly be representative of what was offered in smaller, poorer, or less industrialised areas of the empire.[25]

Orthopaedics and the re-organisation of military medicine

As noted, on the eve of war the Medical Department comprised 2480 MOs and 5043 NCOs.[26] They were quickly overwhelmed. The first year of the war saw the heaviest casualties with 485,900 wounded and 1,047,300 ill; the yearly statistics of sick and wounded soldiers actually decreased with the evolution of trench warfare along the Western Front, although death rates remained high. Not surprisingly the Western Front saw heavier deaths and casualties among soldiers than combat on the Eastern Front.[27] Injuries to the body's extremities comprised the majority of soldiers' wounds. According to one casualty report, of the 2,077,240 battle wounds recorded, 63.5 per cent were to limbs (1,318,473). Of these some 18.9 per cent were bullet fractures and 6.7 per cent were bullet wounds to limb joints, both injuries which required especially complicated surgery and which tested the prowess of Germany's best surgeons.[28]

Pe-war advances in surgery and accident medicine had fostered a conservative approach to trauma treatment, and surgeons used amputation in these cases only as a last resort. Although no complete surgical records for the war exist, one post-war text offered these revealing statistics gathered from individual case studies. Of 504 cases of bullet fractures to the upper arm, 5.5 per cent of the men died from their wounds, 11 per cent underwent amputation, and 83.5 per cent recovered without amputation. Similarly of 1675 cases of bullet fractures to the upper thigh, 23.3 per cent died, 12.5 per cent underwent amputation, and 64.2 per cent recovered without amputation. Still, amputations comprised the majority of operations performed in military hospitals, especially early in the war. According to statistics gathered on twenty-three field hospitals on the Western Front in September 1914, of the total operations performed in a seven-day period, 71 per cent were amputations, the remaining were to the skull, stomach or 'other'.[29] Of all 19,552,696 casualty cases (both injury and sickness) handled by the medical department during the war, 21.1 per cent (4,131,943) were cases in which soldiers had to be returned to the home front for long-term treatment.[30] Thus as orthopaedists had discovered early in the war, a soldier's recovery depended not just on successful surgery, but on the follow-up rehabilitative treatment he received. Orthopaedists argued that they were most useful where they could oversee the long-term physical recovery of the nation's heroes.

Orthopaedists were quick to place their resources in the service of the German military. In August 1914 Biesalski surveyed the 138 existing voluntary and religious organisations dedicated to 'cripple care' regarding their available space and services. At the same time, he suggested ways in which residential institutions dedicated to other populations, such as disabled children or the mentally ill, might find room for taking in severely injured soldiers. These recommendations included moving children to separate rooms within existing structures, temporarily placing civilian patients with relatives, and raising funds from wealthy benefactors in order to construct additional housing in larger complexes. In reply to his survey, Biesalski found that some fifty-four residential institutes could offer a total of 5000 beds for the wounded. He made a subsequent tour of the empire's welfare institutes in order to gather more information and recruit them to his mission.[31]

Whereas the Cripple Census of 1906 had focused on taking stock of the treatments and care being offered to disabled children in Germany, Biesalski's 1914 tour focused on evaluating these resources in terms of their suitability for adult soldiers, and for centralising their services under the umbrella of an empire-wide network. This merging of disabled soldier care with civilian institutes was not without criticism, however. While many orthopaedists agreed that disabled soldiers required the same kind of expert care and attention that only their discipline had been able to offer the empire's disabled children, not everyone agreed that housing and treating severely injured soldiers with this same population was a productive or useful strategy. From his position as head doctor of the military's reserve hospital in Nuremberg, Adolf Silberstein contested this idea, remarking,

> I do not find Biesalski's suggestion to graft the care of war-invalids onto that of crippled Germans appropriate. To take the strongest and most powerful elements of our economy – those wounded now returning from the field – and send them out to cripple homes, in which they'll be placed together with the weakest elements of our society – those dependent upon charity – would have an extraordinarily depressing effect upon a man who up until that point had been in full possession of his strength. … No, soldiers belong in the military hospital, not the cripple home. And the state has enough means to create the necessary institutions for this.[32]

His opinion that the war invalids should be treated separately and independently from the civilian disabled notwithstanding, Silberstein did agree that the care of the empire's wounded soldiers needed to be centralised and overseen by orthopaedists.[33] And clearly military leaders agreed.

In February 1915, as part of a response to the mounting casualties of war, the German War Ministry organised a system of War Medical Inspectorates to supervise the medical organisation of the Corps districts in the home front. Whereas the Deputy Medical Departments were under the command of each individual Army Corps, the Medical Inspectorates reported directly to the War Minister and generally oversaw two or more Corps districts. The duties of the Medical Inspector were to monitor convalescence programmes in the areas under his supervision, and ensure the timely return of recovered troops to their units. This increased the pressure on the Medical Departments of each

Army Corps to speed up the recovery of their troops even more quickly than they already were.[34] When the Surgeon General of the Bavarian 1st Army Corps recalled Fritz Lange from the front in March 1915, it was to put his expertise to use in the Corps' reserve hospitals. By early 1915, the military had become aware of the importance of orthopaedic care to the recovery of the wounded soldier.

Orthopaedics and the rehabilitation of the disabled soldier

When Germany's orthopaedists began organising the rehabilitation of the nation's wounded soldiers, they understood their project to be one of restoring the bodies of wounded soldiers so that they could be returned to civilian life as disabled veterans. They organised their efforts according to their vision of a post-war future in which hostilities had ceased and German society was returned to 'normal'. But returning millions of soldiers to civilian life on such a massive scale – whether wounded or able-bodied – was an unprecedented project in Germany. Neither the imperial government nor the German military had much experience with this sort of economic and social transitioning.[35] In the First World War, men who might have spent years apprenticing as skilled labourers, studying to be teachers, or working in family farms, suddenly found themselves permanently injured through military service. Training programmes existed to give these soldiers 'crash courses' in trench life, weapon use, and military policies in order to prepare them for battle, but in 1914 no programmes or training camps offered them advice on how to return with injured bodies to their pre-war lives.[36] For many, this was not even possible – amputated limbs, closed-down factories, family farms in ruin, jobs now filled by someone else; there were multiple reasons for why the wounded soldier might not easily return to his pre-war life.

Moreover, at the outbreak of war, there was no standardised system of long-term medical care in place for soldiers severely or permanently injured in combat. Although a new system for determining and disbursing pensions to the war-wounded and their dependents had been passed with the Military Pension Law of 1906, these new regulations did not carry with them provisions for the medical treatment and physical rehabilitation that wounded soldiers might need. Furthermore, although a few facilities existed which were dedicated to the long-term care of invalided soldiers, such as the Berlin Invalidenhaus, these institutions offered limited space, and were often reserved for officers. In addition, they focused on long-term or terminal care, not rehabilitation. Therefore although monetary compensation for soldiers seemed rather straightforward (though certainly not uncontested), a clear system of medical care and welfare for disabled soldiers returning from the front was virtually non-existent when the war began.[37]

Thus, although the overarching goal of *Wiedereingliederung* was to return the permanently injured soldier back to his pre-war life – job, family, and community – this was not always as simple as treating the injured soldier and sending him home. Indeed, due to the nature of their injuries, many wounded soldiers had to re-learn the use of arms or legs whose joints were stiffened through injury or surgery. Others had to master the use of artificial limbs that to their wearers often seemed strange, heavy, and awkward. Those whose bodies could not be completely restored, such as the blind, often had to be trained for completely new vocations. This re-training [*Umschulung*] might include mastering new skills, learning to use unfamiliar equipment, or studying new professions. Thus, ultimately the *Wiedereingliederung* of the disabled might necessitate physical therapy, vocational instruction, secondary schooling, or even a combination of all three. Orthopaedists realised that in order to restore the body of the disabled soldier and eventually reinsert him into the workforce, they would have to create the therapies and structures necessary for accomplishing this. In doing so, they drew upon their pre-war experiences with treating the nation's disabled children, adapting the treatments to the needs of the injured soldier.

Most existing therapies for injured workers were deemed inadequate for rehabilitating the war wounded. Sending the disabled soldier back to work, therefore, required a somewhat different approach, and the most common treatment for healing the severely injured was *Arbeitstherapie,* or 'work-therapy'. Different from the therapeutic gymnastics or medico-mechanical therapy prescribed in the nineteenth century, work-therapy combined practical occupational training with bodily exercise in an effort to train the physically disabled body to work. Orthopaedists had used this form of therapy in their institutes for disabled children with the goals of preparing them for life outside the 'cripple home'. The use of repetitive motion was aimed to train existing muscles to overcome growth malformations. Moreover, by linking those motions to productive work activity, Biesalski and other orthopaedists had intended for work-therapy to train these young 'cripples' into workers who might become economically self-sufficient. Orthopaedists applied the principles of *Arbeitstherapie* to their treatment of severely wounded soldiers and used it to help heal their bodies. Through work-therapy the disabled soldier learned to re-use his body by limbering stiffened muscles, overcoming partial paralysis caused by injury, or even becoming skilled with new artificial limbs.

Unlike convalescence, however, work-therapy was not practised in a hospital, but rather in the controlled environment of the orthopaedic workshop.[38]

Common in many orthopaedic institutes before the war, these workshops would have been more familiar to the skilled tradesman than to those visitors of nineteenth-century health spas and institutes. They were especially constructed as spaces where the disabled could recover his skills and earning potential in order to be returned to the workforce. As opposed to the bodies of injured workers which had been manipulated passively by machines in pre-war therapy, in these war-time lazarette workshops disabled soldiers were engaged in active work using the energy of their own bodies to operate tools and equipment for productive ends. These were not the leisurely therapy workshops of the pre-war empire.

The treatment that the disabled soldier underwent in the workshops consisted of more than just physical therapy, however. It included practical vocational training as well. Using the tools and materials in the shops gave men the opportunity to not just sharpen rusty skills, but also learn new ones. Those soldiers with amputated limbs were assigned appropriate work prostheses and then trained with them rigorously in order to restore their bodies. This kind of training could include learning to operate new machinery, studying a new craft or trade, or becoming familiar with new tools. For the blind it might mean learning to read Braille; while for one-handed amputees it might require learning to use a special typewriter, or becoming skilled at more routine activities without the use of a missing limb. For those learning a new trade while using an artificial arm or leg, this practice was especially necessary, for few employers were likely to hire men who were not proficient at their labour.

The benefits of work-therapy could be more than fiscal, however. Soldiers wearing artificial limbs also had to learn how to repair their prostheses as a central part of their own self-care (although self-maintenance is perhaps a better description). The military administration had strict guidelines regarding the distribution and maintenance of prosthetics. Although they were often willing to cover the initial cost of a prosthetic, this did not include repair costs or attachments for the limb. For instance, though the military was willing to provide each disabled soldier with up to two pairs of specially made orthopaedic shoes, they assumed no responsibility for fixing the shoes should repairs become necessary. Moreover, the offer of orthopaedic shoes did not include shoewear for artificial legs, 'normal' shoes outfitted with special orthopaedic braces, or even shoes for soldiers who relied on a partial foot prosthetic but who could wear ordinary footwear. But finding shoes was perhaps the least of many disabled men's worries. The important aspect here is that the military would not cover the costs of repairing the prosthetic device once it had been disbursed to its wearer.[39] Therefore, in orthopaedic workshops many soldiers were also trained in the art of repairing their own artificial limb.[40]

In addition to the practical benefits that work-therapy offered, it was also designed to convey psychological ones. According to many of Germany's orthopaedists, *Arbeitstherapie* was an ideal method for combating an emerging condition among the empire's soldiers – the 'pension-psychosis'. Orthopaedists noted with alarm the lack of enthusiasm among disabled soldiers with regard to their own rehabilitation and attributed this to the loss of the injured man's 'will to work'. The symptoms of this pathological condition were a rejection of physical recovery, a refusal to work, and fear of losing the service pensions. Orthopaedists believed that by re-awakening the wounded soldier's will to work, work-therapy could heal this condition as well.[41]

By 1915 orthopaedists had placed 221 workshops and re-training schools in the service of the military's wounded soldiers. In these shops, they could retrain disabled soldiers in at least fifty-one different occupations, including basketry, carpentry, bookkeeping, agriculture, photography, and bookbinding to name just a few.[42] By arguing that work-therapy was central to the long-term recovery of the severely injured, Germany's orthopaedists were able to buttress their claims of expertise in the rehabilitation of soldiers. As one orthopaedist in Kassel observed just after the war, 'Not until the war did orthopaedic practical therapy become the most obvious and self-evident treatment for injuries nor was it even applied in such wide scope before then.'[43] Thus through these claims of specialised knowledge and skill, by 1915 orthopaedists had positioned themselves as authorities in soldier rehabilitation – authorities whose ideas about rehabilitation reached beyond the walls of their workshops to influence the entire organisation of war-disabled care on the home front.

In response to the promise of success that work-therapy posed, the German Army began to re-organise its home front system of convalescent care. This included not just an expansion of the reserve hospital system, but also the enlistment of local governmental and trade offices into the project of rehabilitation.

Noting the success of orthopaedic therapy in healing the wounded, in late May 1915 the Surgeon General of the German Army sent a missive urging that all Army Corps medical departments should incorporate local orthopaedic workshops into their convalescent system. His letter included a comprehensive list of the available facilities, no doubt handed to him by Biesalski.[44] In Bavaria, military authorities were one step ahead of Berlin and under the advice of Lange had set in motion a plan to build their own medico-mechanical therapy workshop. Erected in the rooms of the National Museum in Munich, the *Ambulatorium Medico-Mechanische Anstalt* was designed to offer convalescing soldiers in Reserve Hospital K direct access to orthopaedic therapies necessary for rehabilitation. It was constructed with an original grant of RM

8000 and opened in late 1915.[45] The Ambulatorium had equipment for administering not just work-therapy, but also water-therapy, heat therapy, electrotherapy, x-ray therapy, and light therapy, as well as facilities for physical and massage therapy.[46] And although it was staffed by a variety of military medical personnel, it was placed under the supervision of an orthopaedist, in this case, Dr Josef Trumpp, Fritz Lange's colleague and co-author of *War Orthopaedics*.

Although no complete statistics regarding the Ambulatorium exist, one 1917 report notes that in a six-month period the workshop had treated roughly 1178 patients with on average 133 men using the institute's facilities each day. In that period, they healed and returned 226 men to battle duty and another 753 to either garrison or work duty. Another 54 were released as wounded, but with no diminished work capacity. Just 80 men were declared disabled or unfit for further duty.[47] Thus, out of 1178 men, 87.6 per cent were returned to work, suggesting that the Ambulatorium was overall successful.

In fact, some considered it too successful. In February 1916 one group of Munich orthopaedists complained that the Bavarian Army was no longer honouring the contract it had with the local therapy workshops. They pointed out that since the construction of the Ambulatorium most of the disabled soldiers were being sent there instead of to the civilian workshops. This was indeed true. But according to the 1st Army Corps' Medical Office this was simply a financial decision and not meant as a slight to them. Contracted civilian therapy for the disabled soldier was expensive, and building a military rehabilitation workshop made economic sense. The Chief Medical Officer noted that the funds spent on paying for the treatment of soldiers in these private institutions had amounted to RM 74,915.50, whereas the construction of their own had cost just RM 8000. He also noted that most private institutions charged on average RM 1 per day for the treatment of each soldier, while the military could accomplish this for just 40 pfg.[48] By 1916 the military was absorbing orthopaedic workshops into its own system of military medicine.

In addition to constructing their own institutions for rehabilitating the wounded soldier, the German Army began organising and distributing soldiers in reserve hospitals according to their rehabilitation needs. For instance, in Munich they created special lazarettes for soldiers with intestinal problems, for dental cases, for 'war neurotics', for one-armed amputees and even one for double amputees. In addition to these recovery hospitals, the medical department created a lazarette designed especially for the purpose of rehabilitating men for agricultural work.

By mid 1915 MOs were becoming increasingly concerned with the fate of disabled soldiers who came from agricultural areas. According to widespread reports, Bavarian farmers 'had little faith in the possibility of recycling amputees'. Whereas the work-therapy institutes concentrated primarily on re-educating men's bodies for work in skilled trades, the farming lazarettes planned for Weihenstephan, Landsberg, and Eglfing – all towns in the surrounding countryside of Munich – were created in order to re-train them in agricultural work. In July of that year Hofbauer, the Chief MO of the Bavarian Army Corps in Munich, ordered all MOs in the city's reserve hospitals to be on the lookout for men like Lorenz Ostermeier, a 26-year old infantry soldier from Mammendorf, who was an ideal candidate for an agricultural lazarette, despite the loss of his right leg. In fact, he pointed out, arm amputees, leg amputees, foot amputees, those with stiffened limbs and joints – all these disabled soldiers – were ideal for farming if they came from that background originally.[49]

Civilian war-cripple care

In addition to their impact on the military's organisation of medical care for the wounded soldier, orthopaedists influenced civilian welfare programmes and policies. Although orthopaedists preferred to rehabilitate soldiers in their own therapy workshops, soon they recognised the value of incorporating more specialised courses or facilities into work-therapy. In Freiburg, Heidelberg, and Karlsruhe, orthopaedic professors developed courses for one-armed soldiers on how to reclaim their physical capacity [*physischen Leistungsfähigkeit*] as part of their attempts to send them back to work.[50] In Württemberg, the city of Ulm founded a School for the Wounded [*Verwundetenschule*] in 1915 which incorporated courses in everything from basketry to metal working to book-binding.[51] In the Prussian province of Westphalia, a similar thought prevailed, and in 1916 an orthopaedic professor and school director together founded the Düsseldorf School for the Wounded. Initially devoted to simply offering the severely injured a place to exercise their bodies, the School for the Wounded eventually evolved into a full-scale institution offering vocational instruction in industrial, clerical, and agricultural work to disabled soldiers.[52]

Upon hearing how other German states were instructing their war-disabled, in Saxony, the Minister of the Interior, Count Vitzthum von Eckstädt, issued a statement urging the trade and vocational schools to open their doors to the disabled soldiers so that they might take advantage of the instructional resources therein.[53] Indeed in Dresden several measures were taken. On July 1,1915 the Streetcar Administration Offices [*Strassenbahn Amt*] placed its own training workshops in the service of rehabilitation allowing disabled soldiers to use their equipment and workspace after working hours in order to practise and recover their bodily strength. By the end of July 1915, a School for

One-Armed War Invalids [*Einarmigerschule*] opened its doors offering courses to disabled soldiers, in both mechanical skills and stenography, as well as left-handed writing. In mid August of that same year, a one-armed school serving the 19th Army Corps opened in Chemnitz. Indeed, by late 1915 all manner of war-invalids were being re-trained and re-educated in Saxony. From carpentry work to bookkeeping, from stenography to machine-operating, Saxony's disabled soldiers had a variety of courses open to them which they could take free of charge if interested.[54]

In addition to launching training courses for disabled soldiers, orthopaedic rehabilitation inspired the creation of a civilian system of 'war-disabled welfare' [*Kriegskrüppelfürsorge*], designed to help re-insert the permanently injured soldier into the social and economic fabric of the nation. This was especially important because if a serviceman could not be restored enough for return to active duty, he was discharged from military service. Indeed, the imperial army had little use for soldiers who could not support the war effort. Therefore, if a soldier could not somehow be made re-usable [*wiederverwendungsfähig*], he was allowed to recover in the reserve hospitals until he was well enough for discharge. Upon release from military service, the care and welfare of these disabled soldiers became the responsibility of civilian welfare organisations. The problem with this, of course, was that there was no organised system of long-term care and disability welfare for disabled Germans – veterans or civilians.

From the outset of the war, orthopaedists had been vocal about the necessity of returning the war-disabled to their pre-war professions. This was not just a way for them to claim superior expertise in their approach to rehabilitation. Orthopaedists were guided by the firm conviction that Germany's last war had resulted in the social dislocation of many disabled veterans and they were determined that no soldier of the current war should experience the same downward mobility. Konrad Biesalski pointed out that after the Franco-Prussian War many medical students who had enlisted voluntarily returned shaken by their war-time experiences. Many of them never got over the war and remained changed men forever. Most of them never returned to their medical studies, and took up jobs which were ultimately unsatisfying, such as business or journalism. Christian Klumker, professor of social welfare, at the Frankfurt Academy of Social and Trade Sciences [*Frankfurter Akademie für Sozial- und Handelswissenschaften*] predicted that disabled skilled workers would sink to the level of the unskilled proletariat. According to Klumker, 'one of the biggest problems that awaits ours [the war-disabled] is occupational change. Many leave their old circle and find themselves not able to return to their old job – especially the war volunteers.' Orthopaedists argued that civilian welfare programmes needed to focus on returning disabled soldiers to their pre-war professions – and orthopaedists were experts in this.[55]

While orthopaedists had been developing and refining treatments for sending the disabled soldier back to work, they soon realised that an institutionalised structure for providing the disabled soldier with practical advice on *how* he might best accomplish this was necessary to ensure the success of *Wiedereingliederung*. They argued that a civilian-run programme should be developed that was geared especially for disabled veterans. *Berufsberatung* was a system of career counselling developed for transitioning the wounded or disabled soldier back to work after his rehabilitation therapy. Orthopaedists deemed it especially important that this system of counselling be conducted independently from the army's administration so that military authorities did not interfere with orthopaedic expertise. To that end they insisted that military personnel limit their role to simply informing soldiers of these services and otherwise refrain from interfering with the process.[56]

By the mid-point of the war, the Imperial Office for War-Disabled Care [*Reichsgeschäftsstelle der Kriegsbeschädigtenfürsorge*] had established guidelines that included defining the parameters of job counselling, how the counselling was to be organised, who was to run the system, and finally clarifying the relationship of this Berufsberatung with other aspects of war-disabled welfare. Once codified, these guidelines were published in *Die Kriegsbeschädigtenfürsorge*, the newspaper of war-disabled care, and subsequently circulated throughout the empire in the official newsletters of each provincial government. Although these guidelines were just that – *suggestions* – most organisations took them to heart and organised the whole of their welfare services around them.[57]

The guiding principle of Berufsberatung was to return the disabled veteran to the same post or position he held before the war. Returning the wounded ex-serviceman to 'his old workplace, his old master, and his old job with the same co-workers' would bring far better results than placing him in an unfamiliar setting. First, if he returned to his pre-war job, the disabled soldier would not require further training. He could simply fall back on familiar knowledge. Secondly, if a soldier did need help, he would find it more easily if he were surrounded by his former boss and colleagues.[58]

If the disabled soldier could not be returned to the job he held before the war, then he was to be placed in a position closely related to his former one. *Berufsberäter* (job counsellors) were to investigate whether the disabled man might be found an auxiliary position or posting in a sub-field of his former profession. If that were impossible, then they were to consider whether there existed a related field or subsidiary occupation for which the disabled man was well-suited. For instance, a locksmith might easily be retrained as a latheoperator [*Metalldreher*]. Alternatively, a carpenter [*Zimmermann*] who was no longer able to work long hours at a construction site might be steered to cabinet-making in a wood shop [*Tischlerberuf*]. Returning the wounded soldier to his pre-war profession or a similar, so-called 'allied' one was a practical choice. If a man had already completed the necessary education or apprenticeship for a particular vocation before his war injury, then returning him to it would require little additional training. His practical experience with the tools and materials of a certain trade would mean a smooth transition to a related one – carpenters were already familiar with the tools of cabinetry and therefore could be placed there more easily than a man who required long hours of training. Finally, given the rigorous training and evaluation that skilled workers had to complete in order to earn their place among their fellow workers, it was surmised that trade unions would more readily accept the return of a 'brother-worker' to their ranks than the assignment of a disabled soldier who had been too quickly or shoddily trained. Only as a last resort were job counsellors to consider directing the disabled soldier to a completely new profession.[59]

In the event that a soldier's injuries made returning to his pre-war profession impossible, however, Berufsberäter were encouraged to follow very specific steps when considering his new occupation. First, job counsellors were cautioned against choosing a vocation for the disabled soldier which was in high demand. Only an occupation that could offer the ex-serviceman a steady supply of work or which had a stable job market was to be placed under consideration for the rehabilitated soldier. Advisors were therefore reminded that these war veterans needed occupations which would ensure their long-term economic well-being.[60]

Second, counsellors were encouraged to seek out job environments which might offer the disabled a variety of tasks or multiple positions as part of ensuring that his employment would remain steady. This would be easy, they concluded, in big, urban areas where enough specialty workshops abounded which could employ a variety of workers. The real challenge, they argued, was finding steady employment for those disabled soldiers who lived in smaller towns or in the countryside. Here it was necessary, they argued, to thoroughly study the employment prospects for specially trained workers.

An ideal solution would be to find a local Berufsberater, one already familiar with the area's economy, industry, and job market. Local Berufsberäter would be able to optimise the relationship between local economy and war-disabled, thus ensuring a smooth transition. Berufsberatung offices were quite concerned with ensuring that the reinsertion of a disabled worker into the workforce took into consideration the local economic conditions and labour needs. To that end they also suggested that each local area be assigned just one single job-counsellor who was to then concentrate solely on matching up disabled workers with local employers of that region. This ensured not just an efficient, well-ordered distribution of rehabilitated workers, but also helped the job counsellor to maintain a more sympathetic and close relationship with 'his' disabled soldiers.[61]

Moreover, in light of the potentially slim number of job opportunities in small towns, the local Berufsberater could even consider whether it might make more sense to train the disabled veteran in a variety of skills. That is, continued the guidelines, it might make more sense for the disabled soldier to be sort of a 'jack of all trades' in areas where steady work in one profession was not always available. For instance, the guidelines suggested that a severely injured carpenter who could not find long-term work in a small town might simultaneously be re-trained as a cabinet-maker [*Tischler*], cartwright [*Stellmacher*], carver [*Schnitzer*], and even – were he dexterous enough – as a barber. Indeed, they noted that although a man in a small town might not be able to support himself through just one of these vocations, the combined incomes that such a handy-man might bring in would more than equal what he had earned before his injury.[62]

In addition to considering whether or not the local job market would be able to absorb an increased number of workers in certain professions, Berufsberäter were also cautioned to take the occupational health and safety of their clients into account. When considering both vocational suitability and job placement for the rehabilitated, job counsellors were reminded that they should be aware of the potential hazards in work environments for the disabled. For instance, soldiers with chronic lung conditions, they were advised, should not be placed in dust-producing factories; those with leg injuries should be kept away from highly combustible environments due to their compromised mobility. Moreover, it was suggested that amputees not be placed in occupations or work areas prone to on-the-job accidents. That is, the guidelines stressed that the extent to which employing the disabled might increase safety risks in certain occupations – for both themselves and their fellow workers – was to also be taken into account. Putting others in danger simply to employ the disabled veteran was not encouraged.[63]

In the main, Berufsberatung was meant to be a 'universal' system. It was not aimed at disabled veterans from a particular vocation or social strata, but rather provided advice to all severely wounded ex-servicemen regarding the work opportunities available to them, regardless of their background, education, or military rank. It was also meant to take a proactive approach. Rather than waiting for veterans to seek them out, Berufsberäter were encouraged to seek out those men not yet registered with their offices and offer them counselling as well. Moreover, job counsellors were advised not to employ a 'narrow-minded interpretation' [*engherzige Auslegung*] of who could be considered 'war-disabled' in any attempt to limit the scope of their counselling.[64] In fact, Berufsberäter were encouraged to visit the reserve hospitals while the soldier was still in recovery and begin counselling as soon as possible.

Orthopaedists insisted throughout the war that early medical intervention was necessary in order to optimise the results of physical rehabilitation, but they also emphasised that early social intervention was crucial to returning a soldier to his workplace.[65] Gaining access to disabled soldiers who were still in military hospitals would allow job counsellors to begin the important work of re-assuring the wounded serviceman that he would remain his 'old self'. It was also another way to prevent the onset of the pension-psychosis. A severely injured soldier who had been left to 'think too long about his future' was more likely to become convinced of his inability to work and sabotage his own rehabilitation. Gaining access to the soldiers while they were still in military hospitals increased the success of sending a man back to work.[66] Of course, it also opened another space within the military administration where doctors – not officers – were in charge of managing the men.

Given their positions as counsellors, Berufsberäter were important to disabled soldiers because they provided them with an economic link to the civilian world. They were not, however, employment agencies for the disabled. Nor were they supposed to allow the personal desires of the injured soldier to influence their counselling. In fact, Berufsberäter were warned that the disabled soldier tended to demand certain employment positions. In response to these demands Berufsberäter were cautioned to remain firm and, if possible, to disabuse the wounded soldier of the belief that he 'deserved' these posts. In this way, Berufsberäter worked as gatekeepers.[67] In particular, they were advised against placing disabled veterans in typical 'disabled jobs' or in the state's civil service bureaucracy. The rehabilitation success of the new orthopaedics made these practices obsolete and they were to be avoided.

Many disabled soldiers expected to be offered a post as concierge, porter, or telephone receptionist upon discharge from the service. Considered by many contemporary Germans to be occupations especially reserved for the permanently injured, these *Verlegenheitsberufe* – 'predicament positions' – had been the fate of some accident victims before the war.[68] Under the national insurance system, those workers who had been injured on the job were often placed in such positions when their accident leave had expired. Because the medical system under the accident insurance did not aim to restore the injured worker's body completely, it was common for railways, industrial concerns, factories, or other manual workplaces to re-employ their disabled workers in less strenuous positions such as these. During the war, many disabled soldiers based their expectations of war-disabled welfare on the practices of the German insurance system and grew to feel entitled to such positions. In fact, orthopaedists often remarked upon the demand among injured soldiers to be assigned such positions rather than to be sent back to their pre-war 'good, old jobs'. Indeed, much like the 'pension-psychosis' which was spreading among the wounded, orthopaedists clearly feared that the demand for the desk job was threatening to become an epidemic as well.[69]

Berufsberäter were cautioned against placing the disabled soldier in such positions, however. First, like all positions left vacant by men called to the war, ideally these jobs were to be held open for their original occupants. However, as it was not always possible to keep vacant posts open or to wait for a particular soldier to be discharged and return, it was acceptable for job counsellors to fill these posts in the short-term with recovering ex-servicemen. As temporary jobs, these positions were ideal for soldiers still recovering from their wounds or surgery. Working temporarily as a porter, for instance, a convalescing soldier might gradually reclaim his strength and agility while also earning his own money and establishing his economic self-sufficiency. Secondly, because the nature of these posts was so undemanding long-term (often requiring little else but opening a door or checking a badge), they were to be reserved for those war-disabled who were permanently incapable of any other work. Therefore, they were best dispensed only as *temporary* posts for recovering veterans or when all other possibilities for re-employment had been exhausted. They were not, however, simply to be handed out to any disabled soldier simply because he claimed to be permanently maimed.[70]

In addition to procedures regarding the *Verlegenheitsberufe*, special guidelines concerning the civil service were established. Berufsberäter were cautioned against placing disabled veterans in the civil bureaucracy, even though many also expected these positions. Wounded soldiers often claimed that their injuries prevented them from competing evenly on the job market and therefore looked to the government for a secure job. Others made claims that 'because they had allowed themselves to be mutilated for the state' they should be rewarded with a job. Because the modern rehabilitation claimed it could return to the men what they had lost, both of these claims were considered spurious. The guidelines characterised some soldiers as hankering for a government post: 'due to a certain laziness, they do not want to re-train'. This last judgment is revealing in that it suggests that some attitudes toward the disabled were less than charitable. Regardless of how they justified their claim on a position in the civil bureaucracy, the guidelines were adamant that disabled soldiers be disabused of the notion that the state was now responsible for providing them with employment.[71]

As with other vacant positions, Berufsberäter were to reserve civil service posts for their original occupants – many of whom might also be injured in the war. Moreover, pointed out the agency, those labourers used to yearly increasing wages on the free market would not be satisfied with the fixed salary of the civil servant. Indeed, because so many Germans were convinced that there would be a labour shortage after the war, Berufsberäter were supposed to emphasise that disabled soldiers would be likely to earn more money in the post-war economy with a waged position rather than a salaried one. Economic arguments were used to sway the disabled from wanting a government position.[72]

Wiedereingliederung *and social order*

Although Berufsberatung was created for assisting the disabled soldier, aspects of it also seem concerned with managing the overall job market in the empire, not simply advising the disabled soldier. Counselling policies included taking into consideration not just the disabled's previous work experience and bodily health, but also the needs of the various regional labour markets, the hiring capacity of the civil service, the displacement of healthy workers called to arms, and co-worker relationships, all suggesting that a larger project of social management was at play in the system of Berufsberatung. This is expressed even more clearly in the following details of the guidelines.

Despite its claims as an equal opportunity system, the Berufsberatung programme for the disabled actually practised strict social segregation between socio-economic groups. The guidelines clearly stated that 'the training and educating of war-disabled from other vocations in order to place them in commercial or clerical positions is to be discouraged.'[73] According to the main office, many disabled soldiers were 'deluding themselves' with the idea that training in bookkeeping or typing would allow them to find an 'easy job'. Although they argued that these professions were already overfilled before the war and thus should be avoided, the language used suggests that Berufsberäter were just as concerned with monitoring access to gateway professions to the lower middle classes.[74] In this sense, they were echoing the sentiments of Germany's orthopaedists who also reported a widespread attempt at social climbing by veterans. Drawing on his experiences in Wurzburg, the orthopaedist Jakob Riedinger, noted that 'Older people take up their previous occupations more happily than the younger ones, who are expecting a betterment in their social position.'[75] Clearly both doctors and welfare workers were worried that the upheaval of war might result in the crumbling of formerly fixed social boundaries if workers were re-trained and placed into the 'easy' white-collar jobs. One sure way, then, to reassert these blurring social boundaries was to guard the gateways into these professions. As one proponent of the new war-disabled care noted,

> Today's war welfare, in the most basic sense of the word ... has reinvented itself in response to this war. It lifts those whom it serves out of the poor house in the sense that it gives the war-disabled not just an assurance of a minimum standard of care, rather it guarantees to him a certain standard of living – according to his status. Indeed, the most important thing about our contemporary war-disabled care is that it does not allow the disabled to fall below his social position.[76]

By regulating the job placement and training of disabled veterans, doctors and welfare workers could prevent skilled workers or farmers from using their injuries to 'better their social positions'. In this way, everyday representatives of the middle classes in Germany – doctors, state officials, welfare providers, and office clerks – were acting as both gatekeepers and managers of the empire's overall social structure.

The second clear marker of large-scale population management being practised under the guise of Berufsberatung was the policy that 'those war-disabled who came from the countryside – either as farmers or as rural workers – were to be redirected back to their previous residences'.[77] Out of a general concern for both the individual and the empire, Berufsberäter were encouraged to relocate those wounded ex-servicemen who were originally from rural areas and backgrounds to their homelands as quickly as possible. Indeed the compilers of the Brandenburg guidelines pointed out that it was obvious [*leicht begreiflich*] that the tantalising attractions of the big city seemed to be exerting too great an influence on those injured soldiers from the countryside. They argued that those war-disabled who convalesced near larger metropolitan areas were regularly 'misled with regard to the supposed pleasures of the city' and too often wished to remain there even after recovery.

However, for two important reasons, Berufsberäter were instructed to counsel their rural clients against this desire. The first was that the urban migration of these rural Germans would put added pressure on the labour market in the city; too many available workers in metropolitan areas would saturate post-war urban markets. The second was that those soldiers who came from the countryside were 'fooled by the superficialities of city life' and had no idea what daily existence in urban areas was really like, especially 'how empty their own existence can turn out to feel in a strange and foreign place'.[78] Back in their hometowns, disabled veterans would be surrounded by long-time, trusted friends who would be more able – and indeed more likely – to help them 'find that inner peace which was so crucially important in the struggle to come to terms with their fate'.[79] Sending the rural disabled back home then was important for multiple reasons, not just in order to manage the urban labour market, but apparently to manage their psychological well-being, as well. Given that the disabled soldier's mental state was considered to be so instrumental in his physical recovery, this is perhaps not very surprising.

What is not mentioned here, but which might well also have played a role in the overall policy to relocate the wounded to the country is the potential housing shortage and political unrest these urban areas faced, as well. During the war rural Germans streamed from the countryside to the cities looking for work in the various war industries. This war-time population shift combined with the larger-scale urbanisation trend in place since the late nineteenth century meant that during the war already overcrowded cities were reaching a crisis point. Housing and other urban commodities were becoming increasingly scarce.[80] Relocating Germans who were not necessary to the war economy through factory work or other auxiliary service away from the cities was a way to remove some pressure on not just the urban labour market, but also that for food, housing, and other commodities, too. Moreover, urban areas had long been considered hotbeds of proletarian unrest by the more conservative middle classes. Huge concentrations of disgruntled industrial workers – and, by 1917, disabled soldiers – appeared to many leaders to be ripe recruitment areas for the Social Democrats.[81] Relocating these men from the cities to the rural countryside could also be a political prophylactic measure, as well. From the outset, then, it appears that Berufsberatung was more than simply job counselling; rather it appears to have marked a serious attempt to rebuild war-time German society, as well.

Ultimately programmes of *Wiedereingliederung* developed along sharply delineated class lines. Despite the claims of impartiality written into the official guidelines for organising the Berufsberatung of disabled soldiers, a deeper analysis reveals clear concerns about the impact that war and widespread disability would have on the social structure of Germany. Moreover, as a response to fears about the dislocation of certain segments of the population, many professional groups chose to organise their own programmes for reintegrating – or 'recycling' – their disabled members, particularly those in the so-called 'intellectual professions'.[82] In fact, many of these seemed especially concerned with the fate of the empire's middle-class disabled soldier. As *Kopfarbeiter* these men were white-collar workers (office clerks, teachers, bureaucrats, and other professionals) whose bodies would ordinarily never have been put at risk in the same way that the bodies of industrial workers or farmers routinely were; this is what made their fate seem so particularly unjust. Therefore organisations that were devoted particularly to the future welfare of the empire's disabled clerks and teachers – even academics – eventually sprang up across the empire.

One such organisation was the German Central Office of Career Counselling for Academics [*Deutsche Zentralstelle für Berufsberatung der Akademiker*, DZBA]. Founded in 1917 in a joint effort by the Academic Auxiliary League [*Akademischer Hilfsbund*] and the German Student Service of 1914 [*Deutscher Studentendienst von 1914*], this organisation was devoted to promoting – through scientific research – career counselling and job placement for academics and research-scientists [*Wissenschaftler*]. Although the DZBA was headquartered in Berlin, the association itself extended throughout the German Empire and included both active members and patrons (i.e. members whose contributions and role was a purely financial one).[83]

In step with the above-mentioned parameters of Berufsberatung, the DZBA firmly maintained that managing the empire's labour resources was crucial to sustaining the national economy. In the founding meeting of the DZBA, the director of the Academic Auxiliary League, Dr Pinkerneil, argued that the war had taken a heavier toll on academics than it had on other segments of society. Indeed, he claimed that the dwindling numbers of both students and academics in war-time Germany meant that the empire could no longer leave vocational choice to chance. Therefore, he maintained, it was crucial to 'now also ration out the intellectual capital of Germany'.[84] What was necessary, he argued, was a more thorough job counselling and examination of all citizens in order to ensure that each German was being directed to that profession which could best make use of his skills.[85] Indeed, as the DZBA codified in its organisational charter, job counselling was important not simply in terms of solving the employment problem. Rather, the group maintained that through vocational choice 'ultimately a person's lifework as well as [his] personality development is determined'.[86] Moreover, the group claimed that the importance of 'professional guidance' – especially with regard to its social, economic and cultural impact – had only become evident during the war.[87]

Clearly to the DZBA, the goals of Berufsberatung extended far beyond just returning wounded academics to work. In fact, the general viewpoint that choosing a vocation (including its subsequent training) included choosing a certain 'lifestyle' as well, suggests that this voluntary association, too, was just as intent on managing German social boundaries as were the officials in charge of rehabilitation. To that end, the DZBA set up courses, such as one offered on September 16–26, 1918, which provided advice and instruction on how to reintegrate the war-disabled academic back into German society. Moreover, in keeping with their overall social goals of regeneration within the academic ranks, these courses were also open to those war-disabled *officers* who wanted to enter the 'intellectual life'.[88] It seems apparent that to the members of the DZBA, certain members of German society were more welcome in academic circles than others.

The DZBA was not the only organisation interested in the future of the empire's disabled officer corps. Founded in the autumn of 1915, the German Auxiliary Union for War Wounded Officers [*Deutscher Hilfsbund für kriegsverletzte Offiziere*, DhkO] was also dedicated to returning disabled officers to the workforce – particularly to the commercial and business enterprises for which they were considered so well-suited.[89] Other organisations included one for consumptive and tubercular war-disabled and another for the independent commercial class [*selbstständiger kaufmännische Mittelstand*].[90] Organisations such as these, which were dedicated to particular social groups within the empire, reinforce the notion that the *Wiedereingliederung* of the wounded was divided along class lines.[91]

The larger project of Wiedereingliederung actually translated into far more than simply rehabilitating disabled soldiers. Guidelines which included as their goals the return of rural Germans to the countryside, re-training veterans according to local or national labour market needs, the distribution of re-trained labour according to employer desires, and the protection of certain socio-economic groups, make it obvious that the job-counselling programmes being instituted under the auspices of veteran welfare were in fact as equally concerned with the social management of the nation as they were with the welfare needs of the wounded veteran. Indeed, when one considers that the design of the various Berufsberatung programmes was ultimately able to control the geographic (re)location of the discharged veteran, his place of future employment, his future employer, *and* his vocational (re)training, the extent of the programme's ability to manage the post-injury life of the disabled soldier appears startling. Indeed, Berufsberatung leaders were not unaware of this aspect, as one notes from the leaders of the DZBA, who maintained that they were not just finding these injured men jobs, they were providing them with 'lifestyles'.

Conclusion

When war broke out in 1914, there were structures in place for the mobilisation of soldiers for war. What was missing, however, were structures for rehabilitating wounded soldiers and re-integrating them back into German society. During the war, military, state and civilian authorities established programmes for treating and healing the severely wounded soldier. In addition to healing him, however, they also developed institutions for re-inserting him back into the social fabric of the nation. Programmes which provided disabled soldiers with career counselling, vocational retraining, and job placement were all part of the larger project of Wiedereingliederung. From the outset, however, these civilian welfare programmes were just as concerned with maintaining the German social order on the home front as they were with providing practical help to the wounded soldier.

Moreover, orthopaedists established themselves at the helm of these rehabilitation efforts. By positioning themselves as authorities in this field, orthopaedists were able to take the lead in the development and institution of these programmes thereby gaining influence over military and civilian policies regarding disabled welfare. By making their expertise indispensable to the managing of Germany's disabled soldiers, orthopaedists were furthering their own interests in specialisation, while demonstrating how crucial they were to the nation at war.

The creation of these new structures for rehabilitating the disabled soldier constituted more than just a new system of welfare for wounded veterans however.[92] Rather, as this chapter has demonstrated, *Wiedereingliederung* eventually developed into a much broader social project of managing the 're-abled' body. Placing the severely injured soldier back into the workforce so that he could earn his 'own bread' was not just an attempt to heal him; it eventually evolved into a system of social engineering, becoming part of a larger attempt to buttress social lines that were in danger of blurring in war-torn Germany. As the representative of an organisation devoted to the social reintegration of disabled academics argued,

> After a lost war and economic impoverishment, the main portion of the German people's national wealth will be its manpower. Reconstruction, therefore, is completely dependent upon the strategic use and allocation of the nation's labour resources as purposefully as possible.[93]

Furthermore, he argued, 'The productivity of work is dependent upon the relationship of every individual to his work. This relationship … is determined by an individual's characteristics, inclinations, and capabilities.'[94] During the economic and social upheaval of war, many Germans realised that the future of the entire nation depended upon the careful management of all the nation's human resources – and orthopaedists gave them the tools for doing so.

Still, before the wounded could be fully re-integrated into society, the orthopaedic community had to convince the majority of Germans that sending the disabled back into the workforce was not only possible, but indeed beneficial – for both the wounded and the nation. The next chapter of this book examines the campaign of 'enlightenment work' that Biesalski and other welfare officials undertook in order to publicise the developments in orthopaedic technology and rehabilitative medicine. This re-education of the general public was instrumental in enlisting popular support and cooperation in the development of broader programmes of social and economic rehabilitation of disabled veterans. By re-casting the image of the wounded veteran as one who was no longer permanently crippled, but rather capable of complete recovery, public perceptions of the so-called 'crippled' began to shift. Ultimately this campaign brought with it the end of *Krüppeltum* in Germany and the invention of 'disability'.

Notes

1 SHAD MdI 7417 fol. 21, 'Industrielle Kriegsbeschaedigten-Fuersorge', *Meissner Tageblatt* (192) August 19, 1916 (archived clipping, not paginated).
2 For more on the development of orthopaedic treatments and their application to the war wounded, as well as the singular expertise therein to which orthopaedists laid claim, see P. Möhring, 'Die orthopädische Übungsbehandlung auf Grund der Erfahrungen des Krieges', pp. 287–310 in Hermann Gocht, ed., *Die Orthopädie in der Kriegs- und Unfallheilkunde* [Deutsche Orthopädie, Vol. 4]. (Stuttgart: Ferdinand Enke, 1921), especially 287, 307.
3 BayHStA, I GenKdo AK, SanA 413. Regarding Lange's re-assignment of duty see von Seydel's directive of March 3, 1915. Regarding the formation of a Fachärztliche Beirat see his directive of February 4,1915.
4 *Wiedereingliederung* is an interesting word. The German root of this compound term, *Glied*, can denote the same meanings as its English counterpart, member. *Das Glied* (member) can refer to a (human) limb or body part, male sex organ, or link among objects. *Das Mitglied* (member) denotes being the member or representative of a group – be it a social, professional, or political organisation, as in being a 'party member'. *Die Eingliederung* refers to the integration of a part into a whole. *Wiedereingliederung*, then, obviously calls up all of these meanings: the re-integration of a body part into the whole body, the restoration/reintegration of the male body, the reintegration of a social group (the disabled) into German society, and finally how it was used by German orthopaedists in WWI to specifically refer to the overall process of medical and social rehabilitation. Therefore this single word simultaneously conjures multiple notions of 're-insertion', the restoration of membership or 're-membering', *and* 'rehabilitation'.
5 Edward M. Hartwell, 'Peter Henry Ling, the Swedish Gymnasiarch', *American Physical Education Review*, Vol. 1, No. 1 (1896), 1–13.
6 Michal Hau, *The Cult of Health and Beauty in Germany: A Social History, 1890–1930* (Chicago: University of Chicago Press, 2003).

7 For more on the broader history of physical therapy – especially with an eye to Krankengymnastik and its role in nineteenth-century German medicine, see W. Heipertz, 'Geschichte der Krankengymnastik', pp. 87–97 in August Rütt, ed., *Geschichte der Orthopädie im Deutschen Sprachraum* (Stuttgart: Enke, 1993).

8 For more on the development of health spas and therapeutic institutions in later nineteenth-century Germany, as well as their overall lack of success in rehabilitating the injured, see Eghigian, *Making Security Social*, 127–45; quote on p. 135.

9 Eghigian, *Making Security Social*, 145–50.

10 Konrad Biesalski, *Umfang und Art des jugendlichen Krüppeltums und der Krüppelfürsorge in Deutschland* (Leipzig: Voss, 1909).

11 Devine, *Disabled Soldiers' and Sailors' Pensions and Training*, 289.

12 Whalen, *Bitter Wounds*, 88–9.

13 When the German Empire initially went to war in 1914, the army consisted of eighteen Prussian, three Bavarian, two Saxon, and one Württemburg Corps. For more on the 1914 organisation and structure of the German army see Hermann Cron, *Imperial German Army 1914–18: Organization, Structure, Orders of Battle* (Solihull: Helion & Co, 2002).

14 Friedrich Ring, *Zur Geschichte der Militärmedizin in Deutschland* (Berlin: Deutscher Militärverlag, 1962), 222.

15 Cron, *Imperial German Army*, 226.

16 D.B. Nash, *Imperial German Army Handbook 1914–1918* (London: Ian Allan, 1980), 66.

17 Generalarzt Dr Paalzow, 'Das Sanitätswesen im Kriege', in *Die Sanitäre Kriegsrüstung Deutschlands* (Dehmigke Verlag: Berlin, 1915), 2–6. Ring, *Militärmedizin*, 227–8.

18 Paalzow, 'Das Sanitätswesen im Kriege', 11–12. Nash points out that initially field hospitals were equipped with 200 beds. Nash, *Imperial German Army*, 66.

19 Paalzow, 'Das Sanitätswesen im Kriege', 13–14. Nash, *Imperial German Army*, 66.

20 Paalzow, 'Das Sanitätswesen im Kriege', 12–13.

21 Ring, *Militärmedizin*, 229–30.

22 Cron, *Imperial German Army*, 293.

23 Devine, *Disabled Soldiers and Sailors*, 295–6.

24 Paalzow, 'Das Sanitätswesen im Kriege', 12.

25 Devine, *Disabled Soldiers and Sailors*, 296.

26 Nash, *Imperial German Army*, 66.

27 Ring, *Militärmedizin*, 221–2.

28 Ring, *Militärmedizin*, 245–6.

29 Heeres-Sanitätsinspektion des Reichskriegsministeriums, *Gliederung des Heeressanitätswesens im Weltkriege 1914/1918. Sanitätsbericht über das Deutsche Heer, Vol. I.* (Mittler und Sohn: Berlin, 1935), 113.

30 Ring, *Militärmedizin*, 244. The medical department counted casualties according to numbers of cases, not soldiers. Thus soldiers could be counted as wounded or ill more than once if they were healed and returned to duty and then injured again.

31 For more on Biesalski's tour of welfare institutes, as well as a list of those resources

he found available, see Biesalski, *Kriegskrüppelfürsorge,* 33–44. For a post-war account, see Devine, *Disabled Soldiers and Sailors,* 289.

32 Adolf Silberstein, *Kriegsinvalidenfürsorge* [Würzburger Abhandlungen aus dem Gesamtgebiet der praktischen Medizin, Vol. 15, No. 6] (Würzburg: Curt Kabitzsch, 1915), 2.

33 Silberstein, *Kriegsinvalidenfürsorge,* 5.

34 Cron, *Imperial German Army,* 293.

35 For a discussion on the lack of experience with large-scale demobilisation, see Bessel, *Germany after the First World War,* especially pp. 49–50, 69–90. For a discussion of the pension system's inability to handle the overwhelming number of war victims, see Whalen, *Bitter Wounds,* especially pp. 95–105.

36 For more on the brief training offered to volunteers and draftees at the start of the war, see Bessel, *Germany after the First World War,* 7. See also Herwig's mention of refresher courses and defensive schools established in early 1916 in order to train new officers and recruits. Herwig, *The First World War,* 249. Of course regular army conscripts received the requisite two years of army training, although Stig Förster notes this 'training' focused more upon the inculcation of militaristic and conservative values, not military skill or weaponry. See Stig Förster's chapter, entitled 'The Armed Forces and Military Planning', pp. 454–88, in Roger Chickering ed., *Imperial Germany: A Historiographical Companion* (Westport, Conn.: Greenwood, 1996), 456.

37 Pensions are discussed further in chapter 4. For more information on the pension systems in place for German veterans of World War I, see the introduction and first chapter of James M. Diehl, *The Thanks of the Fatherland: German Veterans after the Second World War* (Chapel Hill: University of North Carolina Press , 1993), 1–30; and Whalen, *Bitter Wounds,* pp 88–93. For a contemporary account of the history of long-term care and pensions for war-disabled soldiers, see Dr Otto Neustätter, 'Kriegsbeschädigtenfürsorge in früherer Zeit', pp. 329–36 in Artur Baumgarten-Crusius, ed., *Geschichte der Sachsen im Weltkrieg* [Sachsen in Grosser Zeit, 3] (Leipzig: Max Lippold, 1920).

38 Möhring, 'Die orthopädische Übungsbehandlung', 307.

39 BArch R3901/9334. 'Fürsorge für Verstummelte und Sieche', Merkblatt für beinverletzte Kriegsbeschädigte mit orthopädischem Schuhwerk oder Stützapparat.

40 See for example articles from both Biesalski and von Baeyer which include a discussion on the importance of simple artificial limbs which amputees could easily repair themselves. Biesalski, 'Über Prothesen bei Amputationen des Armes insbesondere des Oberarmes', *Münchener medizinische Wochenschrift,* Vol. 44 (1915): 1492–6, 1494; and von Baeyer, 'Prothesen aus Weissblech', 1497.

41 Or so the medical community consistently argued. Ironically, few doctors seemed willing to concede that the disabled soldier simply felt he deserved a pension ipso facto for his injuries and the 'right' to live from its income alone. For more on the pathologisation of the pension psychosis see chapter 4. See also the discussion at the 1916 emergency conference of the DVK in P. Mollenhauer, 'Bericht über

die ausserordentliche Tagung der Deutschen Vereinigung für Krüppelfürsorge', *Zentralblatt für chirurgische und mechanische Orthopädie*, Vol. 10 (1916): 74–81. For a brief discussion on the rise of the pension psychosis in the Kaiserreich, see also Eghigian, *Making Security Social*, 244–5.

42 For detailed discussions of rehabilitation techniques and a list of fifty-one vocations or occupations – including white-collar work and handicrafts – see Biesalski, *Kriegskrüppelfürsorge*, 33.

43 For more on the development of orthopaedic treatments and their application to the war wounded, as well as the singular expertise therein to which orthopaedists laid claim, see Möhring, 'Die orthopädische Übungsbehandlung auf Grund der Erfahrungen des Krieges', 287–310; especially 287, 307. For a look at how other nations used work-therapy to heal their soldiers, see Jeffrey S. Reznick, 'Work-Therapy and the Disabled British Soldier in Great Britain in the First World War: The Case of Shepherd's Bush Military Hospital, London', pp. 185–203 in David A. Gerber, ed., *Disabled Veterans in History* (Ann Arbor: University of Michigan Press, 2000)', especially pp. 192–203.

44 BayHStA, I GenKdo AK, SanA 413. 29 May 1915 Schultzen, KM to all Army Corps Medical Departments.

45 BayHStA, I GenKdo AK, SanA 413. May 2, 1915 from the War Ministry to the Medical Department of the Bay IAK.

46 BayHStA, I GenKdo AK, SanA 335.

47 BayHStA, I GenKdo AK, SanA 335.

48 BayHStA, I GenKdo AK, SanA 414.

49 BayHStA, I GenKdo AK, SanA 1013. Memo from Hofbauer to All Active Duty Doctors in Reserve Troops, Military Hospitals, and Auxiliary Hospitals. Dated 14 July 1915.

50 SHAD AAA 2376. Letter from the Saxon envoy in Munich to Vitzthum dated February 19, 1915, fol. 2.

51 [Ulmer Verwundetenschule], *Die Ulmer Verwundetenschule: Ihre Werkstätten, Kurse, und Einrichtungen der Beratungsstelle für Kriegs-Invaliden* (Ulm, 1918).

52 SHAD LVA 111. See the pamphlet *Die Düsseldorfer Verwundetenschule* (Düsseldorf: A. Bagel, 1916).

53 SHAD MdI 7147, fol. 4. See Vitzthum's request dated April 23, 1915 urging the gewerbliche und sonstige Fachschulen to place their schools in the service of the war-disabled care. For the reports sent to Vitzthum (who was also head of the Foreign Office in addition to being Minister of the Interior) from various Saxon envoys to other German states see SHAD AAA 2376.

54 Dresden Stadtarchiv: Schulamt III: File 813: 'Einarmigerschule'. See the June 24, 1915 protocol of a meeting held in the Dresden Rathaus regarding courses and schools for the war-invalid. See also the correspondence between the Strassenbahn directors and the founders of the one-armed school as well as the advertisement posters and newspaper articles collected in the same file.

55 Biesalski, 'Die ethische und wirtschaftliche Bedeutung', 12.

56 BArch R 86/2310, 'Berufsberatung (1902–1926)'. According to the Berufsberatung guidelines, the relationship between the superior and subordinate – regardless of its quality – was too likely to inhibit quality advising. Indeed, as they pointed out, 'Career-advising, especially with regard to older people, demands close interpersonal contact, while with a superior officer – as is implied already in the relationship – there will always remain a certain distance.' *Amtliche Mitteilungen der Brandenburgischen Kriegsbeschädigtenfürsorge* 6 (September 16,1916), 85.

57 BArch R 86/2310: Berufsberatung (1902–1926). See the *Amtliche Mitteilungen*, 85. This official newsletter from the Landesdirektor of Brandenburg was distributed to all offices and people to whom war-disabled care was entrusted. Not only was it meant to be archived and used as a reference, but according to its masthead, was also meant to be confidential [*vertraulich*].

58 *Amtliche Mitteilungen* 6, 92–3.

59 *Amtliche Mitteilungen* 6, 93.

60 *Amtliche Mitteilungen* 6, 93–4.

61 *Amtliche Mitteilungen* 6, 88.

62 *Amtliche Mitteilungen* 6, 93–4.

63 *Amtliche Mitteilungen* 6, 94.

64 *Amtliche Mitteilungen* 6, 86.

65 *Amtliche Mitteilungen* 6, 86.

66 *Amtliche Mitteilungen* 6, 86

67 *Amtliche Mitteilungen* 6, 89.

68 The term *Verlegenheitsberuf* is not a term of contemporary use, nor is it found in any historical dictionary. The term clearly refers to a certain group of occupations (*Berufe*), however, the descriptive itself – *Verlegenheit* – is not easily translated. In general, it can mean 'embarrassment', 'awkwardness', 'difficulty', or 'confusion'. To bring or put someone 'in Verlegenheit' can mean to place a person in an awkward, difficult, or even embarrassing position, so a 'Verlegenheitsberuf' could be a position found for someone in an 'embarrassing' or 'difficult' situation. This definition, however, does not connote for whom the job is awkward or shameful – the job-holder, the employer, or society. The term definitely does, however, appear to be a negative or pejorative one, especially in its use here. For more on Verlegenheitsberufe see the discussion in chapter 4.

69 *Amtliche Mitteilungen* 6, 94–5.

70 *Amtliche Mitteilungen* 6, 94–5.

71 *Amtliche Mitteilungen* 6, 95.

72 *Amtliche Mitteilungen* 6, 95.

73 *Amtliche Mitteilungen* 6, 95–6.

74 *Amtliche Mitteilungen* 6, 96.

75 Dr Riedinger (Würzburg) in 'Bericht über die ausserordentliche Tagung der Deutschen Vereinigung für Krüppelfürsorge' (February 7, 1916), 77–8 in *Zentralblatt für chirurgische und medizinische Orthopädie*, Vol.10 (1916).

76 R. Hans Roeseler, 'Deutsche Kriegsfürsorge', *Wegweiser fuer das werktätige Volk*. 5, No.1 (January 1918), 11
77 *Amtliche Mitteilungen* 6, 96.
78 *Amtliche Mitteilungen* 6, 96.
79 *Amtliche Mitteilungen* 6, 96.
80 For more on urban migration and the lack of affordable housing in Germany in the second half of the war and the immediate post-war period, see Susanna Magri's chapter, 'Housing', pp. 374–417 in Jay Winter and Jean-Louis Robert, eds, *Capital Cities at War: Paris, London, Berlin 1914–1919* (Cambridge: Cambridge University Press, 1997). See also Bessel, *Germany after the First World War*, 166–94.
81 For more on the increased social democratic agitation in Berlin, as well as the participation of disabled veterans therein, see Adrian Gregory, 'Lost Generations: The Impact of Military Casualties on Paris, London, and Berlin', pp. 57–103 in Winter and Robert eds, *Capital Cities at War*; especially pp. 100–1. For more on the fear of political conservatives that disabled soldiers would be seduced by the Left and their social and political groups, see Diehl, 'The Organization of German Veterans, 1917–1919', especially pp. 147–58.
82 Germans were not forbidden to create specialised offices. In fact, the Brandenburg office for war-disabled care noted that specialised offices for particular vocations could be created when these were deemed absolutely necessary. These 'special offices' [*Sonderstellen*] were to be constructed adjacent to the 'general' ones if they dealt with so-called 'sharply delineated' professions which required separate counselling. Specifically these might include agricultural work and the so-called 'intellectual professions', which due to both the specialised nature of the work, as well as the operating conditions [*Betriebsverhältnisse*] of each region, required more expert advice. *Amtliche Mitteilungen* 6, 89.
83 BArch R86/2310. Satzungen der Deutschen Zentralstelle der Berufsberatung der Akademiker, e.V.
84 Although Pinkerneil offered no statistical evidence to support his claim that the war had taken a particularly heavy toll on 'academics', Charles McClelland has noted that the war did drain universities of both students and teachers, as well as doctors and other civil servants. See Charles McClelland, *The German Experience of Professionalization: Modern Learned Professions and their Organizations from the Early Nineteenth Century to the Hitler Era* (Cambridge: Cambridge University Press, 1991), 137, 170–1.
85 BArch R1501/113089/6. 'Zentralstelle für Berufsberatung heimkehrender Krieger und Internierten', 83.
86 BArch R86/2310. Leitsätze der Deutschen Zentralstelle der Berufsberatung der Akademiker, e.V., 2.
87 Leitsätze der Deutschen Zentralstelle der Berufsberatung der Akademiker.
88 'Zentralstelle für Berufsberatung heimkehrender Krieger und Internierten'.
89 BArch R3901/36070: 8866 'Vereine und Stiftungen für Kriegsbeschädigten und

deren Hinterbliebenen'. See 'Geschäftsbericht des Deutschen Hilfsbundes fur kriegsverletzte Offiziere für das Jahr 1916'.

90 BArch R86/2310. For more on the organisation devoted to the job counselling and placement of war-disabled lung patients, see the minutes of the 21st general meeting of Das Zentralkomitee zur Bekämpfung der Tuberkulose (May 23, 1917). For more on the guidelines designed to protect the self-described 'neu Mittelstand' or commercial middle class from being overcrowded with war-disabled see SHAD MdI 7417. *Kriegsfürsorge für die Angestellten in Handel und Industrie* (Essen: Verband kath. kaufm. Vereinigungen Deutschlands e.V., 1917).

91 What would be useful here is a discussion of how the trade unions and guilds reacted – or even contributed – to the overall project of *Wiedereingliederung*. For instance, did they support training courses and independent programmes designed to integrate the wounded soldier into their ranks? Or did they see these as competing sources of second-rate labour which would eventually dilute their own wage-earning potential? Unfortunately such an analysis lies outside the research of this current study.

92 For an example of such an analysis see, for instance, Cohen, *The War Come Home*. Cohen's focus is on the role of the state in creating and managing welfare programmes for the disabled, rather than offering an in-depth analysis of these actual programmes themselves; therefore her study misses the veteran's actual experience within the system. Moreover, her study primarily looks at veteran care *after* the war, not during it. Therefore she also fails to see how this care was part of the larger social organisation of war. The impact of orthopaedic medicine and the role of rehabilitation in the empire's mobilisation for 'total war' will be discussed further in chapter 5.

93 BArch R86/2320. 'Leitsätze' Deutsche Zentralstelle für Berufsberatung der Akademiker (DZBA).

94 'Leitsätze' DZBA.

4

INVENTING DISABILITY: RE-CASTING THE 'CRIPPLE' IN WAR-TIME GERMANY

> Through a tireless campaign of enlightenment it has been possible in the past year to plant in the minds of those even in the remotest regions of the nation, the crucial importance of the physical training of the disabled. Throughout the land sentimental pity for them has yielded to our campaign, even among the wounded themselves. (Konrad Biesalski, 1916)[1]

In 1915, the same year that Fritz Lange issued *War Orthopaedics,* his medical guide for military doctors, Konrad Biesalski published a short pamphlet for the empire's injured soldiers and their families: *War Cripple Welfare: An Educational Word of Comfort and Warning.* Biesalski penned the booklet with the intention of alleviating the fears that many contemporary Germans held, as trainloads of severely injured soldiers returned from war. Aware that many in the empire were concerned about the welfare of these men and the economic security of their families, he wrote the brochure in order to educate the public on the ways in which modern medicine could ensure that the war-disabled would still be able to 'earn his daily bread'. Within the brochure's forty-four pages, Biesalski used medical explanations, a wide variety of diagrams and photographs, and several case studies to detail how any disabled soldier could be physically restored and returned to his pre-war occupation. He outlined the advances in fracture care, methods for repairing damaged nerves, techniques for relaxing stiffened joints, and even how artificial limbs could replace lost ones. In fact, Biesalski comforted his readers that the widespread concern regarding the economic fate of the war-disabled (and their dependents) was really unnecessary because with the recent developments in modern orthopaedics all the essential conditions for restoring these men were present, except for one – the 'correct perception of the bodily capacity [*körperliche Leistungsfähigkeit*] of the maimed'.[2] Indeed, according to Biesalski what threatened the rehabilitation of the wounded patient most was *not* the severity of his injury, but rather the manner in which he was perceived and treated by the general public.

The previous chapters have examined the war-time innovations in disabled care and welfare. They have detailed the re-orientation of Germany's orthopaedists and their focus on the physical rehabilitation of the nation's severely injured soldiers. This shift in orthopaedic medical goals was coupled by a revolution in artificial limb design and the re-organisation of disability welfare services – developments which were both guided by a mission to send these men back to work. In short, what orthopaedists had been inventing during the war was a modern system of medical rehabilitation.

But many Germans did not believe that it was possible to heal the so-called 'war cripple' and send him back to work. Many considered the physically disabled incapable of basic self-care, let alone productive labour. Others did not believe that such a goal was fair or necessary – given the enormous bodily sacrifices these men had already made in defending the empire. The disabled themselves complained about a system that appeared to dismiss the severity of their injuries and there is evidence that at least some of these men resisted attempts to restore their bodies. Thus despite their war-time medical advances, orthopaedists still faced the formidable task in rehabilitating the disabled of bringing the rest of the nation on board.

Therefore in addition to revising the medical treatment and social services for disabled soldiers, German orthopaedists also launched a broad public relations campaign designed to shift popular attitudes regarding the severely injured body. Through a series of newspaper articles, public lectures, educational pamphlets, films, and medical exhibitions, orthopaedists and their allies in rehabilitation carefully re-cast the public image of the wounded soldier, depicting him as a useful, capable member of society, who should no longer be viewed as a helpless, pitiable victim. Indeed they argued that the nation's disabled ex-servicemen could be just as self-sufficient as able-bodied Germans, and urged their compatriots to dispense with their 'old-fashioned' attitudes regarding 'cripples'. This re-imagining and re-locating of the disabled soldier within German society thus could be called the *cultural invention of disability*.[3]

This chapter examines this invention of disability in Germany. It begins with a look at pre-war attitudes toward those permanently injured members of society and explains how and why these attitudes prevailed in the empire. It then examines how orthopaedists re-conceptualised the disabled soldier within the larger social and economic fabric of war-time Germany. Finally it traces how orthopaedists then began to systematically re-educate all segments of society – not just fellow medical professionals, but the general public, the German state, and even the disabled themselves.

Re-imagining the cripple: the medicalisation of disability

To Germany's orthopaedists, the resignation and fear with which both the wounded veterans and the general public accepted the dependent, helpless state of the permanently injured soldier was a source of great concern. Throughout their war-time publications and meetings these emergent leaders in disability care repeatedly emphasised that it was old-fashioned to think that the wounded veteran was someone to be pitied or coddled. They argued that this attitude that the disabled were incapable of taking care of themselves or earning a living was out of date, the product of both archaic medicine and an undeveloped social consciousness. Rather, orthopaedists contended that the recent innovations in disability care and welfare called for revised social and cultural expectations for the 'crippled'. Biesalski characterised these new cultural attitudes that Germans should adopt in the pages of *War Cripple Welfare* when he wrote,

> Only the sentimental sop says: 'How can anyone be so heartless as to expect a poor man who has lost his hand for the fatherland and who has endured so much pain to go back to work – especially when it is clear that a one-handed man can't do anything.' Whereas the healthy, socially conscious mind responds rather: 'The maimed man should return to earning his own bread – not just for himself but also for the sake of dependents – so that he doesn't end up doubting on both God and mankind and fall victim to misery and poor relief. Because the heroes of this war deserve more than that, rather, they should become once again upright, economically independent members of our national community [*Volksgemeinschaft*].'[4]

One of the important aspects of Biesalski's brochure on the new welfare for Germany's permanently injured soldiers is that, although he wrote in order to allay the economic anxiety that soldiers and their families were experiencing about the future, he did this *not* by describing the welfare which had evolved under the empire's path-breaking social insurance programme, nor by detailing the revised pension system that the military had passed in 1906. Rather, Biesalski did this by minutely detailing how the interventions of modern medicine – specifically orthopaedics – could help the disabled soldier to overcome his injuries and return to his proper place in the workforce. Indeed, in this and countless other war-time outlets orthopaedists stressed that returning to work was important not only so that the disabled soldier might secure his own economic future, but also in order that he might continue to contribute to the economic prosperity of the nation. In fact, a closer look reveals that not only did orthopaedists believe that the severely injured *could* be returned to work, but also that, in fact, these men had a patriotic obligation to do so.

This idea – to re-create economically and physically self-sufficient Germans from those who in previous eras would have been labelled 'useless cripples' – was actually a fairly radical one in Imperial Germany. To repair and return the permanently injured body to the workforce, rather than to simply compensate its 'owner' with a monetary pension, challenged the practices within the empire's social insurance system as well as the military's own pension programme. Before the Great War, the German social insurance system had relied upon insurance courts and panel doctors to determine how much future income an invalided worker was likely to lose due to his injury – whether permanent or temporary – and then financially compensate him accordingly. Instituted by Bismarck in the 1880s as part of a series of measures to quell the restless urban proletariat, German social insurance was more oriented toward maintaining social order, not healing the wounded populace. Even the medical care offered by workplace doctors was geared toward healing the injured worker, but not toward complete rehabilitation. Pensions, not rehabilitation, were the order of the day in Imperial Germany.[5]

Given the established nature of the pension system, it is perhaps not surprising that a culture of 'entitlement' had arisen in the empire, one in which popular understandings of social justice held that bodily incapacity deserved immediate and lifelong monetary compensation.[6] And even though some permanently injured Germans found work as front-desk men in government offices or private businesses, these so-called 'predicament positions' [*Verlegenheitsberufe*] were generally offered by employers to their own 'deserving' disabled employees. These positions were filled internally by firms and were not guaranteed. Regardless of the nature of injury, however, the point here is that in the pre-war German Empire, the onset of permanent bodily incapacity was considered reason enough for lifelong government allowances, even if generally meagre. And, in the twenty years before the war, applications for invalidity pensions had increased nearly five-fold from approximately 30,000 to nearly 180,000.[7]

Disabled soldiers felt especially entitled to compensation for their injuries because of the manner by which they had sustained them. As defenders of the empire, these men had risked life and limb in battle to protect Germany. They expected that the 'thanks of the fatherland' [*der Vaterlanddank*] would include not just patriotic parades or ceremonies in their honour, but also lifelong financial support. And they had good reason for these expectations. For in fact, the experience of disabled veterans had always been somewhat different from that of the permanently injured civilian. Whereas accident victims or so-called 'industrial cripples' might have been pushed to the margins of imperial society and become dependent upon poor relief and the social insurance system, disabled veterans of earlier wars had had access to military pensions, posts in the civil service, and even 'Heroes' Homes' – residential homes providing long-term medical and social care for the invalided war hero; before 1914 few veterans had been expected to continue earning their livings as work-a-day civilians. Indeed their time was most often spent meeting with their fellow veterans in associational meetings or regaling younger generations with their war stories. Of course, those wars had resulted in far fewer disabled ex-servicemen and even fewer of those were still around in 1914. Still, disabled veterans had never belonged to that category of 'useless cripple' because in the authoritarian and militaristic structure of imperial German society, the injured war hero was imbued with – indeed physically embodied – a high level of national and social capital.[8]

Beyond the lingering popular memories of disabled soldier care, however, firm guidelines for awarding pensions to the empire's wounded soldiers were set in 1906 – eight years before Europe plunged into war. The 1906 Pension Law established three compensatory systems for war veterans: one for officers, one for enlisted soldiers, and one for military dependents of fallen soldiers. Pension amounts for disabled soldiers were determined according to their military rank, war injury, length of military service, and military pay grade. These amounts could be further adjusted for meritorious service or skill. In addition, military officers received a 'service allowance', meant to pay for lodging, any hired servants, and hospital fees.[9] Therefore soldiers with exactly the same injury could be awarded vastly different pension sums. In 1914 the German military's pension system was designed not to equitably compensate soldiers for similar injuries, but rather to reinforce its own social hierarchy.

Furthermore, over the course of the Great War, these systems were revised in response to the changing social and soldier demands. A 1916 Pension Capitalization Law permitted soldiers to apply for a lump-sum pension settlement if they met the necessary criteria. In 1917 the pension systems were revised once more to take into account a disabled soldier's pre-war salary and social status as well. By then Germans had recognised the social injustice of pensioning off a highly skilled worker (who had commanded top wages before the war) as a lowly private with little time in the service. The pension of the lowly enlistee would hardly have replaced the lost 'future income' of a senior metalworker. Although the soldiers of the Great War would not get rich from the meagre pensions offered as 'the thanks of the fatherland', they did view pensions as their just reward for their war-time sacrifice.[10]

However, by 1914 Germany's orthopaedists did not share this opinion. While they did not advocate eliminating pensions for disabled soldiers, they were widening their understanding of what form the 'thanks of the fatherland' could take. In developing methods for restoring and rehabilitating the injured body, orthopaedists understood their work as returning to the nation's injured soldiers exactly 'what the war had taken from them' – their bodily capacity.[11] That is, to orthopaedists the re-construction of the soldier's body was more than just medical treatment, they saw it as an additional aspect of the state's restitution to the injured warrior. In physically rehabilitating the disabled soldier and restoring to him his pre-war civilian life, orthopaedists interpreted their efforts as the ultimate 'thanks of the fatherland' – not just compensation for what the veteran had sacrificed, but the return of it. Through modern medical intervention they could re-enable the disabled soldier, if not erase his injuries.

But, as they had realised in the reserve hospitals, in order for rehabilitation to be fully successful, the injured soldier had to take part in his own recovery. Troublingly to orthopaedists, however, his participation was not always eagerly forthcoming. Given that both the civilian and military pension systems determined financial restitution based upon a person's loss of work capacity, it is perhaps not surprising that some soldiers might have had qualms about recovery. E.P. Hennock has noted that before the war, injured German workers tended to resist medical rehabilitation programmes 'because they had a bad reputation among workers as *Rentenquetschen*, places for the reduction of pensions'. In fact, most workers resented them and only participated if their receiving a financial pension depended upon it.[12] Many soldiers probably shared this belief and feared that regaining any ability to work might compromise their pension claims. As a soldier increased his work capacity, he simultaneously diminished the amount of future income he could claim as 'lost' due to his war injuries – or so many thought. Thus any malingering in recovery was in many ways the expression of an individual soldier's concern about his future pension.

Although orthopaedists did not report any specific instances of resistance to their rehabilitation efforts, their concern regarding the 'pension psychosis' among their disabled patients is evidence that many soldiers were not always willing participants in their own recovery.[13] Orthopaedists not only pathologised this condition (as noted in chapter 3), but considered it to be one of 'epidemic' proportions. They argued that this feeling of pension-entitlement had infected the psyche of the wounded soldier, turning men who had once been confident, self-sufficient, and patriotic into helpless, dependent, self-centred victims. Moreover, they added, the German public was in part responsible for this phenomenon. According to the empire's new rehabilitation experts, by avoiding, pitying, or otherwise treating the permanently injured as if they were no longer capable of being 'productive members of society', healthy, able-bodied Germans were reinforcing precisely these sentiments in the mind of the wounded soldier. What was necessary, they thus concluded, was the re-education of them both.

Orthopaedists were agreed that the greatest obstacle to war-time physical rehabilitation was not the injury itself, but rather the soldier's own lack of sufficient 'will to work' [*Arbeitswille*]. Too often, they noted, the injured were allowed to believe that they could not resume their pre-war lives and were thus encouraged by others to become dependent on welfare and charity. Biesalski contended that these injured men were choosing to remain disabled in order to continue collecting their pensions. This wilful refusal to return to work was symptomatic of the pension-psychosis, a phenomenon doctors believed to be widespread among Germany's disabled veterans. This pension-psychosis manifested itself as the neurotic desire of the disabled soldier to surrender himself to his injury and thus embrace helplessness and economic dependency by expecting to be supported and cared for by others. However, the pension-psychosis was not 'chronic' and according to Biesalski, through vigilance and effort on the part of all those around him, the pathology of the disease could be reversed. As he explained in the pages of *War Cripple Welfare*,

> We cannot force anyone, rather we can only educate and try to prevent a man from becoming infected with, and falling victim to, the delirious thought that he can no longer work and has to be compensated with his pension – a pension for which he naturally depends upon his very crippledness [*Krüppeltum*] to receive. Doctors call this pension-psychosis and they can relate astounding stories about the mental devastation that it exercises upon its victims.[14]

All around him, he claimed, severely injured soldiers rested in their convalescent beds, having already withdrawn from both social and economic life. In his 1915 speech at *The Exhibit of Wounded and Sick Care in the War*, Biesalski explained to his audience that this pension psychosis often took precedence over a war victim's thoughts and feelings about his family. When the war-disabled were allowed to fall victim to this delirium, he continued, they often clutched even tighter at their pensions, holding them above more important things. 'When it comes down to it [his pension], he'll let his family, house, and garden perish first, because he thinks he must hold on to his pension, that is has become the sole focus of his life.'[15]

Importantly, however, the 'battle for pensions' [*Kampf um die Rente*] was not solely a phenomenon among disabled solders. It ran rampant throughout German society, Biesalski lamented, and not just among the empire's lower classes. Indeed, despite the widespread and popular misconception that only members of the working classes demanded pensions, Biesalski did not believe that only those impecunious soldiers were in danger of becoming 'infected' with the pension-psychosis. Rather he argued that this addiction was endemic to contemporary society and that one could find Germans from all classes demanding this compensation.

> The millionaire who has suffered a shock to the nerves in a train accident fights the railway office for a pension to the same degree as a train conductor whose little fingers have been run over. This is a purely human condition, and we must save our wounded from it – cost what it may![16]

To Biesalski, the nation's war-injured were not the only Germans suffering from the pension-psychosis. Indeed his criticisms were intended for all Germans – war-disabled or not. Eliminating the reliance of modern society on the welfare of the state appears to be his larger goal.

Biesalski was not alone in thinking that the empire's population had become all too eager to collect pensions. In a 1915 speech, Adolf Silberstein complained that one outcome of the German social insurance system had been an increasing greed on the part of many citizens for state pensions. Indeed, in his opinion what had started as a blessing for his fellow countrymen, had gradually begun to show its darker side. In elaborating upon this sentiment, Silberstein protested,

> It has become typical for the state, the commonality, to step in for the individual, when he is no longer – because of disease, accident or invalidity – able to care for himself. ... [B]ut gentlemen, this coin has another side! The social welfare has brought us an abundance of greed, which is culminating in the perception that the state must now take care of everything – today and for all time, and I fear that the 'pension hysteria' [*Rentenkampfhysterie*], which we ran into often enough in peacetime, will make itself rather unpleasant when the time for determining the [war] pensions comes about.[17]

As of 1915 then, orthopaedists were beginning to reconsider the value of the pension system. Now that modern medicine could return to these men what the war had taken from them – the ability to work and earn a living – it seemed unnecessary to many of them to award injured soldiers with invalid pensions. Indeed, as Biesalski himself pointed out, the war-invalid must no longer expect the German state to financially support him simply because he had lost an arm or leg. This compensatory practice was outdated, belonging to a past when it had not been possible to replace lost limbs or fully restore the working capacity of disabled men. Repeatedly, he argued, that instead of becoming a financial burden to the state, the war-injured ought to say to himself,

> Yes! I don't need to remain a useless cripple, I may once again eat my own bread [*Eigenbrot*] with my family and I will be the same man that I was before, even up to the little injury I have endured and that I accept – for the sake of the fatherland – as a sign of honour.[18]

Here Biesalski is clearly identifying working and earning one's 'own bread' as part of the disabled veteran's continuing responsibility – even duty – to his nation and its future well-being. Whereas before the war, the severely injured might have been considered a 'useless cripple', Biesalski is suggesting now that patriotism and individual pride ought to inspire the wounded man to overcome his 'little injury' and continue living his life as he had before the war. Indeed, that the orthopaedist compared the a severe battle wound to a 'little injury' suggests not only that the soldiers themselves should not exaggerate their sacrifices, but that these injuries perhaps deserved less attention from the public as well.

It is precisely this shift in the perception of the disabled soldier which was perhaps the most radical war-time medical innovation of all. Whereas before the war, the severely injured were considered permanently and irrevocably incapacitated by their bodily damage, the war-time revolutions in medical treatment for the so-called 'cripple' were initiating a wholesale re-conceptualisation of the maimed. Indeed what had once been perceived as an immutable bodily state was now being re-imagined as a conditional one.

In re-conceptualising the damaged body as one that could be healed by medicine, orthopaedists medicalised physical disability in the empire – transforming it from a social concern to a medical one. That is, over the course of the war, what had previously been a condition 'treated' by social welfare via the disbursements of pensions was transformed into a medical one that could be healed by doctors. Moreover the medicalisation of disability did not simply place orthopaedists at the forefront of this treatment, it also transformed the bodily state of the 'crippled' into a transitional one. As German orthopaedists invented therapies and devices for restoring to the wounded what the trauma of war had taken from them – their ability to work – they no longer considered severe bodily injury (even amputation) reason enough to label these men 'permanently incapacitated'. Quite the reverse; the technological revolution in artificial limbs combined with the invention of rehabilitation meant that for the first time in German medicine these injuries were temporary conditions which could be overcome.[19]

This phenomenon was not surprisingly of increasing interest to the state, for orthopaedists were not the only Germans concerned with the nation's disabled citizens. The growing pension demands among injured workers had been a source of concern for the government in the decades before the war.[20] The pension-psychosis was not a war-time phenomenon – as Germany's orthopaedists well knew – and they had found a cure. By demonstrating that it was not bodily injury that kept the war-disabled from recovering, but rather the patient's own lack of sufficient will to overcome his affliction, orthopaedists were simultaneously demonstrating their importance to the peace-time state, as well. This shift in claiming that bodily recovery depended as much upon the individual as it did upon the medical procedures designed to heal him exerted significant influence on the ensuing nation-wide educational campaigns.

Awakening the 'will to work'

Sending the disabled soldier back to work thus required not only physically restoring his body; it also had a psychological aspect. Orthopaedists became concerned with restoring or 'awakening' the serviceman's 'will to work'. According to their pathology of the pension-psychosis, the shock of injury and the fear of permanent disability had only superficially effaced what they considered an innate desire of all healthy and patriotic Germans: the desire to work. Orthopaedists were convinced that once fully enlightened about the national importance of economic self-sufficiency, the war-disabled would eagerly take up their old professions. Thus the re-education of the disabled soldier included not only convincing him that it was possible for him to overcome his injury, but indeed that it was his patriotic duty to do so. Therefore throughout their recovery, disabled soldiers were provided with literature reminding them of the broader significance of their recovery.

One good example of this re-education is a 1915 pamphlet entitled *The Carefree War Invalid*. Written by Walter Salzmann, this short volume discussed the welfare programmes available to the war-disabled while stressing the importance of the wounded's responsibility in his own recovery.[21] While acknowledging that the German state played a significant role in caring for injured soldiers, Salzmann pointed out that 'the state alone is not responsible, but also the entire German people, including the invalid soldier himself.'[22] He assured his reader that the German people were just as indebted to the extraordinary sacrifices of the wounded soldier as the German state was. However, he maintained, the repayment of this debt had to include not only caring for the war-wounded, but also promoting the continuous economic and cultural development of the fatherland. In making this point, he informed the reader that

> The invalided soldier belongs to the entire German people. However, he should not and will not be treated as an object, not even within the welfare system. Yes,

> as we already know, he has an incontestable right to this welfare, but he also has responsibilities. He must not just passively take what he is offered, but rather actively participate in this welfare – and not just for his own individual interest, but in the interests of all invalids and the entire German nation.[23]

Thus to paraphrase Salzmann, a wounded soldier's duty to his nation did not end with his injury, but rather was only transformed by it. In the remainder of his pamphlet, Salzmann described the new disability welfare as deriving from the nation's present economic circumstances. This modern welfare therefore came not just in a pecuniary variety, such as a pension, he explained, but also took the form of restoring the work capacity of the injured. Maximising the labour potential of the wounded, Salzmann clarified, was not simply a way to contribute to the national economy by increasing the productivity of the disabled, but would also return to the wounded 'a greater joy for work [*Arbeitsfreudigkeit*], an ever-increasing belief in his remaining energy, and a confident joy for life [*Lebensfreude*]'.[24] Clearly to Salzmann this emerging aspect of war-invalid welfare – sending the wounded back into the workforce – would have enormously positive consequences for the disabled, not only by increasing his earning potential and his ability to serve his country, but also by restoring his *joie de vivre*, as well.

In the pages of *The Will Conquers All*, another such educational book, recovering soldiers could read stories of men who had not simply recovered from their wounds, but continued to defend their country through future service. This volume by Hans Würtz, educational director of the Oskar-Helene-Home in Berlin, aimed to inspire Germany's disabled through descriptions of real men who had overcome their injuries sustained in war. Thus he included not just tales of those battle legends such as Marcus Sergius and Götz von Berlichingen, warriors who had lost arms and returned to fight with artificial ones, but also the first-hand account of Heimbrod, a hero from the Franco-Prussian War (1870/1871) who withstood painful battle injuries because he was too proud to admit to being wounded. Even when finally overcome by his injuries and forced to undergo surgery, it was through his focused will that Heimbrod finally recovered, or at least according to the story.[25]

In addition to these 'historical figures', however, by the third edition of *The Will Conquers All*, soldiers could read accounts of their disabled compatriots from the present war who had been healed by the new orthopaedic treatments. Stories of leg amputees, one-armed men, double-amputees and the war blind – who had not just recovered from their wounds but were actively supporting the war effort – were proof positive that all damaged bodies could be restored. Captain Brunck, who had returned to active service despite losing his leg, and Sergeant Elisath, who had learned stenography at the One Armed School in Zehlendorf, were but two examples from the nineteen object lessons in recovery that the book offered its readers. And if that were not enough inspiration for his readers, Würtz included a 'Wake-Up Call to the War-Disabled' in the final pages of the primer which informed the men not only of the current advances in prosthetic technology, but also reminded them that they were 'men just like everybody else'.

> You don't need to let yourself be fed by father or mother or even strangers, you don't have to buy yourself an organ and traipse around from place to place, door to door! You can remain a farmer or wainwright or carpenter or whatever else you were. You can do that, which to most utterly stupid [*stockdummen*] people seems like a punishment, but what is in fact the best thing on this Earth, the thing that makes life right: work, work, work![26]

As these educational materials for the disabled make clear, what I am calling the 'cultural invention of disability' did not simply mean providing the medical means by which the war-disabled could be returned to work. It also necessitated a broad shift in the way Germans conceptualised the post-injury relationship of the wounded soldier to the state. In addition to convincing him that he could return to work, orthopaedists were convincing the disabled that he *wanted* to do this, as well. By educating the war-injured on how his return to the labour force had important repercussions for his own physical and mental health, the maintenance of his family, his relationship to the greater German population, and even the national economy, men such as Salzmann and Würtz hoped to be able to re-awaken the disabled's spirit. In their eyes, no self-respecting, patriotic German would sit back 'passively' taking from the war-time state, when he could still be contributing to it. The inventors of the new rehabilitation were certain that once fully aware of the consequences of failing to return to work, the war-wounded would embrace the opportunity to continue serving their country.

Just in case re-educating the injured was not enough to staunch the pension epidemic threatening the nation, this enlightenment campaign also targeted those people surrounding the disabled veteran. According to orthopaedists, it was up to the general public, the disabled's family, and – most importantly – the orthopaedic specialist to practise a kind of vigilance against the injured man's propensity to sulk in self-pity and descend into uselessness.[27] Therefore those around the wounded soldier were encouraged to not only act as a psychological bulwark against the pension-psychosis which lay latent in all disabled soldiers, but also to persuade him to take an active part in his recovery and return to work as soon as possible.

'There is no crippledness!'

With these words, orthopaedists claimed to have averted the medical emergency threatening the war-time Empire and every wounded German's future.[28] Whether delivering lectures to the public, organising medical exhibitions, or outlining the latest rehabilitation therapies in the empire's illustrated press, German orthopaedists spent the war years repeatedly emphasising that their specialty could eradicate disability among the war-injured. Indeed, Biesalski, Lange, and others assured the public that with their new therapies and devices, any injured soldier could be fully restored. Moreover, they argued, those who had lost a limb or suffered significant damage to their senses could be mechanically rebuilt as well, so that even these disabilities could be ultimately overcome. According to them, no injury was too severe to be healed, no body too damaged to not work again. So confident were the nation's orthopaedists in the capacity of modern medicine to heal the war-disabled, that they could see only one potential obstacle to their success: the failure of either the public, or the wounded themselves, to cooperate with and support the national project of rehabilitation. Thus, in addition to the re-education of the injured soldiers, German orthopaedists also began to systematically re-educate the public regarding the proper treatment of and future expectations from the disabled.

According to Biesalski, this 'enlightenment work' [*Aufklärungsarbeit*] was of the utmost importance if orthopaedists were going to be successful in their mission to send the disabled back to work. In his eyes the rehabilitation of severely injured soldiers was a project of national importance; therefore he called for a systematic campaign to re-educate all Germans. So beginning in 1915 orthopaedists also engaged in broad canvassing of the war-time empire with newspaper articles, medical pamphlets, public lectures, films, medical exhibitions, design contests, and public demonstrations. Through a careful project of re-casting the popular image of the war-disabled, Biesalski and others hoped to revise the 'misperceptions' in the general public regarding the disabled body.[29]

In outlining this public 'enlightenment work', Biesalski knew that Germans would have to be convinced that the disabled body was not just healed, but fully restored. This was crucial because so long as those around the disabled soldier continued to coddle or dismiss him, all the medical and therapeutic treatments created for the disabled would be of little use. Thus this educational campaign was to target the popular and academic press, as well as the weekly news magazines. They would also have to offer public lectures and tours of welfare homes, distribute educational literature, and organise medical exhibits touting the success of the new disability care. Moreover, although he insisted that orthopaedists lead this campaign, he urged cooperation with state and local organisations, as well. Only through the use of every form of modern communication would orthopaedists be able to reach every German. Moreover, he suggested the use of large, widespread organisations, such as the Red Cross, whose reach extended from reserve hospitals to small towns, as well as government offices, insurance companies, trade unions and fraternal societies.[30] As one pamphlet asked rhetorically, 'How many authorities, teachers, nurses, and doctors (with the exception of orthopaedists) are there, who know something about the ethical, national, and economic meaning of disability care?' Although it may have stemmed initially from the private desks of a few men, this enlightenment work eventually incorporated aspects of both commercial advertising and public health campaigns in order to radically re-educate the German public about the disabled body.[31]

Biesalski was concerned that the German public's deep-rooted pity for the disabled would thwart medical efforts to restore the soldier's body. In the minds of orthopaedists, the public's coddling of the injured would only promote the pension-psychosis by reinforcing feelings of physical impotence within him. They considered this particularly true in the case of those disabled soldiers whose dependents feared their own economic futures were being adversely affected by his injuries. Therefore orthopaedists directed certain components of their educational campaign specifically towards dependents.

One of the most important aspects of re-educating the general public was the distribution of medical literature directed at a popular, lay audience. Here Biesalski's own pamphlet, *War Cripple Welfare,* serves as an excellent example. As already noted, he published this booklet with an eye towards alleviating the anxiety that both the disabled and their dependents might be experiencing. The book contained information about the latest medical and rehabilitation procedures, examples of restored men, a list of the professions to which they could be returned, as well as a catalogue listing the broad disability resources of the German Empire. All this was meant to convince readers not just that physical recovery was possible, but also that there were multiple institutions in place to guide this process. Written to enlighten all those in contact with the disabled, the booklet was aimed at the broadest, general audience in Germany – and it reached them. Advertising leaflets promoted the booklet as available to all for just 35 pfg apiece or at reduced rates in bulk amounts (25, 100, and 1000) for those organisations or offices that might want to keep a steady supply on hand.[32] Within eight months some 120,000 had been printed; by August 1916 this number had reached 140,000. According to one source the pamphlet was quickly translated into Hungarian; translations into Slovenian, Polish, Bulgarian, and Turkish were planned but never realised.[33]

In *War Cripple Welfare* Biesalski argued that it was of paramount importance that the German public dispense with its pity and sentimentality for the maimed, lest many be tempted to feel sorry for him.

> You, young lad or lass of the decadent, refined luxury of yesteryear, tear off the trappings of your selfishness, grip that mutilated hand and shake it heartily – it was lost for your sake. And you, hero of the holy war, get used to the idea that you are a 'little bit' crippled, but still the same old person. ... There is no crippledness [*Krüppeltum*], if the iron will is there to overcome it. ... And if everyone who is a part of this work can re-learn this from the ground up, then, and only then, will it be possible to eradicate this terrifyingly serious danger of war-crippledness both for the individual and for the entire nation [*Volk*].[34]

Biesalski proceeded to argue how important it was for the general public to overcome its misconceptions regarding the permanently wounded. Indeed, as he noted in this section, 'The lay-person must impress upon himself the notion that there is hardly any mutilation so severe, that the affected man is made completely and permanently incapable of work.'[35] He related to the reader many examples of soldiers who had lost arms, legs, hands – even all four extremities – while simultaneously pointing out how easily these men had been sent back to work. Extreme examples of men who had lost multiple limbs or one (or more) of their senses were clearly the more persuasive and Biesalski made the most of them. He reminded readers of the 'Höftmann Mann', a successfully restored quadruple amputee and one of Biesalski's more favourite success stories. Touted also at the 1915 *Exhibit of Wounded and Sick care in the War*, the so-called Höftmann Mann was a carpenter who had not only survived his injuries, but had become the manager of the carpentry workshop in the welfare home where he now lived. His real identity concealed, this orthopaedic wonder was now generally known by the surname of the Königsberg orthopaedist who had restored him.

Biesalski used other case studies to illustrate the success of modern rehabilitation, as well. For instance, he pointed to the example of a man who had lost his right hand in an industrial accident and later studied orthopaedic technology in one of the welfare institutes. In the pages of *War Cripple Welfare*, the public could learn that as part of his training, the patient fastidiously constructed a complex piece of orthopaedic machinery in order to fulfil the requirements of his post-injury vocational schooling, eventually submitting it in order to pass his journeyman's test. Another example cited a young apprentice, who was not only missing his left arm, but had lost half of his right hand, as well; yet still, noted Biesalski, he had a smart prosthetic that could bend at various angles, and with it he was now busily employed as a basket-weaver.

Finally, he observed, there was the example of the patient who had lost one of his legs at the hip. After studying orthopaedic engineering, this young man was now hard at work, proving that despite the loss of a leg, he was capable of working at even those professions whose practice did not allow workers to sit down on the job. As Biesalski triumphantly concluded,

> Never again must the unworthy images of the war-disabled organ-grinder or street peddler appear on our streets! With unanimous cooperation between the orthopaedic experts and the German employment community it could now be possible to accord to every amputee employment [*Verstümmelten*].[36]

Beyond Biesalski's own writings, other publications discussing the new methods of restoring disabled soldiers were circulated as well. Salzmann's *The Carefree War Invalid* and Würtz's *The Will Conquers All,* both of which were made available to the general public, also made a point of depicting the permanently injured soldier as one who could be easily and joyfully returned to work through the new programmes and new direction of the welfare system. In 1917, Baroness Alice von Bissing wrote a booklet titled *Women in War-Disabled Welfare,* in which she outlined how Germany's female social workers could aid in rehabilitation.[37] That same year, the Saxony's Heimatdank mailed out small pamphlets entitled *Work from the War-Wounded,* which were supposed to offer an account of the ways in which the war-invalids were being put to 'tasteful' work in the hospitals and recovery homes. Concerned that the wounded might elsewhere be encouraged to produce and sell the sort of 'tasteless kitsch' with which other destitute vendors often peppered the streets, this organisation assured the public that the war-wounded did not have to succumb to this fate. As the director of the work programme put it, 'More and more one begins to realise that the proper employment of our invalids, be it plain and simple, turns out to be a blessing.'[38]

Disability on display

In addition to using medical and welfare publications to impress upon the public the importance of new attitudes regarding the disabled, orthopaedists partnered with other welfare groups to organise large-scale exhibitions to educate Germans about the rehabilitation of the wounded. Through displaying medical innovations alongside images of dexterous disabled soldiers restored to work, war welfare circles hoped to sell the nation on the new success of rehabilitation. If patriotic speeches and scolding could not convince the empire's citizens that the severely injured could be returned to work, the irrefutable visible display of medical technology and the re-abled body was to convince the rest. Two such

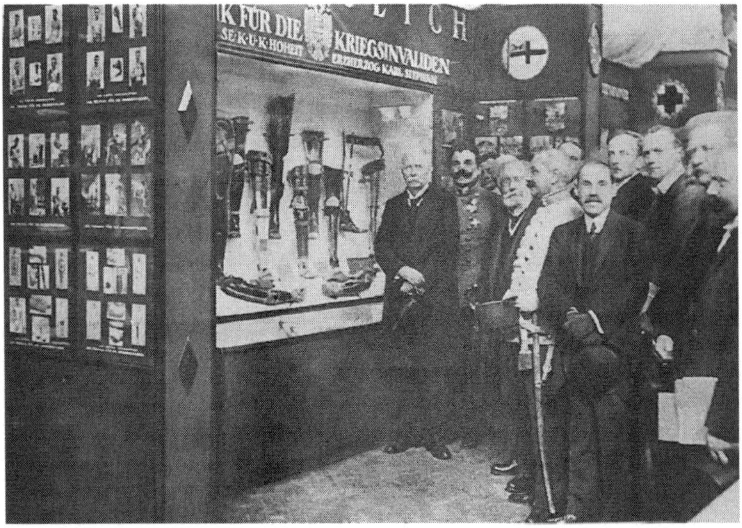

18 The Exhibit of Artificial Limbs and Working Tools for the War Injured. January 6, 1916.

shows were *The Exhibit of Wounded and Sick Care in the War* and the *Artificial Limb Exhibit*. At the first, Biesalski delivered his seminal speech on the ethical and economic ramifications of war disability welfare. Held in the entrance rooms of the German capitol building, the Berlin Reichstag, this exhibit aimed not just to inform the public of the efforts being made to restore the wounded soldier, but also to convince them that this was a project of national importance. The *Artificial Limb Exhibit* was also held in Berlin. Organised by the Centre for Artificial Limb Testing, the show displayed the technical advances in prosthetic design and how these devices re-abled soldiers' bodies. These and other exhibits in Germany and its allied lands offered proof positive that the wounded were not only well cared for, but that through the intervention of modern medicine, they were being fully restored, as well.

In 1915 *The Exhibit of Wounded and Sick Care in the War* travelled to Saxony and took up residence in the kingdom's capital. Although the exhibit originated in Berlin, through the concerted efforts of the Saxon War Ministry, the Deputy War Office in Dresden, the Red Cross, the Dresden Association of War Organizations, and the National Hygiene Museum, the exhibit was brought to the halls of the Royal Art Academy in Dresden. As Dr Karl Lingner, renowned amateur hygienist, industrial entrepreneur, and municipal philanthropist, acknowledged in his introduction to the exhibition catalogue, the heavy casualties and injuries suffered by the Saxon Army in the course of the war were the root of much worry among the kingdom's populace.[39] In fact, his opening comments suggest that there was widespread concern – indeed panic – among German citizens regarding the medical treatment of the skyrocketing numbers of wounded. As he noted, 'Reports from the field about all sorts of inconveniences and descriptions of the suffering of the wounded, complaints regarding insufficient methods of, or opportunities for, transporting the wounded, stories about deficient care in the field hospitals have all only sharpened and darkened this concern.'[40] He told his readers that in order to determine which reports were gross exaggerations, which were completely false, and which were accurate accounts, committees of experts had investigated these concerns in order to determine the actual circumstances in the field. Most of them, it turned out, were exaggerated – if not fantastic. Moreover, Lingner continued, the Saxon Army's medical corps had in the meantime adapted to the 'extraordinary' circumstances of war, learning new treatments which enabled them to respond now to even the most severe cases of injury.[41]

The exhibit before them today, Lingner informed museum-goers, was the result of these all-encompassing expert investigations conducted into war-time medical care. Apparently a huge success in Berlin, the show had been expanded extensively from its original design and brought to Dresden with the specific intention of allaying the local fears regarding the medical handling of the wounded. Here in the models and demonstrations set out in the Academy's halls, the Saxon public was encouraged to see for itself how the military and civilian medical communities were responding to the crisis of war. To that end, the exhibit showcased the complete professional activity of the army's medical corps. In addition to this, the public could inspect the entire run of medical arts and techniques being deployed not only by the military's medical units in the field, but also the civilian sick relief found behind the front lines [*Etappengebiet*] and on the home front. Finally, especial care was given to demonstrate the treatment and rehabilitation of the war-disabled. Part of the Dresden organisers' expansion efforts lay in the inclusion of film and photographic representations of severely injured soldiers returned to work.[42]

Lingner encouraged all members of the public to inform themselves regarding the wide-ranging care available to wounded soldiers so that they might take comfort in the knowledge of how much was being done for Saxony's disabled. But it also seems obvious that he meant to overcome any popular misunderstanding of – even mistrust in – the German state's responsibility to them. Given Lingner's high regard and influence in the Dresden medical, health, and philanthropic community (the result of the widespread public renown he had gained through his organisation of the 1911 International Hygiene Exhibit just four years earlier) it is not surprising that he became the spokesperson for this medical exposition in Dresden.[43] Clearly he commanded respect among those Dresdeners already concerned with matters of health and hygiene; words coming from him might carry more weight than those coming from officials outside the local community or who were direct representatives of the military or the state. At any rate, his introductory remarks to the exhibit's attendees focused rather on assuaging their concerns about the wounded's future, than on more technical or medical explanations; moreover, he ended his words by underlining once again what he wished the public to take from the display: 'The curators of this exhibit hope that its presentation here in Dresden will also serve to spread calm and comfort throughout all circles of the population.'[44]

Whereas Lingner's remarks in the exhibition catalogue focused on assuring the public that the German medical community was expending every possible effort to meet the demands of the wounded, the brief foreword written by Dr Martin Kirchner concentrated on the emotional and patriotic importance of medical care for the wounded, as well as detailing the various segments of German society involved in this work. As a professor of medicine, as well as Ministerial Director of the Supreme Medical Council [*Ministerialdirektor des Obermedizinalrats*] in Berlin, Kirchner was well-informed of the situation of Germany's wounded.[45] His main purpose in his introductory remarks was to enlighten the German people regarding the parameters of care and treatment being made available to the injured soldier. Although Kirchner opened his discussion espousing the honour inherent in dying for the fatherland on the field of battle, he also pointed out that those wounded in battle were just as deserving of respect and honour. As he put it, 'suffering for the fatherland, when wounds or disease are the fate of the brave soldier' was equally praiseworthy.[46] Now, he argued, it was up to the rest of the German nation to come to the aid of those men who were suffering in their name. Indeed in Kirchner's opinion, the welfare of the wounded fell not solely to the German state, but also to local communities and indeed every individual German – especially the nation's womenfolk.

Although Kirchner took pains to point out how recent advances in medicine (such as bacteriology and epidemiology) were of great service in treating the wounded, he argued that the civilian volunteer effort on the home front was just as important to ensuring their recovery as that of organised medicine. Here he especially made note of the relief work of the various hospitaller orders, including the Knights of St John, St George, and Malta [Johanniter-, Malteser-, and Georgsritter], the German Red Cross Association, the Vaterländische Frauenverein and the Samaritervereine as specific – but by no means the only – examples of volunteer organisations contributing to the care and welfare of the sick or injured soldier. It was this voluntary relief work, such as the reception posts and medical way-stations [*Labungsstationen*] set up at various train stations, the mobile 'hospital trains' set up for transporting the wounded, the union hospitals and convalescent homes that were made available for the soldiers and staffed by volunteer organisations, that Kirchner also highlighted in the exhibition catalogue. Indeed, the exhibit itself was not only to showcase the great progress made in medical technology and treatment, but also to demonstrate the breadth of care being offered – by both official and civilian authorities – to the wounded. Indeed, as Kirchner concluded,

> *The Exhibit of Wounded and Sick Care in the War* is supposed to display all of this [military, medical, and volunteer efforts] before your eyes. It should awaken the comforting conviction in the hearts of all who have had to send their dear ones into the battlefields that everything possible is being done for them should they become sick or wounded.[47]

Clearly Kirchner was not convincing the German public that the wounded could be made fit to work again as much as he was convincing them that all was being done to treat and heal the wounded. Still his discussion – especially the great detail he included – reflects perhaps not only the amount of panic coursing through the average German, that the wounded would be useless for future work, but also that the medical community – be it military, state, or volunteer – was going to great lengths to not just treat the wounded but also instil in the nation's home front population confidence that they could do this successfully. It is therefore perhaps not surprising to learn that the public flocked to the new exhibit and the show was quite successful. Whether it was in order to allay their fears or out of sheer curiosity or both, we may never know for sure. Still, according to the annual report of the National Hygiene Museum, in the four weeks during which the material was on display, some 103,000 patrons visited the exhibit. Moreover, the show itself was crowned a glowing success, not simply in fulfilling its mission to 'calm the people regarding the care of the war-wounded', but apparently also financially as well.[48]

In addition to this exhibit, a similar one detailing the care for Bavarian soldiers circulated in that kingdom, as well. A collection which outlined disability welfare – a permanent exhibit at the Workers' Museum in Munich since 1915 – was ready by early February 1916 to travel throughout Bavaria, educating its citizens on the rehabilitation of the wounded. According to one source, the show was 'supposed to give the public an overview of current welfare being offered by the Bavarian government in this area'.[49] In addition to demonstrating the medical treatment offered to the wounded, the exhibit also combined slide shows, films, and lectures, each coordinated to inform the public regarding the social programmes for restoring the wounded. Moreover, the show was especially designed to encourage public participation in these efforts by demonstrating how local voluntary organisations were contributing to the care of the wounded (as noted already in chapter 3). As the official report noted,

> this exhibit should entice [the public] to cooperate and ultimately popularise the idea that it is a holy duty to both the fatherland and its defenders to help in paving the way for the war-invalids to return again to the ongoing work of the German people and eventually find once more their joy for life.[50]

Clearly the sort of enlightenment at work in the Bavarian exhibit, which combined both education and national propaganda, was part of a larger effort to not just re-educate the public regarding the medical treatment of the wounded, but indeed enlist their aid in this work, as well. And given the initial *lack* of organised medical care for disabled soldiers, it is perhaps not surprising that these exhibits were simultaneously suggesting to civilians ways they could help with the rehabilitation of the war wounded, and also actively recruiting them in these programmes.

A second exhibit in Dresden detailing the care of the wounded was held two years after the first. Organised this time solely by the National Hygiene Museum, the 1917 exhibition, *Care and Treatment for the War-Disabled in Germany,* opened at the newly constructed pavilion directly outside the museum. As with the other shows, this one was designed to update the public on the state of medical and social care for the wounded, as well as to display the progress being made on the efforts to re-train the disabled's body in order to secure his future employment in civilian life. Organised into two major parts, this show focused on providing its patrons with an overview of the history of war-invalid care, followed by a detailed display of the modern welfare developments of the present war.

The second, much larger section on modern welfare for the war-wounded was in turn split between a first segment that focused on the medical treatment of specific war-related injuries and a second that detailed rather the economic and social care of the wounded. The medical displays included not just information on treatments for shattered limbs or their prosthetic replacements, but also specifics on how to treat brain and nerve injuries, wounds to the face and jaw, diseases of and damage to the eye, malaria, war neuroses, tuberculosis of the lung, and ear and throat conditions. Its economic and social counterpart, the other half, focused rather on detailing the pension and medical laws, defining the scope and limits of the military and civilian welfare programmes, and outlining the job training and placement programmes for the rehabilitated disabled.[51]

In addition to educating Germans on the progress made in soldier care through the display of medical instruments, artificial limbs, pictures of convalescent homes and workshops, and even photographs of the disabled back at work, the organisers of the Hygiene Museum's 1917 exhibit handed each patron a booklet of short, easy to understand articles describing each arena of treatment pictured in its halls. Rather than 'burden' their visitors with a typical exhibition catalogue, which included a map to the various museum stations or reproduced images of the objects on display, the exhibition team argued that this collection of essays, written by experts, was clear and easy to read, 'therefore making it of long-lasting use to those lay-persons who wished to instruct themselves on the subject'.[52] Indeed, in their eyes, the exhibit stations were already easy to navigate, each object was clearly labelled, and signs pointed the way through the museum's rooms. To them, a map or description of the exhibit was unnecessary; what was more important was the knowledge which a visitor might take away from the display. Therefore, each patron received upon entry a 'guidebook' to educate them along their tour of the world of disabled soldier care and welfare.[53]

The Guidebook through the Entire Field of War Wounded Care was a 102-page collection of essays on the various medical, social, and welfare aspects of caring for the war wounded.[54] Edited by Dr Karl Sudhoff, medical advisor to the National Hygiene Museum (and the so-called 'father of medical history' in Germany), the book contained articles written by orthopaedists and other medical professionals from across the empire. Their contributions ranged from essays on facial surgery and jaw reconstruction to the use of radiation for both diagnosing and treating bodily injury. One essay specifically discussed the military pension and welfare programmes of the 12th and 19th Army Corps, the two Saxon armies subsumed within the larger German Imperial Army. Another focused on the treatment and after-care for the blind, with an addendum devoted particularly to the care of blind academics (a social group which as the previous chapter pointed out evoked especial concern among some). Two other essays outlined the post-injury professional re-training of the war-disabled for future work and detailed the agencies responsible for finding them employment. All in all twenty essays were included in the guidebook.[55] More than simply supplementing the exhibit, this collection marked a serious attempt to educate visitors about the goals, progress, and organisation of war-injured care in Germany and its essays were significantly more detailed than anything Biesalski had penned for the public.

The Hygiene Museum's exhibit opened on December 15, 1917 and ran for close to three full months before closing on February 10, 1918. In addition to the permanent displays, visitors were also invited to lectures and film screenings that were held in conjunction with the exhibit and which further detailed the processes of rehabilitation. One such film recorded at the Jakobsberg Orthopaedic Hospital of the 20th Army Corps in Allenstein (East Prussia) depicted soldiers using their prostheses at industrial work, such as welding, and agricultural work on the farmlands surrounding the hospital. Another film showcased the Walking School at the Ettlingen Reserve Hospital in Baden and depicted re-built soldiers as they walked and exercised with their artificial legs.[56] Unlike the static images in the exhibits photographs, these films allowed their viewers to see these re-abled bodies and their mechanical devices in action as they worked happily and productively – albeit hundreds of miles away. They might also be more appealing to those who did not feel compelled to read through the exhibit's educational literature. And although the museum's final report did not include attendance records, it did mention the huge crowds which attended the exhibit and accompanying programmes, suggesting that the number of patrons for this second exhibit exceeded that of their earlier one in 1915. Moreover it mentions that special invitations were extended to local charity and volunteer organisations.[57]

Countless other exhibits were organised throughout the Empire including ones in Breslau (1915), Magdeburg (1915), Kassel (1915), and Cologne (1916). Exhibits also travelled to Germany's war-time allies in an effort to educate those publics as well. Some examples include ones in Budapest (1915) and Bratislava (1917).[58] However one final exhibition deserves particular mention: the 1917 *Heimatdank Exhibit on the Welfare for the War-Disabled.* Held in the Crystal Palace of Saxony's trading centre, Leipzig,[59] this massive show was sponsored by Saxony's most important organisation for veteran care, the Home Front's Thanks [*Stiftung Heimatdank*]. The Home Front's Thanks was founded on June 11, 1915 as Saxony's chapter of the empire wide Reich Committee for War-Disabled Care [*Reichsausschuss der Kriegsbeschädigtenfürsorge*]. Formed and administered under the auspices of the Saxon Interior Ministry, the Heimatdank was a coordinating organisation that aimed at bringing together the various military, state, and voluntary agencies attending to the war victims. The Heimatdank understood its contribution toward war-disabled care not as a financial one, but rather as an administrator and distributor of in-kind services which would support the war-disabled (or his surviving family members) in their efforts to return to the workforce.[60] As such, these contributions included the provision of artificial limbs, work implements, bodily rehabilitation, and job re-training.[61] To that end, the organisation's 1917 exhibit concentrated on displaying all aspects of the services and care which the Heimatdank systematically made available to the wounded and their families, as well as evidence of their success.

The Heimatdank Exhibit was perhaps the most comprehensive of all the war-time medical displays. In addition to a permanent exhibit which was open to the public daily, the organisers made available a wide variety of supplementary materials: an evening lecture series, daily films, postcards, books, a raffle, and even offered goods for sale to patrons which had been produced by the disabled. According to its curators, the exhibition aimed to provide an overview of the measures being taken to help the wounded 'win back' their health as well as to ease their return to civilian life. Therefore the show displayed not only a history of disabled care, but also detailed the local process of *Berufsberatung* discussed in chapter 3. Moreover, it included an on-site workshop where rehabilitated soldiers demonstrated how they were able to operate industrial machinery despite the loss of a limb or other severe bodily injury. The show also set up a book display that made visitors aware of the breadth of medical, military, and popular publications available regarding the care and rehabilitation of disabled soldiers. Finally, it included a room dedicated to showcasing the various housing options offered to the permanently injured, including welfare apartments and a variety of settlement colonies. The organisers of the Home Front's Thanks exhibit considered it to be a practical, useful one that displayed all aspects of rehabilitation.[62]

The show's curators included an exhibit catalogue which focused on detailing the display objects and auxiliary aspects of the exhibition. In addition to a map of the Crystal Palace's rooms, forty pages of advertising notices, and a calendar of the public lectures, the 135-page catalogue included a lengthy list of sponsors, advisors, and an honorary advisory committee comprising medical doctors, judges, university professors, the police director, army officers, and the heads of the chamber of commerce in Leipzig and neighbouring cities – the participation of whom are a testament to the wide-ranging social interest in disabled care. The exhibit catalogue detailed in great length the medical advances on display and the chapters on job training and re-education courses for the war-injured were quite detailed. And, although the exact dates of the exhibit are unknown, the catalogue notes public lectures being held from August 13 to September 1, suggesting these as likely dates for the exhibit's overall run, too.[63] The massive size and scope of the 1917 Heimatdank exhibit reflects the extent to which war-disabled welfare had evolved since 1914, as well as the increasing popular interest in the subject.

Consuming disability

In addition to educating patrons on the rehabilitation and welfare programmes for the disabled soldier, these exhibits typically included two other features of note: items manufactured *by* the disabled and consumer goods designed *for* him. These aspects of the disability welfare exhibits were particularly important for convincing the public that newly restored soldiers could lead independent and self-sufficient lives when they returned to civilian society. This buying and selling of goods – either designed by or for the disabled – demonstrates what I consider to be the creation of a 'consumer culture of disability'.

In addition to the display objects and consumer products at the Heimatdank exhibition, the 1916 travelling exhibit in Bavaria included writing samples of men who were using artificial hands, documents typed by the war-blind, and even models of specially modified machinery designed to facilitate the integration of the disabled into the workplace. Baskets, books, woodwork, and glass objects – all crafted by the war-disabled and put on display – testified silently and irrefutably to the ability of each and every one of them to return to hard, honest work. In addition to these displays, publications depicting these wares, such as Oskar Seyffert's *Works from the War Wounded,* were printed and distributed to patrons, as well.[64]

In 1916, the Dresden chapter of the Home Front's Thanks sponsored an exhibit devoted solely to displaying the handiwork of the war blind. Held November 18 to December 4 in one of the capital's concert halls, the *Exhibit of Work by the Blind* specifically targeted Saxony's industrial and business leaders in an effort to convince them of the valuable labour remaining in blinded soldiers. Its organisers divided the exhibit into five departments:

1 Goods for sale which were produced by the blind,
2 Intellectual contributions of blind poets, authors and composers,
3 Aids for learning and living,
4 Practical demonstrations of objects created by the blind,
5 Dresden's blind workers as managers or businessmen.[65]

According to their report, special attention was paid to the fourth exhibit category: the craftsmanship of the disabled. Here all those who toured the displays could see for themselves the high quality work being produced by the blind. These goods included not only handiwork such as macramé, brushes, and baskets, but also products from the carpentry workshop, bookbindery, and cigar manufactory. In addition to inspecting these products, those present could actually witness blinded men at work using sewing machines, typewriters, and phones, or reading and writing Braille. This exhibit was not just meant to show off the successful rehabilitation of the war-blind, however. In a letter to the Saxon Chamber of Trade and Commerce, the deputy minister in charge of farming and commercial industry in the Ministry of the Interior encouraged

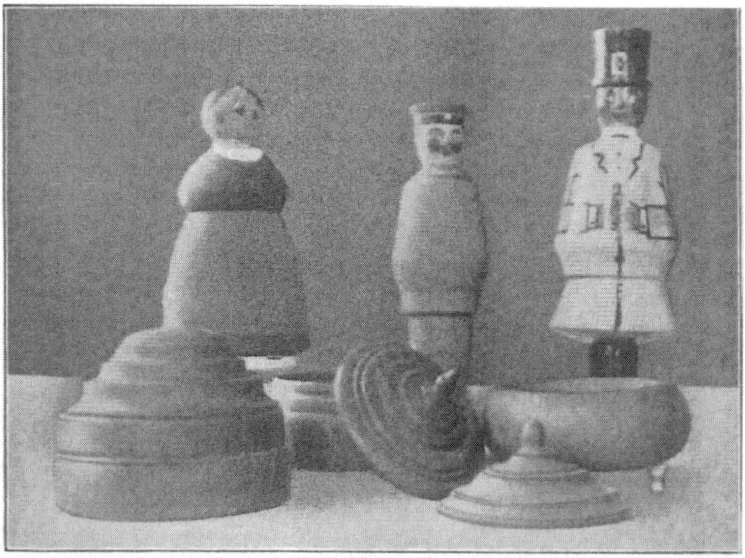

19 Objects crafted by a one-armed wood turner at the Nuremberg Field Lazarette.

factory managers to tour the exhibit and seriously consider hiring these men in their manufacturing works.[66] These exhibits therefore worked not only to inform and educate the public, but also to promote disabled soldiers as an emerging, highly skilled, and competent source of labour.

Dr Adolf Silberstein also used photographs of the goods produced by soldiers recovering at his reserve hospital in Nuremberg in order to convince the public of the wide-ranging success of rehabilitation. In his published works, he consistently maintained that once adequately trained and outfitted with the correct prosthesis, the war-disabled were capable of producing outstanding handiwork. These opinions he underscored with images of woodworking, technical drawings, and wicker furniture – all designed and produced by the disabled soldier (see Figure 19).[67]

Alongside these kinds of consumer products constructed by the disabled, museum visitors might also find special products, devices, and technology invented in order to ease the daily life of these re-abled men. Although not always necessary – or even designed – for their working lives, these products became part of a larger consumer culture which targeted this newly restored and self-sufficient population. Flyers and catalogues advertised devices which might help the severely injured accomplish routine tasks like eating with the help of specially designed cutlery, such as a fork-clamp which could hold meat

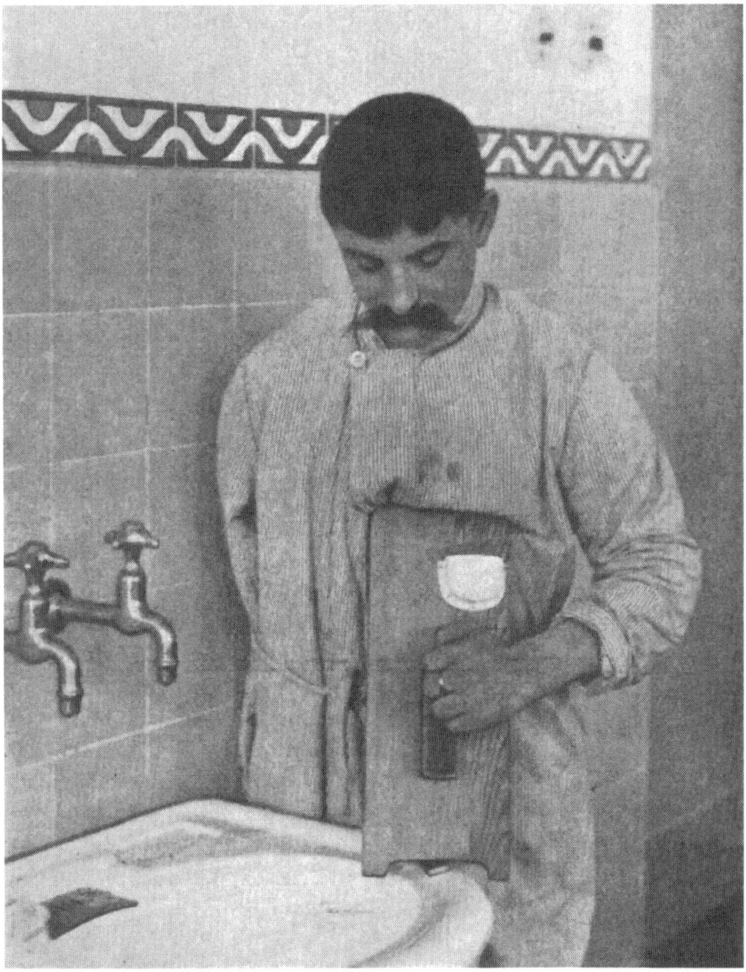

20 and 21 Orthopaedists also worked with inventors to create devices for helping soldiers to carry out routine tasks in daily life independently.

(or other food) on a plate thus allowing a one-handed wearer to use his healthy hand to hold a knife.[68] One medical resident in Munich developed a set of so-called 'finger cutlery' for one-handed men. This was composed of a thumb ring which held a small-tined fork and a knife which was worn like a blade across the back of the hand and attached to both the index and little fingers. This set of so-called 'universal cutlery' could be attached to the fingers of one healthy

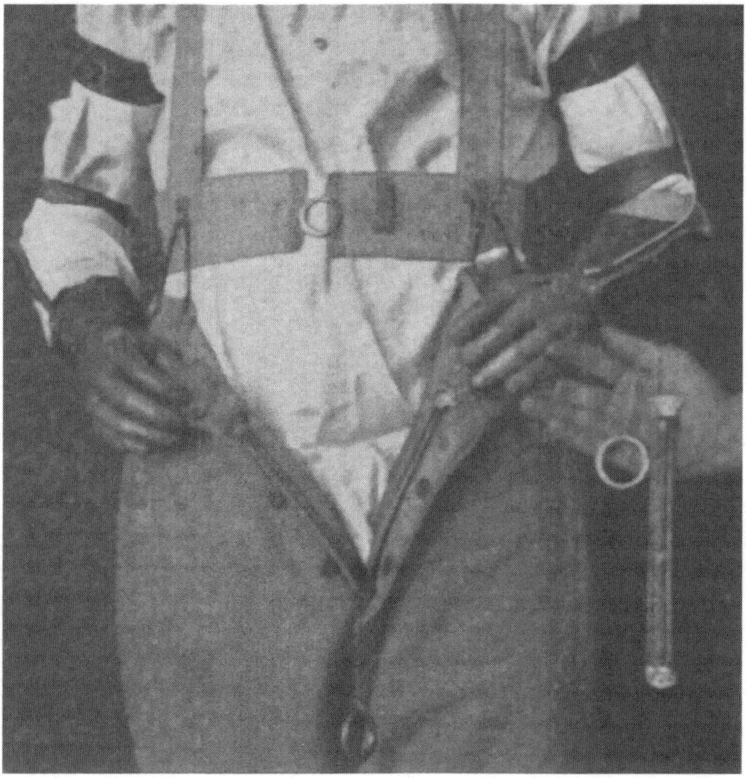

hand and through dexterous use allow its wearer to cut, hold, and eat his meal without assistance.[69] Other devices aided wearers in personal grooming, such as a washboard modified to help a one-armed man independently wash and clean his hand by affixing a nailbrush and soap holder to a wooden panel (Figure 20).[70]

In addition to these products for everyday eating and grooming, specially designed clothing, such as trousers, work aprons with pockets designed to hold the 'working hands' needed for artificial limbs, and even a 'prosthesis-jacket' which could be laced and fastened by a double-amputee were marketed to these emerging consumers (Figure 21).[71] Advertisements in the back pages of the museum exhibit catalogues promoted modified typewriters and drilling machines for one-armed men or hand-inserts which could be specially ordered for those men wishing to have more variety in their artificial limbs. In the catalogue for the Home Front's Thanks Exhibit, advertisements enticed readers to buy expensive cosmetic limbs, such as the Sunday-arm advertised by Hermann Steiner's Institute for Fine Mechanics, or machinery for disabled entrepreneurs, such as A. Hogenforst's rapid printing press for the graphic arts which had been modified for one-armed workers.[72] Though it would be interesting to know to what extent these particular products were actually used by disabled Germans, it seems abundantly clear that many manufacturers and product marketers eagerly embraced and supported these emerging consumers by vying for both their attention and their Reichsmarks. Obviously, the disabled consumer who bought these kinds of products would not just be participating in his own recovery, but ideally contributing to the overall growth of the national economy, as well.

Medical literature, travelling exhibits, and permanent museum displays, as well as their accompanying catalogues, are obvious aspects of this public re-education, but one could argue that these attempts at enlightening Germans were capable of reaching only a limited, even self-selected, population. Only those citizens already looking for this information were likely to attend a museum exhibit or buy a medical pamphlet. However, orthopaedists were aware of how myopic it might be to expect the public to come to them; and, therefore they also marshalled the popular press in their campaign. Photo essays in the illustrated weeklies informed Germans of the latest developments in orthopaedic technology, while also demonstrating how these devices sent soldiers cheerfully back to work in the factories and fields.[73] Other articles such as the one in Figure 22 depicted the recovery hospitals, surgical stations, and convalescent homes – especially those housed in spas resorts such as Bad Elster, Bad Tölz, and Baden-Baden, places where the German bourgeoisie had gone for health cures and nerve treatments before the war.[74] In the pages of these magazines, those resorts not officially commandeered to hospital or recovery service for wounded soldiers offered their rooms and 'cures' at discounted rates to those wealthier soldiers who might need rest and recovery from the trials of combat. Indeed, in one 1914 issue of the *Illustrirte Zeitung*, readers saw photographs of the military hospital recently set up at the Empress's request in the orangery of Sans Souci, the imperial palace in Potsdam.[75] Images such as these suggested that war-time recovery and rehabilitation were not only successful, but indeed might even resemble a vacation.

Pictures of one-armed men exercising and re-training their bodies convinced Germans of the sturdy, healthy nature of these newly rebuilt soldiers. Magazine pages were also filled with articles extolling the virtues of the new artificial limbs and the agility with which their wearers could now function again, and included images of these men climbing stairs or marching on uneven ground.[76] But of course, all work and no play might make 'Jupp' a very

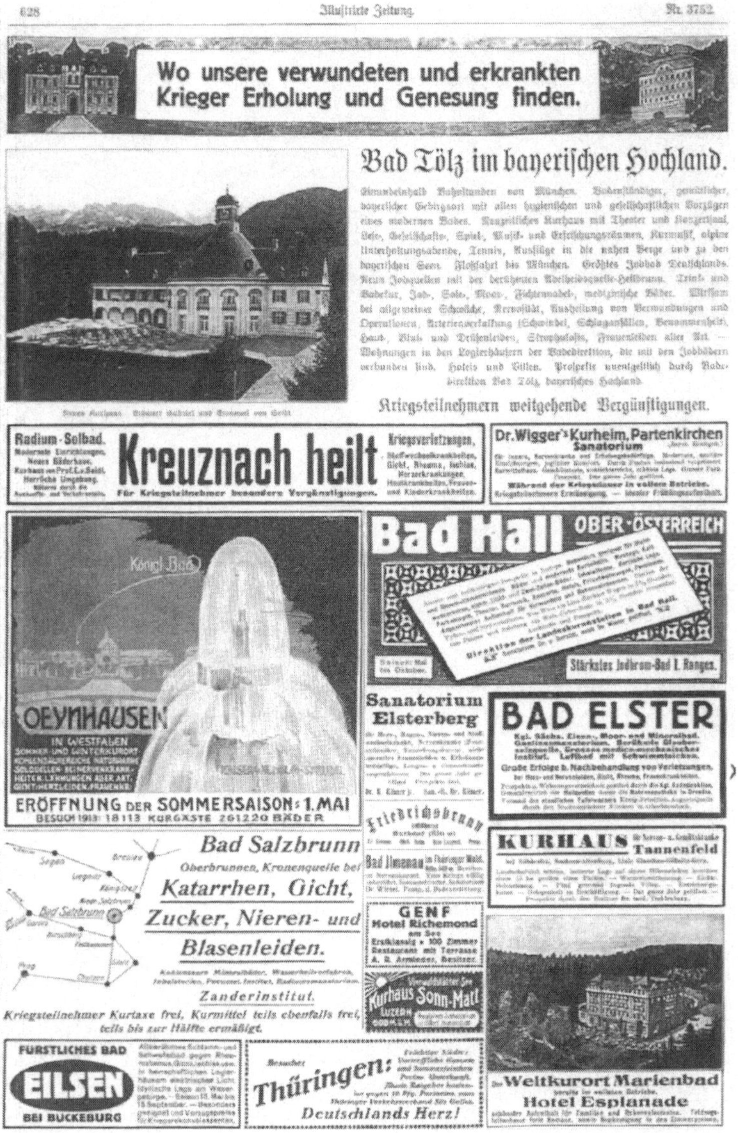

628 Illustrirte Zeitung Nr. 3752

Wo unsere verwundeten und erkrankten Krieger Erholung und Genesung finden.

Bad Tölz im bayerischen Hochland.

Kriegsteilnehmern weitgehende Vergünstigungen.

Radium-Solbad. Kreuznach heilt

Für Kriegsteilnehmer besondere Vergünstigungen.

Dr. Wigger's Kurheim, Partenkirchen Sanatorium

Bad Hall OBER-ÖSTERREICH

Stärkstes Jodbrom-Bad I. Ranges.

Oeynhausen in Westfalen

Eröffnung der Sommersaison: 1. Mai

Besuch 1913: 18113 Kurgäste 261220 Bäder

Sanatorium Elsterberg

Bad Elster

Große Erfolge b. Nachbehandlung von Verletzungen.

Friedrichsbrunn

Bad Ilmenau

Kurhaus Tannenfeld

Bad Salzbrunn

Oberbrunnen, Kronenquelle bei Katarrhen, Gicht, Zucker, Nieren- und Blasenleiden.

Zanderinstitut.

Kriegsteilnehmer Kurtaxe frei, Kurmittel teils ebenfalls frei, teils bis zur Hälfte ermäßigt.

Genf Hotel Richemond am See

Kurhaus Sonn-Matt Luzern

Fürstliches Bad Eilsen bei Bückeburg

Besuchet Thüringen: Deutschlands Herz!

Weltkurort Marienbad Hotel Esplanade

22 Every week the popular newspaper, *Illustrirte Zeitung*, reminded Germans of the various resort spas and vacation towns 'Where Our Wounded and Sick Soldiers are Resting and Recovering'.

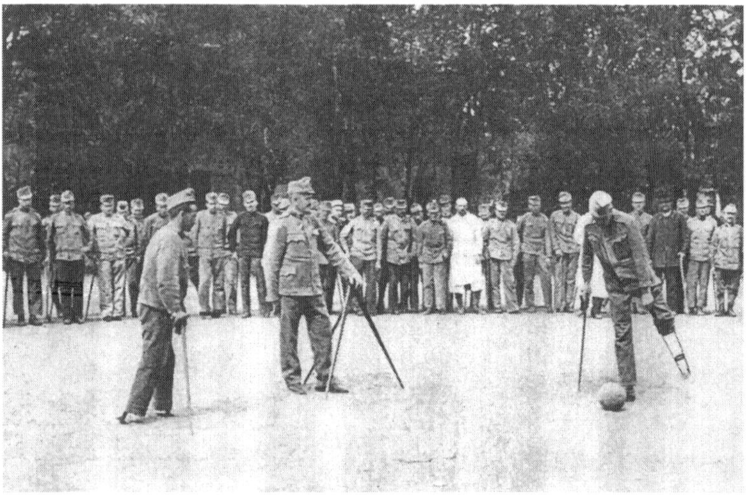

23 and 24 Newspaper articles with images such as these reassured Germans that medical innovations could not only send disabled soldiers back to work, but also enable them to enjoy life's leisurely pursuits.

dull boy, and so these newspapers also included photos of the wounded simply enjoying themselves at football and other sporting contests as in Figure 23.[77] Naturally, these images of the disabled at sport were never used to suggest that they were simply idling about enjoying their recovery. In keeping with the ideology of rehabilitation programmes designed to re-awaken the wounded soldier's will to work, articles accompanying these photographs always explained the serious business of rehabilitation. In fact, as one army general noted in an article on the relationship between war-disabled care and gymnastics, this kind of bodily exercise had a clear goal in mind and was closely partnered with other sorts of welfare for the wounded. In describing the new healing regimens being used, he informed the magazine's readers that,

> The goal of this kind of care culminates in the attempt to awaken new lust for life [*Lebensmut*] and creative power [*Schaffenskraft*] in the war wounded through properly directed body exercises which put them in such a state that – freed from the downtrodden feeling of being a cripple dependent upon the charity of their fellow citizens – they might once again become useful and independent members of the nation [*Volk*].[78]

Publishing images in the *Illustrirte Zeitung* which displayed the newly restored as they deftly exercised, alongside an article entitled, 'Modern Care for the

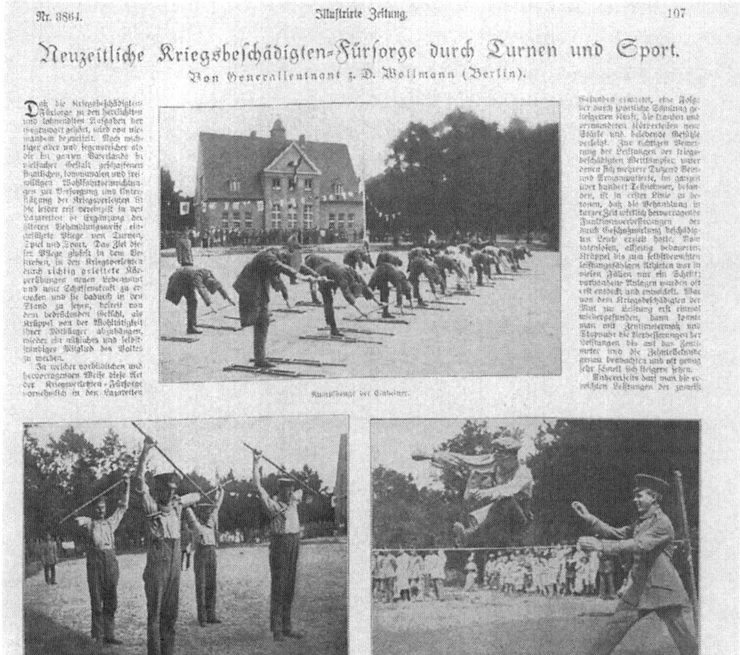
Nr. 3864. Illustrirte Zeitung. 107

Neuzeitliche Kriegsbeschädigten-Fürsorge durch Turnen und Sport.

Von Generalleutnant z. D. Wollmann (Berlin).

War-Disabled', was all part of convincing readers that everyday life would soon be back to normal for these wounded soldiers.[79] Photographs of these injured men busily engaged in industrial, farming, or sporting 'work' was irrefutable evidence to many Germans that the bodily wounds of these soldiers, however severe, were not permanent enough to incapacitate them for long. And in fact, it is not hard to imagine that as many soldiers on the front or civilians at home suffered from lack of food, adequate clothing, or heating fuel, some Germans might have considered that these convalescing soldiers had it comparatively easy in their resort hospitals and weekly sporting tournaments.

Conclusion: from the state's body to the body's state

This chapter has argued that a cultural invention of disability occurred in World War I Germany. In medicalising disability and re-conceptualising the severely injured body as one which could be successfully healed and restored, German orthopaedists and their rehabilitation allies fundamentally transformed the epistemology of 'crippledness' [*Krüppeltum*]. Whereas before the war, 'bodily incapacity' and the inability to work could be blamed on injury, with the invention of disability, the blame shifted to the recovering soldier himself. Disability shifted from being a material condition of the body to being the sign of a weakened will.

By pointing to the success of orthopaedics at restoring the body of the disabled soldier, the medical community around him strove to reduce the war-injured's dependency on others. If the disabled body could be returned to work and economic self-sufficiency, then the state would not be responsible for his life-long care. Beyond the importance of work to the wounded soldier's own recovery, however, the rehabilitation community maintained that returning him to work was a part of his continuing obligation to the nation – not only as a soldier, but as a private citizen, as well. Therefore, this new 'disabled body' was not a body dependent upon the state, but rather was conceived as one which was obligated to *support* it through contributions to the armed forces, labouring industries, and national economy. Indeed, precisely because it had been made whole again, the re-abled body was supposed to be a body dedicated to upholding the state, not undermining it.

This invention of disability was more than just the medicalisation of 'crippledness', however. It also necessitated the general re-education of the German people in order to correct their 'misperceptions' about the body. As this chapter has argued, it was through a tireless campaign of so-called 'enlightenment' [*Aufklärung*], that German orthopaedists, rehabilitation allies, and civic leaders gradually re-cast the image of the wounded soldier in the public sphere. As the war progressed, they published countless articles extolling the virtues of their technological progress in the nation's medical journals and popular press. Orthopaedists included discussions of artificial limbs in their internal pamphlets aimed at professional development, as well as for those in related health fields, voluntary associations, and the lay public. In addition to this kind of academic 'enlightenment', they sponsored public exhibitions of these limbs, held design competitions to encourage further innovation, published catalogues and even made films of this progress – all of which they shared with the German public. By the end of the war, German doctors had cultivated a shift in public perception of the maimed, replacing older pre-war notions of crippled bodies with modern images of disabled one.

Thus, this invention of disability was constituted by: a revolution in artificial limb technology and the material culture of medicine; the re-education of the German people in order to correct their 'misconception of the bodily capacity of the injured'; and the creation of a disabled consumer identity through the material culture which he both produced and consumed. Whereas before the war, 'crippled' Germans in the empire were considered helpless beings – largely incapable of work and dependent upon others – the disabled body emerging in war-time was depicted as one which could be made independent and self-sufficient thanks to the intervention of modern medical technology. Thus, this invention of disability was a cultural and sociological shift in the national perception of how the injured body should be understood in the era of modern medicine – a new bodily *Dasein* (the body's being-in-the-world) that was created during World War I.

As news of the progress in rehabilitating the disabled soldier spread throughout the far reaches of the German Empire, other groups grew interested in the national project of rehabilitation. Their interests stemmed not just from a desire to aid it, however, but a desire to benefit from it, as well. The previous chapters have already outlined how voluntary associations, schools, and other civic groups developed their own programmes for aiding the recovery of the disabled. However, as the war continued and the demand for fit, healthy men in the war-time economy increased, two groups in the empire took a much greater interest in the disabled soldier. The next chapter examines how military and industrial circles who were already facing an acute labour shortage found ways to recycle these men as the nation plunged into total war in 1916.

Notes

1 Mollenhauer, 'Bericht über die ausserordentliche Tagung der Deutschen Vereinigung für Krüppelfürsorge', 74–88, quote on p. 75. This quote from Biesalski is from Mollenhauer's published proceedings of the emergency meeting of the DVK on February 7, 1916.

2 Biesalski, *Kriegskrüppelfürsorge*. Quotes from pp. 14, 13.

3 Here I am using the phrase the 'cultural invention of disability' to refer to the creation of a set of cultural values and social norms regarding the injured body. This

phrase reflects the influence of Eric Hobsbawm on my own thought and it was he who coined the phrase 'the invention of tradition' with regard to the creation of practices and behaviours which sought to root themselves in the past. However, although like Hobsbawm I am trying to dissect and analyse a 'set of practices, normally governed by overtly or tacitly accepted rules and of a ritual or symbolic nature, which seek to inculcate certain values and norms of behaviour by repetition', I am not suggesting that these practices in any way mark a continuity with the past. Rather they were clearly invented in the present. For more on the 'invention of tradition' see Eric Hobsbawm and Terence Ranger, eds, *The Invention of Tradition* (Cambridge: Cambridge University Press, 1983).

4 Biesalski, *Kriegskrüppelfürsorge*, 13–14.

5 Eghigian locates the birth of the social entitlement state in Germany between 1884 and 1933. He argues that this period marked '[t]he development of a popular sensibility of social entitlement and how it emerged out of disability insurance'. For more on the creation of the social insurance system and the pension culture, see Eghigian, *Making Security Social*, quote on p. 20. For a discussion of military pensions and pension culture see Whalen, *Bitter Wounds*.

6 For more on the emergence of a culture of entitlement in Imperial Germany, see Eghigian, *Making Security Social*, especially chapter 3, 'Embodied Entitlement: The Policy, Practice, and Politics of Disability, 1884–1914', 67–116.

7 E.P. Hennock, *The Origin of the Welfare State in England and Germany, 1850–1914: Social Policies Compared* (Cambridge: Cambridge University Press, 2007), 203.

8 In previous wars, wounded soldiers who did not die of their injuries were generally granted lifelong pensions under the various army corps' own insurance programmes; for long-term medical treatment, they were usually turned over to the voluntary care of civic and religious welfare organisations. In the Prussian Army military disability had been revisited and codified after the wars of unification under the Pension Law of 1871, which made clear and distinct provisions for officers, medical officers, non-commissioned officers, and enlisted men. According to this law, a wounded soldier, depending on his rank and length of service, could expect to receive a disability pension, various supplementary pensions, a certificate entitling him to civilian welfare services [*Zivilversorgungsschein*], might be offered a place in an institute for invalids, be reassigned light duties in garrison, or any combination of these benefits. These benefits were so described in the Pension Law of 27 June 1871. Supplementary pensions were dedicated to those who lost limbs [*Verstümmelungszulage*], who were wounded in war service [*Kriegszulage*], or who had served more than eighteen years. For more on the Prussian system, see Ottomar, Freiherrn von der Osten-Sacken und von Rhein, *Preussens Heer von seinen Anfaengen bis zur Gegenwart. Vol. III* (Berlin: Mittler und Sohn, 1914), 337–8; 341–2. In the kingdom of Saxony, whose army was administratively separate yet remained under the command of the Kaiser, the Military Health Office [*Militär-Gesundheitsbeamte*] was responsible for the care of disabled Saxon soldiers. Similar to the Prussian system, this included the issuing of pensions based upon the level of

disability and rank while also sometimes including provisions for long-term convalescence or care. In the early modern period pensions might have ranged from 40 Thalers per year plus institutionalisation in one of the 'poor relief' facilities for those invalids who required constant attention, to a small *Gratifikation* of between 10 and 20 Thalers with no medical care for those who experienced little to no loss of work capacity. In addition to this monetary compensation by the Saxon government, supplementary funds were provided by voluntary organisations such as the Freemasons and bourgeois women's groups; this mirrored the care in Prussia, as well. Long-term convalescent care might be provided in 'Heroes' Homes' [*Heldenheime*] or 'invalid homes' [*Invalidenhäuser*], hospice-like institutions which were run and supported by charitable associations and private noblewomen, but which were more often designed as universal homes for the unwell indigent. One such institution was the invalid home founded by Frau Simon in Loschwitz-Sachsen for those soldiers wounded in the 1870 wars of unification. More usually, however, these soldiers found themselves relegated to the general welfare homes, such as the Waldheimer Versorgungshaus, which confined the care of disabled veterans within the same rooms as those of the poor, convicted, mad, and orphaned. For more on the history of war-disabled care in Saxony see Otto Neustätter, 'Kriegsbeschädigtenfürsorge in früherer Zeit', pp. 329–36 in Artur Baumgarten-Crusius, ed., *Geschichte der Sachsen im Weltkriege* [Sachsen in Großer Zeit, 3] (Leipzig: R. Max Lippold, 1920).

9 For a contemporary American perspective on the German system, see Devine, *Disabled Soldiers and Sailors*, 281–7.

10 Robert Whalen's study on the pension system for German veterans of the First World War and its subsequent reform in the Weimar Republic and early Nazi period remains the authoritative account of the pension struggles. See Whalen, *Bitter Wounds*. Moreover, as James Diehl has pointed out, there was also much resentment and distrust regarding the allocation and distribution of veteran's benefits once these were subsumed into the 'more mundane' welfare programmes administered by the Labour Ministry. See the first chapter of Diehl's book on German veterans in the post-war period for a discussion of the importance of the state's administration of veteran's benefits, as well as the in-kind contributions of voluntary organisations to these 'official' ones. Diehl, *The Thanks of the Fatherland*, especially pp. 11–14.

11 Quote from Lange, 'Eine neue Kunst-und Arbeitshand'.

12 Hennock, *Origin of the Welfare State*, 114–15.

13 I have found no medical or military reports of soldier resistance to war-time recovery. There are letters of complaint and reports of soldier dissatisfaction with war welfare in the post-war period of the Weimar Republic (1919–1933), but these shed little light on soldier resistance *during* the war. Given that soldiers were still under military orders during medical treatment and rehabilitation, however, it is not surprising that they did not resist so much that they would be noticed. For more on post-war veteran dissatisfaction with pensions and welfare see, Whalen, *Bitter Wounds* and Cohen, *The War Come Home*.

14 Biesalski, *Kriegskrüppelfürsorge*, 17–18.
15 Biesalski, 'Die ethische und wirtschaftliche Bedeutung', 9.
16 Biesalski, 'Die ethische und wirtschaftliche Bedeutung', 9–10.
17 Silberstein, 'Kriegsinvalidenfürsorge', 3.
18 Biesalski, *Kriegskrüppelfürsorge*, 17.
19 For more on the medicalisation of bodily conditions, the invention of diagnoses, and the discovery of old diseases, see the collection of essays on medicalisation in contemporary America by Peter Conrad. Although Conrad does not examine the medicalisation of disability in these essays, he does outline the broader concept. More interestingly, perhaps, he notes the movement among late twentieth-century disability rights activists in the U.S. to de-medicalise disability and transform it rather into a societal condition. Peter Conrad, *The Medicalization of Society: On the Transformation of Human Conditions into Treatable Disorders* (Baltimore: Johns Hopkins University Press, 2007).
20 Hennock, *Origin of the Welfare State*, 202–4.
21 BArch R1501/113045. Walter Salzmann, *Der sorgenfreie Kriegsinvalide: Die Hinterbliebenenversorgung* (Cassel: Friedr. Lometsch, 1915), 162.
22 Salzmann, *Der sorgenfreie Kriegsinvalide*, 6.
23 Salzmann, *Der sorgenfreie Kriegsinvalide*, 7–9.
24 Salzmann, *Der sorgenfreie Kriegsinvalide*, 14.
25 Hans Würtz, *Der Wille Siegt!* [Beiträge zur Invalidenfürsorge 1] (Berlin: Reichsverlag Hermann Kalkoff, 1916). For more on the Oskar-Helene-Home founded by Konrad Biesalski see chapter 1.
26 Würtz, *Der Wille Siegt!*, 137–40, block quote on 140. For more on the significance of work in defining the German character, see Joan Campbell, *Joy in Work, German Work: The National Debate, 1800–1945* (Princeton: Princeton University Press, 1989).
27 Biesalski, *Kriegskrüppelfürsorge*, especially 12–19.
28 See for instance Biesalski, *Kriegskrüppelfürsorge*, 4; Lange, *Kriegs-Orthopädie*, 182.
29 Biesalski, *Kriegskrüppelfürsorge*, 15–16. For Biesalski's own description of this campaign, see Mollenhauer, 'Bericht über die ausserordentliche Tagung', 75.
30 Biesalski, *Kriegskrüppelfürsorge*, 15–16.
31 Biesalski, *Kriegskrüppelfürsorge*, 16.
32 SHAD AA 2389. 4-page advertisement for *Kriegskrüppelfürsorge*.
33 Klaus-Dieter Thomann, 'Die medizinische und soziale Fürsorge für die Kriegsversehrten', in Wolfgang U. Eckart and Christoph Gradmann, eds, *Die Medizin und der Erste Weltkrieg*, (Pfaffenweiler: Centaurus, 1996), 183–96, 192.
34 Biesalski, *Kriegskrüppelfürsorge*, 4.
35 Biesalski, *Kriegskrüppelfürsorge*, 19.
36 Biesalski, *Kriegskrüppelfürsorge*, 20.
37 Alice, Freifrau von Bissing, *Die Frau in der Kriegsbeschädigtenfürsorge* (Leipzig: Leopold Voss, 1917).
38 SHAD MdI 7417. Letter H.226/17 from the Unterausschuss für kunstgewerbliche

Betätigung in den Lazaretten und Genesugnsheimen, Stiftung Heimatdank to Geheim Rat Ministerialdirektor Roscher dated April 14, 1917.

39 National Hygiene Museum, *Ausstellung für Verwundeten- und Krankenfürsorge im Kriege* (Berlin: J.J. Weber, 1915), iii. Karl Lingner made his fortune developing and manufacturing Odol Mouthwash. He was also instrumental in the founding of the National Hygiene Museum in Dresden and its 1911 path-breaking travelling Hygiene Exhibit. For more on Lingner, the National Hygiene Museum and the International Hygiene Exhibit, see Paul M. Weindling, *Health, Race, and German Politics Between National Unification and Nazism, 1870–1945* (New York: Cambridge University Press, 1989.)

40 Karl Lingner, *Ausstellung für Verwundeten* (Dresden), iii.

41 Lingner, *Ausstellung für Verwundeten* (Dresden), iii–iv.

42 Lingner, *Ausstellung für Verwundeten* (Dresden), iv. For a brief discussion of the Dresden expansion of the Berlin exhibit, see the yearly reports of the National Hygiene Museum, DHMD Archiv. Sig. 837. *Jahresbericht, 1912–1918*, 7

43 For more information on Karl-August Lingner (1861–1916) and his popularisation of health and hygiene in Dresden as well as the rest of the German Empire, see Weindling, *Health, Race, and German Politics*, 228–30, 378.

44 Lingner, *Ausstellung für Verwundeten* (Dresden), v.

45 *Ausstellung für Verwundeten* (Dresden), vii.

46 Kirchner, *Ausstellung für Verwundeten* (Dresden), 6.

47 Kirchner, *Ausstellung für Verwundeten* (Dresden), 6–7.

48 DHMD Archive. Sig. 837 Jahresbericht 1912–1918.

49 SHAD AAA 2376, f. 31. Article clipped from the *Bayerische Staatszeitung*, 35 (February 12, 1916). 'Bekanntmachung, die Ausstellung der bayerischen Invalidenfürsorge betreffend'.

50 SHAD AAA 2376, f. 31. 'Bekanntmachung, die Ausstellung der bayerischen Invalidenfürsorge betreffend'.

51 DHMD [National Hygiene Museum], *Die Kriegsbeschädigtenfürsorge in Deutschland*. Exhibit Catalogue (Dresden: National Hygiene Museum, 1917), 1–3.

52 DHMD *Die Kriegsbeschädigtenfürsorge in Deutschland*, 2.

53 DHMD *Die Kriegsbeschädigtenfürsorge in Deutschland*, 2.

54 [National Hygiene Museum], *Führer durch das Gesamtgebiet der Kriegsbeschädigtenfürsorge* (Dresden: National Hygiene Musem, 1917).

55 See Inhaltsverzeichnis in *Führer durch das Gesamtgebiet der Kriegsbeschädigtenfürsorge*, 5–6.

56 DHMD-Archive. See for instance *Ansichten aus dem Lazarett Jakobsberg, orthopädisches Lazarett des XX.A.K., Allenstein O.pr.* (1918), and *Reserve-Lazarett Ettlingen i. Baden, Turnübungen der Amputierten (Gehschule)* (1918). These are also located in the Bundesarchiv-Filmarchiv (Berlin).

57 National Hygiene Museum, *Jahresbericht, 1912–1918*, 7.

58 See for example the report of the historical department of the National Hygiene

Museum which kept records of those war-wounded exhibits to which it loaned materials. DHMD-Archive. 837. 'Die geschichtliche Abteilung', *Jahresbericht, 1912–1918*, 17–18. See also the exhibition poster for the Poszony exhibit drawn by the Budapest artist, Pal Sujan in 1917. A digital copy can be found in the on-line poster collection of the World Digital Library. 'National War Relief Exhibition', World Digital Library, www.wdl.org/en/item/250/ (accessed November 8, 2013).

59 Leipzig was an important centre of commercial trade and exposition in Germany and it is not surprising that it would have an exhibit hall called the Crystal Palace [*Krystalpalast*], no doubt inspired by the British Crystal Palace of the nineteenth century. It continues today to be known as Germany's *Messestadt* [trade fair city].

60 For more on the relationship between the Heimatdank and the Reich Committee for War-Disabled Care see August Stocker, *Kriegshinterbliebenenfürsorge: Ein Handbuch der sozialen Fürsorge für die Hinterbliebenen der im Kriege Gefallenen* (Macklot'sche: 1918), 17–34. For a brief discussion of the Heimatdank (in Sachsen and Baden), see Cohen, *The War Come Home*, 66–70.

61 SHAD, MdI 177742, f. 81. Unaddressed letter from the Chemnitz office of the Heimatdank,. October 23, 1917.

62 *Heimatdank Ausstellung für Kriegsbeschädigten-Fürsorge* [Exhibition Catalogue] (Leipzig, 1917), 19–20.

63 The eleven exhibit departments were: history of the medical corps, medical care in the field, medical care at home, transportation, reserve hospitals, artificial limbs, courses of instruction, literature, organisations and statistics, training in industry and craft, settlement colonies and apartments. *Heimatdank Ausstellung*, 15, 5–6.

64 See for example one pamphlet printed and distributed by the Heimatdank: SHAD MdI 7417. O. Seyffert, *Arbeiten Kriegsverletzter*. Seyffert was a professor at the Royal Art Academy in Dresden as well as a folklorist. See also 'Bekanntmachung, die Ausstellung der bayerischen Invalidenfürsorge betreffend'.

65 SHAD MdI 7417. Letter dated November 10, 1916. No. 1357 III M from MdI to Handels- und Gewerbekammern.

66 SHAD MdI 7417. Letter dated November 10, 1916. No. 1357 III M from MdI to Handels- und Gewerbekammern.

67 Adolf Silberstein, *Ergebnisse der Kriegsinvalidenfürsorge im Reserve-Lazarett Nürnberg* (Würzburg: Curt Kabitzsch, 1916), 145–6.

68 Silberstein, *Ergebnisse der Kriegsinvalidenfürsorge im Reserve-Lazarett Nürnberg*, 22.

69 See for instance, Kurt Wiener, 'Fingerbesteck für Einhändige', *Münchener medizinische Wochenschrift*, Vol. 93 (1916), 1442.

70 Silberstein, *Ergebnisse der Kriegsinvalidenfürsorge im Reserve-Lazarett Nürnberg*, 23.

71 Gocht, *Künstliche Glieder*, 378–9.

72 Adverts run throughout the exhibition catalogue; however, the ones mentioned above can be found here: *Heimatdank Ausstellung*, 105, 115.

73 See for instance the untitled article on artificial limbs and the special exhibit on artificial limbs in Berlin-Charlottenburg in *Illustrirte Zeitung*, 146 (1916),

256–7; An article on the professional occupation of the war-invalids showed disabled men busily making baskets, tailoring, making shoes, woodworking, and metal-smithing among other occupations. See 'Die berufliche Beschäftigung der Kriegsverwundeten und Invaliden', *Illustrirte Zeitung*. 2 (1916), 157–8.

74 See for instance, 'Wo unsere verwundeten und erkrankten Krieger Erholung und Genesung finden', *Illustrirte Zeitung* 144 (1915), 628; and 'Die Behandlung Verwundeter im Landesbad Baden-Baden', *Illustrirte Zeitung* 144 (1915), 658.

75 *Illustrirte Zeitung* 143 (1914), 689.

76 Untitled article in *Illustrirte Zeitung* 2 (1916), 263–4.

77 Untitled article in *Illustrirte Zeitung* 147 (1916), 263–4.

78 LAB. Generalleutnant z.D. Wollmann, 'Neuzeitliche Kriegsbeschädigten-Fürsorge durch Turnen und Sport', *Illustrirte Zeitung* 149 (1917), 107–8.

79 Wollmann, 'Neuzeitliche Kriegsbeschädigten-Fürsorge durch Turnen und Sport'.

5

RECYCLING THE DISABLED: THE MOBILISATION OF THE WOUNDED IN WAR-TIME GERMANY

> The welfare of the war-wounded is indisputably a concern of the state and it will be administered by the state, first through the maximal healing of the wounded and then through the awarding of pensions. ... But the healing and pensioning of the war-wounded does not fulfil our obligations to the war-wounded. Steps should be taken to ensure that the war-wounded resume the solid economic professional activity that they had before the war. (Friedrich Syrup, 1916)[1]

> Due to the desperate circumstances, the exploitation of all manpower – even the slightest – is hereby ordered. Therefore all war-disabled soldiers who are capable of even the slightest amount of useful work are being commandeered for duty. Even those who have been labelled as 'severely injured' that is, evaluated at a medical disability of 50% or more, are still capable of work. Moreover, every public and private workplace must be informed that severely injured workers are better than none at all. ... The war-disabled must be informed that he is not being healed out of pity, but rather because his labour is crucial for the collective good. (General Hermann von Stein, Imperial German War Ministry, 1918)[2]

In 1916 Friedrich Syrup, an engineer working in the Prussian industrial inspection office, published a pamphlet regarding the best and optimal use of labour in the nation's factories. In this pamphlet he offered guidelines on how to maximise the efficiency of worker movements and also best distribute workers – according to their physical fitness or bodily capacity – around the factory floor. His goal was clearly to help mitigate the war-time labour crisis that German factory managers were experiencing, but also to ensure that each worker was placed in a position which most suited his needs. What makes Syrup's pamphlet noteworthy is not its focus on increasing worker efficiency, nor is it unique in its description of how to increase war-time production. By 1916, most belligerent nations in Europe had developed programmes and founded governmental agencies dedicated to the efficient and rational production of war materials. What makes Syrup's pamphlet remarkable is that his suggestions, strategies, and studies were geared not toward optimising the labour of new factory recruits, but rather disabled Germans.

Syrup's war-time pamphlet, *Welfare for War-Disabled Industrial Workers,* was written to instruct factory managers on how to maximise the 'bodily capacity' of disabled soldiers and civilians. Not only did it focus on how the remaining limbs of amputees or the senses of the blind might best be exploited for industrial gain, it also pointed out for which positions a one-legged man or double amputee was ideally suited. He noted the prosthetic devices invented for facilitating this work and he argued passionately that nearly every disabled soldier was still capable of earning his own living. But, he added, it was up to the leaders of German industry to hire these men. In the pages of the pamphlet he dismissed the claims of foremen and floor managers that hiring the 'sickly' might increase accident risk or endanger others. In response to these concerns he informed readers that 'the war has necessitated that we un-learn things in certain areas'. Part of this un-learning included re-evaluating the employment of war-disabled. Hiring the disabled, he argued, was crucial to the national economy.[3]

The previous chapters have focused on the expansion of orthopaedists' knowledge and authority into various spheres of German war-time society. Orthopaedists re-defined the scope of their field to include trauma victims; they incorporated artificial limb design into their expertise; they moved beyond 'the clinic' to shape both military and civilian care for wounded soldiers; and they even re-defined the cultural meaning of disability in the German imagination. Moreover in each of these arenas, orthopaedists were positioning themselves as experts and argued for exclusive authority in these matters. By 1916 they were ready to take stock of their efforts. In February of that year, the DOG and the DVK convened a joint 'emergency congress'. Thus, it is not surprising that for three full days in Berlin, German doctors from across the empire as well as from its ally Austria-Hungary debated strategies and compared notes on the best ways to heal and restore the rapidly increasing number of 'war-cripples'. What is surprising, however, is that the community of medical professionals at these specially convened conferences included not only orthopaedists and surgeons, but also representatives of the military, heavy industry, private cripple-homes, insurance officials, school administrators, agricultural commissioners, architects, engineers, and the German Empress and an Austro-Hungarian Archduke. By early 1916 the organised rehabilitation of the war-disabled was well underway and Germany's orthopaedists were in charge of it.

But when the war radicalised that same year, the twin pillars of modern warfare – army and industry – became increasingly interested in exploiting rehabilitation goals for their own needs. What had begun as a medical project to rehabilitate Germany's soldiers for a post-war future was enlisted into war-time efforts aimed at the total mobilisation of society. This militarisation of medicine as part of the management of modern war marked a significant shift in the rehabilitation of the disabled. Whereas the previous chapters outlined the medicalisation of rehabilitation and the growing authority of orthopaedists during the conflict, this chapter examines their militarisation by industry and army under the extreme conditions of 'total war'.

This chapter begins with an elaboration of the significance of the year 1916 in the German war effort. It then turns to an examination of how German social reformers grafted their ideas of national expansion and regeneration onto the body of the disabled soldier. Next it looks at how German industrial circles interacted with the disabled soldier: first, by taking advantage of his newly reclaimed labour and then, by conducting workplace studies to determine how best to exploit this manpower reserve. The chapter then ends with an investigation into the ways in which military officials re-mobilised severely injured soldiers into various war-time industries in order to meet their own increasing materiel demands.

1916 and the emergence of 'total war' in Germany

By 1916 the shortage of labour in Germany had reached crisis proportions; and industry and army were locked in a struggle over manpower. Indeed by then it was clear that the victors in this new war of attrition would be determined not by superior military strategy, but rather by troop endurance and the supply of war materiel. Early battles in the conflict had signalled the importance of outlasting the enemy. However, at Verdun in early 1916 Eric von Falkenhayn, Chief of Staff of the Imperial German Army, revealed his new strategy of engaging the French army in a war of attrition designed ultimately to 'bleed the enemy white'. By then fit, able-bodied men – whether factory workers or soldiers – were at a premium and the successful management and exploitation of the empire's material *and human* resources would soon become an all-encompassing goal in the economic mobilisation demanded of 'total war'.[4]

Indeed when Generals Paul von Hindenburg and Erich Ludendorff took over the Supreme Army Command (*Oberste Heeresleitung*, OHL) of the German war effort in 1916 after Falkenhayn's dismissal by the Kaiser, the pair made the economic mobilisation of the empire's economy one of their top priorities. The War Raw Materials Office (*Kriegsrohstoffabteilung*, KRA) – created in August 1914 – already provided for the empire-wide collection, storage, and distribution of important raw materials in order to ensure that industrial production of munitions did not suffer due to scarcity of goods. One of the first steps toward centralising military planning was the creation in late 1916 of the Supreme War Office (*Kriegsamt*) – an office which aimed to centralise the military's economic planning by subordinating all other mobilisation offices under it. Headed originally by Wilhelm Groener, the Kriegsamt eventually came to administer the War Raw Materials Office as well as military recruitment, exports, and labour exemptions. Moreover, in addition to managing the human and material resources of the empire, the newly created office also continued re-organising Germany's consumer economy for war.[5]

At the same time that Ludendorff and Hindenburg were restructuring the empire's military organisation, the OHL also introduced the so-called Hindenburg Program – the complete re-organisation and total harnessing of the German economy for the more efficient production of war. Under the aegis of the OHL and the Kriegsamt, the Hindenburg Program aimed to double the stores of munitions, triple the supply of artillery and machine guns, and eventually mobilise another 3,000,000 workers into war-related industries.[6] Indeed, the aim was to concentrate every available resource – human and material – into munitions production. At the same time, the programme placed a moratorium on the manufacture of consumer and other 'non-essential' goods and all those resources – human and material – were diverted to the arms industry. Finally, the Auxiliary Service Law (*Vaterländische Hilfsdienstgesetz*), passed on December 5, 1916, marked the institution of a wholesale civilian (male) labour draft in the German Empire, under which all men between the ages of seventeen and sixty who were not already on military duty were to be mobilised for the war effort in some sort of patriotic service.[7] Clearly, the organisation and enlistment of all the nation's resources – especially healthy bodies and materials – to the state's war-time needs had become all but routine (if not smooth) by the winter of 1916.

Eventually, however, the demands of industrial warfare created a kind of manpower paradox. On the one hand, the military's demand for able-bodied soldiers – those recognised by the military as fit for active service (kv) – seemed insatiable. On the other hand, the factory demand for labourers increased as industry struggled to meet the munitions and materiel demands of the army. In short, there simply were not enough fit men to fulfil both industrial and military demands. Moreover, as the battles continued, the numbers of severely disabled returning from the front continued to mount. Thus, as the war progressed, the German war economy faced an increasingly desperate labour shortage.

Colonising the disabled

At the same time as military authorities were re-organising German society for the war effort, employers, workers, and social reformers began to found organisations and develop guidelines for returning the disabled soldier to work. No doubt these developments were due in part to the re-educational campaign designed to inform Germans on the proper treatment of and expectations regarding the disabled body. However, this change in the treatment of disabled soldiers was also influenced by the scale of the war. Indeed, the massive number of disabled soldiers returning from the front was too overwhelming for the sort of welfare offered to wounded veterans of 1871. Moreover, although originally understood as a system of social care for the war-injured, many soon realised that the programmes of disability welfare could have advantageous consequences not only for the wounded veteran, but, as Biesalski had repeatedly emphasised, also for the German nation.

As the news of the re-abling of the wounded spread, other social and political groups became interested in broadening the scope of *Wiedereingliederung* by enlisting disabled soldiers and their labour into other national regeneration projects. While some *Berufsberatung* organisations, such as the German Central Office of Career Counselling for Academics, sought to protect the economic futures of particular social strata, other groups wanted to enlist disabled soldiers in the economic development of particular regions of the empire. Through the creation of settlement societies and soldier colonies, some voluntary organisations hoped to re-settle the disabled in rural areas of the empire and any newly conquered territories to the east, while also using their labour to reclaim agricultural wasteland in order to supplement the empire's food supply.

In March of 1917 the rural settlement society 'Saxon Home' [*Landessiedlungsgesellschaft 'Sächsisches Heim'*] formed in Dresden with the purpose of resettling the Saxon countryside with disabled soldiers and war widows. The organisation aimed at once to both combat the shortage of affordable housing in the empire, while also providing for the long-term care of disabled soldiers, by creating homes for them. These so-called Soldier Homesteads [*Kriegerheimstätten*] were small housing communities designed and built for disabled war veterans and their dependents. In accordance with a law passed in Saxony on May 5, 1916, that provided for the re-settling of veterans in the rural countryside as part of their overall welfare benefits, Saxon Home had been founded to coordinate and assist in this programme. In addition to being substantially subsidised by the state, it also received support from the Saxon state insurance institution; this allowed the company to guarantee loans and credit to the disabled veterans.[8]

Together with the 1916 Capitalization Law (which provided for disability pensions to be paid in a lump sum), Saxon Home and other organisations were able to help disabled soldiers buy property, thus ensuring their long-term security.[9] For instance, the settlement company, Saxon Land [*Sachsenland*] acquired a feudal estate of 900 Morgen (approximately 270 hectares) which was subsequently divided into individual lots for war-invalids. According to one announcement small plots of land equivalent to roughly 3–4 Morgen each (approximately 1 hectare) were to be allotted primarily to war-invalids for the purpose of raising fruits and vegetables. Moreover, the notice mentioned that the ideal location of the farms – close to both Leipzig and Halle – meant that the settlers would have easy access to city markets for selling their produce.[10] In Dresden the disabled veterans welfare organisation, Heimatdank, built a settlement at Weinböhla just outside the city limits. Their leaders argued that the quietude, healthy forest air, and relative seclusion would be an ideal place not just for the wounded veteran to recover his strength and independence, but also to secure his own existence through the cultivation of fruits and vegetables. Moreover, any surplus fruits of his labour, they added, could be conveniently jarred at a nearby cannery or sold at market.[11]

While clearly such settlement programmes were designed to ensure that disabled soldiers and their families enjoyed the security and stability that homeownership offers, a closer look suggests that at least some of these re-settlement programmes, or 'inner colonisation' [*innere Kolonisation*] programmes as they were called, also contained social agendas, as well. Indeed, along with providing for the welfare of disabled veterans, they looked to repopulate the rural countryside, manage the re-distribution of dislocated Germans, and perhaps most importantly, annex new territory to the empire. Although these programmes were developed especially for disabled soldiers, they were clearly grafted on to larger nationalist and annexationist programmes which emerged during the war.[12]

Take, for instance, the mission of the welfare organisation the Settlement Help Society for German Soldiers [Verein 'Ansiedlungshilfe für deutsche Krieger']. In its newsletter, *Der Osten*, the group argued that the 'thanks of the fatherland' should include making the disabled independent by providing him with his own home and farming land. However, they also linked this project to nationalist visions of territorial expansion and reclamation. Indeed in their opinion the resettlement of German soldiers in the eastern borderlands on the Baltic Sea [*Kurland*] was necessary: 'to create a national bulwark [*Volkswall*] to the East in order to improve the security of our borders against the land-hungry Muscovites'.[13] In addition to reasons of national security (which resonate strongly with later Nazi ideas of racial and territorial expansion), however, they also argued that resettling the east would: help in the agricultural training of new farmers; benefit industry by increasing available manpower reserves; and provide jobs to those Germans willing to relocate.[14] Surely the addition of 'free' land to the empire (and its citizens) was not lost on the readers of *Der Osten* either.

Of course, the principles of this particular association were clearly being expressed in ultranationalist language, but the writers and readers of *Der Osten* were not alone in holding these sentiments.[15] In early 1916, the chief architect and head of the housing authority in Saxony gave a speech to the state's economic society on the social politics of inner colonisation. In this talk, 'Rural Settlement Politics in Saxony', he argued that the war had highlighted the significance of social and population management.[16] Indeed, he pointed out the importance of reversing the trend towards urban migration, and the preservation of agricultural labour and society, and – in accomplishing these first two objectives – ultimately safeguarding the national food supply.[17] In addition articles abounded in the popular and specialist press which advocated 'recycling the disabled' into rural areas in order to not just ensure their own food needs, but those of the entire nation, as well. Indeed, according to the empire's national economics office [*Zentralstelle für Volkswirtschaft*], sending the disabled soldier into the countryside would not just offer him the health benefits of fresh air and the psychological well-being of an independent existence, it would ultimately also contribute to increasing the overall nourishment of the nation.[18]

Industry and the rationalisation of the disabled

Whereas social reformers sought to graft the medical treatments and welfare for disabled soldiers onto their own programmes for regenerating the war-torn nation, industrial circles looked for ways to enlist the disabled into their works. Syrup's publication, mentioned at the beginning of this chapter, on how to maximise the labour potential of disabled soldiers in German factories is a prime example of this effort. Published as part of a series issued by the German Association of Shop Foremen, *The Welfare for War-Disabled Industrial Workers* was a booklet that outlined ways to re-use the severely injured in German industry because, as Syrup pointed out, 'The goal must be for the war wounded to take up a full economic role in the work-world through their own jobs just as they did before the war.'[19]

Although the first half of the pamphlet reiterated the familiar points regarding the administrative divisions in war-disabled care and the importance of returning the disabled to his previous post or similar occupation, the second half focused on the practical use of the disabled as workers in industrial concerns. However, whereas the Berufsberatung guidelines developed by the war welfare community focused on the importance of taking advantage of the existing knowledge, technical training, and learned skill which remained in every injured soldier when assigning to him his new profession, Syrup argued that it was the nature of the injury itself – not the injured's pre-war training-which should be considered when returning the disabled soldier to the workplace.[20] Indeed, his discussion of returning the wounded to the workplace concentrated largely on mapping out the best ways for maximising the productive abilities of the disabled *body*, not individual persons, in the workplace.

As a factory inspector and engineer – not an orthopaedist – Syrup was well-positioned to evaluate the practical uses of the disabled in the industrial workplace and he drew upon his own experience in Gleiwitz, Upper Silesia (East Prussia). In the pages of his booklet, he expertly weighed in on the challenges facing these soldiers – amputations, impaired vision, nervous disorders, degrees of paralysis – and then outlined which occupations, workstations, and equipment were best suited to each of the varieties of injured men who now peppered the labour market. He noted, for instance, that the new models of artificial feet and legs now available to the disabled were so perfectly constructed that 'strong-willed' men who had lost just one leg seemed to have little problem returning to work. Walking, taking the stairs, riding bicycles and horses, even climbing ladders were all everyday movements, Syrup observed, which created little trouble for such men with determination once they had become accustomed to their new limbs. In fact, his booklet included lists of professions for which one-legged soldiers were particularly suitable – plumbing, masonry, and quarry work were just a few. Moreover, Syrup contended, a man who had lost both legs could still ably carry out most occupations while sitting provided he still had the use of two healthy hands. So long as he had the assistance of factory machinery and the ability to sit steadfast at his post, Syrup assured his readers that most double-leg amputees could be returned to industrial work.[21]

Injuries to the upper extremities were not as easily overcome, conceded Syrup, but certainly men who had lost fingers, hands, and arms could be returned to work. Cramped, contorted fingers actually created more difficulty in operating machinery and holding objects than the loss of digits, Syrup observed, therefore he recommended that skilled surgeons simply 'help' these men by removing these useless fingers. Those men with severed fingers or palms were better off, however, if directed to new professions. Syrup maintained that with the aid of new prosthetic devices and a little tenacity on the part of the wounded, most arm amputees could be returned to their work, as well. Indeed, by either re-learning to practise his craft with his able arm or through the use of his stump, knee, chin, or teeth, some might even be returned without the help of an artificial limb at all. Finally even those injured soldiers who had lost an eye might be returned to their former professions – except perhaps to those which necessitated the accurate judging of distance or depth, a skill which required both eyes (such as the work done by railway workers).[22] Clearly for Syrup, there were few injuries so disabling for a man that he would not be able eventually to find a place in German industry.

Although the claims that the disabled soldier could easily be returned to work sound familiar, the arguments in *The Welfare for War-Disabled Industrial Workers* are noteworthy for several reasons. What is different about Syrup's pamphlet is that he was addressing not the injured men themselves or their families, but rather factory employers and industrial managers. Rather than convincing the public that the wounded could be restored (as the orthopaedic community had), Syrup's aim was to convince the leaders of German industry to hire these men. As mentioned above, he countered arguments that hiring the disabled might be inefficient or hazardous, by pointing out that hiring the disabled would actually aid the soldier's physical and economic recovery by providing him with the necessary work-therapy to retrain his body. If that were not enough incentive, however, he added that it would also stimulate the national economy.[23] Of course, providing the wounded veteran with an income would also reduce the pressure on the pension system and it is easy to see how this kind of reasoning would benefit Syrup in his later career in the Labour Ministry.[24]

Syrup outlined the ways in which factory foremen and managers could aid in the recovery of the severely injured. First, as employers they could be instrumental in reinforcing the 'will to work' by exerting pressure on them and refusing to allow an injured man to give up or quit when his body felt tired. In addition, he argued, managers and supervisors were in a prime position to 'clarify' for soldiers why filling the so-called 'easy posts' in industrial firms with younger, less severely injured men was not possible. For, in step with the *Berufsberäter*, Syrup maintained that such positions as doorman, guard, custodian and the like were to be reserved for the older, more severely injured soldiers – and clearly not to be offered to men who were capable of industrial work. Moreover, disabled men who were closely monitored and disciplined while on the job would have a more difficult time trying to argue they were incapable of work that they were already performing – no matter how slowly or inefficiently. In addition to spelling out for the disabled man which type of job was open to him, a manager could also exercise control over the worker's behaviour. Indeed, Syrup noted that sometimes the disabled worker had to be reminded not only to comply with routine general factory regulations, but also to not expect any 'special treatment'.[25] Clearly to Syrup the floor manager played a crucial role in rehabilitation because of his position as taskmaster and worker-disciplinarian. Indeed this closer reading of Syrup's comments reveals that in his experience, sometimes work-therapy was a treatment which had to be forced upon its 'patients', echoing the concerns already voiced by orthopaedists.

But while industrial managers could help promote physical rehabilitation and the re-integration of disabled soldiers into the work environment, Syrup also emphasised that they had certain responsibilities in this project, as well. First and foremost, managers were compelled not to think 'asocially' and let a wounded man's disability pension influence his wage rate. What he meant, of course, was that supervisors should not try to save money by paying disabled veterans less than their fellow workers. Indeed the issue of wages would become a sore point between disabled soldiers and their able-bodied co-workers who feared that employers would rationalise paying lower wages to veterans because their incomes were being supplemented by their war, injury, and/or service pensions. Able-bodied workers and their trade unions feared that their disabled competition in the workplace – like women – would ultimately drive down overall wages. Clearly aware of this, Syrup sought to circumvent this tension by urging wage equity from the outset.

Additionally Syrup argued that workplace supervisors could protect disabled soldiers from being shut out of piece-rate teams by their co-workers. This was important given that many industry wages were paid according to the piece-rate system, that is, wages were paid not by the hour, but rather paid according to how many items or 'pieces' each worker produced. Because it often took a team of workers to complete the production and assembly of a single item, each team was dependent upon the timely and skilled coordination of every member's role in the group. Syrup's admonition suggests that many workers were balking at having to accept a disabled man on their teams as his slower pace might hold up their rate of production and perhaps lower the entire team's wages, as well. Foremen and managers, however, were to monitor this sort of co-worker harassment and ensure that the disabled encountered no difficulties in joining work-teams.[26]

What is interesting about Syrup's pamphlet is not so much that he puts forth additional arguments for why the disabled should be returned to work or even that it represents yet another layer of the educational campaign which sought to re-orient German attitudes regarding the disabled body. Rather, what is remarkable here is the degree to which the management of the post-injury welfare of the disabled soldier also fell, to a certain extent, to his employers and co-workers. In addition to the military superiors, doctors, nurses, and Berufsberatung officials, workplace supervisors and employers represented another level of control and administration in the Wiedereingliederung of the disabled. Moreover, unlike the social welfare organisations, whose pamphlets and guidelines seem genuinely concerned with the re-integration of the disabled in society and work, Syrup's brochure is clearly aimed at employers, instructing them on how to maximise the labour potential of the disabled and minimise any negative impact of their hiring. Indeed, guidelines which included denying 'special rights' to injured workers and outlining the optimal productive use of each injured body, not individual, implies that as much consideration was being given to employers as to the disabled worker himself, suggesting that perhaps not all employers were moved enough by patriotism to hire the war-wounded. Moreover, the caution to monitor the equity in co-worker relationships suggests that at least some Germans were not pleased to have the disabled returned to the workforce. Indeed, as this study's conclusion points out, after the war a hiring quota was established to promote and ensure the employment of the disabled.

By the midpoint of the war many firms were experimenting with the use of disabled labour. In 1916 Felix Krais, one of Stuttgart's leading industrialists published an even more comprehensive guide to using the disabled soldier in the workplace. More detailed than Syrup's booklet, *The Employment Possibilities for the Disabled in Industry, Trade, Handiwork, Farming, and the Public Works* included over 450 pages and more than 100 photographs minutely detailing how war amputees could be returned to work – and which prostheses were most helpful in those endeavours.[27] By 1917 disabled soldiers were at work in firms across Germany including: AEG (Apparatefabrik II); Bergmann Elektricitätwerke AG, E. Zweitusch & Co., GmbH; Dr Paul Meyer AG; Deutsche Telefonwerke GmbH; H. Aron Elektrizitätszählerfabrik GmbH; Ehrich & Graetz, and the Siemens-Schuckert-Werke.[28] The next section of this chapter examines more closely the way in which disabled soldiers were recycled into German industry using the Berlin-based Siemens-Schuckert Works as a case study.

Recycling the disabled in industry: the case of Siemens

As news of the medical programmes for reclaiming the labour of the disabled for industrial and agricultural uses spread, some firms and organisations jumped at the chance to make use of this emerging source of reserve labour. One such firm was the Siemens-Schuckert Works in Berlin, whose engineers had designed the universal work prosthesis which bore its name. Although

Siemens had gained recognition in the medical community for its artificial limb design, the firm's various companies were more well-known among contemporary Germans for their production of military munitions and war materiel. Indeed in 1904 the company had created a Department of War and Shipbuilding Technology [*Kriegs- und Schiffbautechnische Abteilung*] which primarily fulfilled contracts for floodlights and other electrical materiel for the imperial navy's war ships. According to Wilfried Feldenkirchen's 1997 study of the firm, Siemens's pre-war military revenues for 1905/06 came to roughly five million Reichsmarks and had more than doubled by 1914.[29] As one might expect, munitions orders skyrocketed during the war and Siemens along with other industrial firms profited enormously from military contracts.[30] In the first year of the war alone, company revenue from munitions and materiel production totalled over fifty-four million Reichsmarks. By 1915, the firm was delivering not only on long-established contracts for typical electro-mechanical devices, but also telephone and telegraph materials, grenade fuses, submarine motors, and machine-gun parts.[31]

This dramatic increase in military contracts meant that over the course of the war Siemens needed to retain all its industrial workers – and even hire more – if the firm were to meet the munitions contracts being negotiated with the War Ministry. Looking for alternative sources of labour, many companies turned to women, children, and those men too old for combat duty hiring them on as 'ersatz labour' until the war was over.[32] In step with other industrial firms, the Siemens-Schuckert Works turned to these under-tapped sources of labour; however, in addition to drawing on women and children, the firm looked toward an emerging new component of this reserve labour force: the disabled soldier.

In the spring of 1917, the chief engineer at the Siemens-Schuckert Works in Berlin, Paul H. Perls, published an article entitled, 'Employing the War Blind in the Workshop: Job Opportunities in the Mass Production of Electrical Army Materiel'.[33] In this essay, Perls took stock of the efforts being made since 1916 to re-think the treatment of the blind and specifically the ways in which this segment of the disabled population might be made useful and eventually re-employed in industry. Although he noted that before the war Germans had been content to house such unfortunates in state run asylums and busy them with typical 'blind jobs', the war had prompted significant developments in and changes to the treatment of the blind. As an 'educator' [*Krieg als Erzieher*], the war was teaching Germans that rather than simply pitying the blind, now they should return the 'joy for work and life' to those who had sacrificed their sight in the service of the fatherland. Returning the blinded veteran to work, argued Perls (much like Carl Salzmann), would not only restore to him his 'courage for life' but could also return to him the excitement and animation which had been lost with his vision. To that end, Perls proudly noted, industrial and technical firms – who had already proven themselves to be such helpmates to the state's production of war – had also busied themselves with the 'Rehabilitation Question' [*Frage der Wiederertüchtigung*] in the workplace.[34]

Indeed since the onset of the war the Siemens-Schuckert Works in Berlin had been engaged with the question of how to employ the war blind. Initially conducting employment studies using residents of the city's municipal Blind Home in order to test the viability of such an option, Siemens had begun making use of the war blind in its factories in 1916. Within a year, the firm had realised that war-blinded soldiers were well-suited for the production of war and munitions materiel. Particularly optimal occupations had proven to be testing gauges, assembling cartons, packing fuse plugs, assembling parts, testing bolt threads and fuses, and running certain motorised machinery. Such machinery included operating equipment for metal glazing, making fuse jackets, drilling and/or pressing metal, and trimming fuses.[35]

Blind veterans might not initially seem best suited for manufacturing munitions, but experiments at Siemens had demonstrated that as ex-soldiers, they had practical experience with the materials they were constructing. Unlike civilian workers who had never seen or used these devices, ex-soldiers – even blind ones – had a more intimate and personal knowledge of the objects they were manufacturing. But looking beyond their military familiarity with such objects, Perls also argued that it was in fact their blindness that gave them an 'edge'. As he pointed out, 'often the blind worker earns more than his seeing counterpart because he is not distracted from his work'.[36] So diligent and efficient were the blind ex-servicemen, that he noted that some 'particularly gifted' workers were able to work two machines simultaneously. Here Perls is revealing not just how 'usable' blinded soldiers were in Siemens' factories, but that their labour was more efficient and preferable than those able-bodied Germans still on the home front. At Siemens blinded soldiers were not just recovering, they were busy producing war materiel for the military's use. And, as the following discussion elaborates, Perls' analysis of the employment of the war-blind was one informed by the practical economics of industrial production, not social welfare.

The successes with recycling blinded soldiers at Siemens notwithstanding, there were a few difficulties the firm needed to overcome. For instance, although those sightless soldiers still convalescing in military hospitals might be guided to work by their sighted co-workers, blind soldiers who had been already discharged from these facilities had more trouble finding an escort. Perhaps somewhat optimistically, Perls offered a solution to this: wives or female co-workers should be encouraged to take on this task as a 'good deed'. But, he lamented, because these men were completely dependent upon their escorts they were often 'left in the lurch' when these guides were unavailable. These instances were apparently common, for Perls next listed sick days, household duties, and 'differences of opinion' as reasons for why some men had already been 'abandoned' by their female guides. Their inability to show up to work on a regular, predictable basis, therefore, might be a drawback with which employers would have to reckon, but it also seems clear from his language that Perls considered this problem to be as much the fault of co-workers who were failing to do their duty as it might have been of the disabled soldiers themselves.[37]

In addition to highlighting the importance of securing reliable guides for the blind, Perls also advised his readers to limit their working hours (at least initially) and to pay them wages, as well. According to Perls, while the war-blind were still undergoing medical treatment, doctors advised limiting their work shifts to a maximum of six hours per day. This was to ensure a gradual acclimation to their labour without too much stress – an especially important issue, he noted, because those with severe head wounds often suffered nerve damage in addition to their blindness. Gradually, however, once the blind had been medically discharged, they could be expected to work the full eight and a half hour day of the 'normal' worker.[38]

Perls also recommended that firms pay the blind for their work – an indication perhaps that many employers did not, which would explain Syrup's similar admonition. The reasons for offering them financial compensation were twofold: to ensure that they did not lose their zeal for work, but also to underscore to them that the work they were doing was important. The men started off with a guaranteed wage of 35 pfg/hour; however, given the nature of the piece-rate wage system, many were soon earning up to 55 pfg/hour, a wage far higher than their blind compatriots working at home or in the blind schools. Moreover, many blind soldiers eventually were earning more than their female co-workers, no doubt a causal factor in Perls's final suggestion: that due to resulting conflicts, it had proven unsuccessful to form teams of blind soldiers and female co-workers and therefore he did not recommend it.[39]

But despite the obvious gender struggles in the war-time workplace, Perls found the experiment of taking on war-blind workers to be a successful one that he recommended highly. By 1917, Siemens was employing twenty blind soldiers, in addition to ten male and seven female residents of the Berlin municipal blind home and one blind female home-worker. Certain precautions were of course necessary for avoiding on-the-job accidents, but advice thereon had been easily gleaned through the industrial inspections and the employer accident insurance programme [*Berufsgenossenschaft*]. And while he noted with some surprise the overall positive attitude with which the severely disabled set about their tasks, he attributed this happiness to their being surrounded by healthy, able-bodied co-workers who no doubt were having a good influence on the men.[40] Thus, while some feared that the pension-psychosis could be contagious, apparently *Arbeitsfreudigkeit* (an eagerness to work) could be, as well.

Perls did have one suggestion, however, for easing the long-term employment of blind workers, one which he hoped that his readers would seriously consider. Employing blinded veterans in huge, city factories might not be practical, he admitted. Encountering many dangers on the route back and forth to work everyday, navigating the stairs and hallways with thousands of other workers, negotiating the narrow passages between various machinery, and dodging the vans and trucks delivering raw goods and materials – these were all difficulties which the blind would face when working in a big city. For Perls, the ideal solution would be for larger factories already located in outlying areas to build nearby settlements with small homes for the war-blind and their families. In the midst of these housing areas, the firms could place a communal workroom with all the necessary machinery and equipment for blind workers and there, under the supervision of older, retired experts in the trade, the war blind could perform their work safely and ultimately more efficiently.[41] As the section above revealed, this idea of creating 'disabled colonies' for blinded or severely injured war veterans where they might live and work together – yet also remain somewhat removed from the outside world – found favour in a variety of circles during and after the war. However, while the colonies of the Heimatdank were clearly aimed at restoring economic independence to the disabled, the colonies in Perls's imagination were obviously meant also to benefit German industry.

The experiments at Siemens with employing the war-disabled did not focus solely on the blind, however. The firm also employed amputees and other physically disabled soldiers in order to research their suitability for work. In a second article on these labour experiments, Perls outlined how Siemens had skilfully re-integrated a variety of disabled veterans into its works in an attempt not just to find them gainful employment, but also to help heal their bodies through the application of work-therapy.

Perls opened his article with a sweeping judgment on the impact and responsibility of technology in this war.

> Until today technology has opened up unimagined possibilities, but in this war it has also brought about horrors unimaginable. This is no longer a struggle of man

against man, but rather the exploitation of all the most fearsome weapons which industry and technology can spawn. As quickly as industry and technology put themselves in the service of the Fatherland in order to create all these weapons, so is it now their duty to mitigate the damage which they have caused.[42]

Aware that amputees and others who were permanently wounded by the war would face the greatest challenges in the workplace, Siemens had taken on the project of helping to restore them. Using photographs and corresponding case studies of the disabled soldiers they depicted, Perls outlined in his essay the variety of ways in which these disabled soldiers had been recycled into the workplace.[43]

Siemens had employed and physically 're-trained' a wide variety of disabled men. Take for instance the case of 'B'. B was a travelling salesman who had been shot in the right arm and who as a result of his injury suffered from partial paralysis in the same limb. B had been designated a 'packer's assistant' [*wurde einem Packer zur Hilfe gegeben*] and while assisting in the packaging of goods was forced to use his right arm and hand in the process, thereby providing him with his necessary work-therapy. In order to facilitate the use of his otherwise limp and useless hand, engineers at Siemens had constructed a special kind of brace which both steadied his arm and also doubled as a packing tool. Perls noted that the movements necessary for loading goods and packing materials in the boxes replicated that of the medico-mechanical apparati used by orthopaedists to promote healing in stiffened or partially paralysed limbs. In the case of B, then, the work that he was performing at Siemens, Perls argued, would also help to regenerate his nerves and tendons and ultimately aid in his recovery.[44] Moreover, the by-product of his physical therapy actually benefited the firm's production of war materials and thus aided the empire's war effort, as well.

Other men had suffered more debilitating injuries and required an artificial limb in order to be returned to work. 'St' for example was a coachman [*Kutscher*] whose left arm had been amputated as a result of severe injury from machine gun fire. Following his injury, St worked at a mechanical metal press [*Stanzerei*] wearing a prosthetic arm. The metal press ran on a simple mechanised spindle which could be turned on and off with a lever that he operated with his healthy arm while his artificial one actually ran the press.[45] Perls mentioned several other cases of arm-amputees who had been returned to work.[46] And although the majority of the case studies were of men with injured or amputated arms, there were also a few with leg injuries, including the butcher 'L' whose left leg had been amputated below the knee and who now operated a modified metal drill which allowed him to work while sitting.[47] In total Perls outlined thirteen specific case studies of men successfully recycled into various occupations in the Siemens-Schuckert Works; he then turned to a more general, overall assessment of the programme.[48]

In his evaluation, Perls found that the factory at Siemens was an ideal workplace for re-training the disabled. As a firm which focused on the mass production of goods – not specialty items – the majority of the jobs in question either involved sitting at machinery or were considered 'easy women's work' [*leichte Frauenarbeit*]. That is, as positions which relied on simple, repetitive movements, they were the ideal work activities for the severely injured. As jobs that required little training, skill, or precision, they were also positions rewarded with lower pay. Subsequently, these were jobs in lower demand among healthy war workers – or being performed by women. It is easy to see how filling these jobs with the disabled might free up able-bodied workers for either positions requiring more skill or the armed forces.

Indeed, an early 1918 internal company report took stock of the on-going experiments with war-invalids at Siemens. According to the brief, at the time, the factory employed 3400 workers: 2600 women and 800 men. In addition to these workers, the firm also employed 789 war-disabled of which there were 194 arm amputees, 309 leg amputees, 57 fully blind, and 70 half-blind men. The rest were simply defined as 'miscellaneously wounded or sick'.[49] Perls argued that with the proper training and prosthetic device, these severely wounded soldiers could easily take on the 'light work' which the women were currently performing, thus replacing them in the factory.

A brief look at one of the labour comparison studies between disabled soldiers and German women conducted at Siemens supports this conclusion. Take for instance, the case of disabled soldiers 'Ko' and 'We'. Ko was a soldier who had lost his lower right arm at the elbow as the result of a grenade explosion and who was now employed at the metal press on the factory line. According to the study, Ko was able to reach the production wage of the average female worker (81 pfg/hour) by Week 17 of his employment. He then exceeded her wage rate in Week 19. Although he was not able to maintain this level of productivity consistently, Ko did earn on average 91 per cent of the typical female wage. The soldier We, however, was somewhat more successful. We had also lost the bottom third of his right arm, but through diligent application had managed to reach the typical female wage by Week 2 of his arrival at the firm. Moreover, by Week 4, he had exceeded his female co-workers earning on average 84 pfg/hour – 103.7 per cent of the average female wage. The study noted, however, that part of We's success also needed to be attributed to the prosthetic arm which he wore – one especially designed for his work. What is particularly revealing about the experiments with Ko and We (and others) is that they are evidence that Siemens was not simply concerned with evaluating the usefulness or efficacy of 'work therapy' on the disabled soldiers. Indeed, studies which sought to 'prove' the greater efficiency and usability of disabled men over able-bodied women suggest that on some level engineers such as Perls were also concerned with re-asserting the traditional gender hierarchy in the war-time workplace.[50]

In addition to having the ideal posts for injured workers, Siemens also had access to a steady supply of subjects on which to experiment. The firm had volunteered its own infirmary to local authorities and it had been incorporated into the Prussian Army's system of recovering military hospitals. As word of the successful rehabilitation and re-use of disabled soldiers in their factory spread throughout the region, other military and civilian hospitals had begun sending their wounded to Siemens for work-therapy.[51] By placing their services at the disposal of the military, the firm had not just found a way to help heal the disabled, they had apparently also figured out how to circumvent labour problems.

Indeed, Perls stressed the importance of cooperating with the medical community in the project of recycling workers, especially the doctor in charge at each reserve hospital. Although the general goal at Siemens had been to return the disabled soldier to an occupation closely related to his pre-war one, Perls admitted that this had not always been possible (as the case studies above clearly demonstrate) and often severely injured men were assigned positions at various machines. And although Perls conceded that doctors – as medical men – knew nothing regarding the machinery which the men were operating, he found their knowledge to be crucial in evaluating the injured body's performance. Therefore it was his opinion that ideally engineers and doctors should work together to determine the appropriate work therapy for each soldier.[52] In this manner, Perls's suggestions echoed those included in the recently issued guidelines of the Berlin Electrotechnical Association for rehabilitating war-disabled industrial workers.[53]

This examination of the use of disabled soldiers in the Siemens-Schuckert Works suggests that overall it was both a successful and profitable endeavour for the firm. However, Perls felt compelled to note one minor downside – that the disabled needed much encouragement and convincing in being returned to work. Indeed, given what these men had already endured, he argued, it was not surprising that they might want to give up when their bodies faltered. Or, he alternately admitted, many men seemed to misunderstand the nature of work-therapy and therefore resisted working for fear that their pensions might be reduced.[54] However, Perls stressed that only a legal re-evaluation of a soldier's disability could reduce his pension; any wages he might be earning had no effect upon pension adjudication whatsoever and the reluctant disabled soldier should be reminded of this. He agreed that the wounded should be sent to work-therapy as soon as they were physically able to withstand the labour for 'only work will offer him satisfaction and help him to overcome his spiritual and physical pain'.

Like Salzmann and other rehabilitation advocates, Perls believed in the rejuvenating powers of physical labour and therefore he remained confused when the disabled worker chose another occupation over factory work, as they apparently often did. In fact, one-armed workers proved especially difficult for the factory to retain. Perls noted that they constantly demanded positions as messengers, porters, and elevator operators, and, once offered these, resigned their factory positions immediately. By 1917 already fourteen arm amputees had left the factory floor. As an antidote to combating the recalcitrance evident among some disabled soldiers, Perls recommended that those men severely injured but still on active duty be commandeered to work-therapy if their attending doctors deemed them fit enough. 'After all', he justified, 'it was in the soldier's own best interest'.[55]

Although these studies conducted at Siemens illustrate the variety of ways in which the disabled were recycled into the war-time economy of labour, it is really the second half which is more pertinent to this chapter. The fact that some men resisted returning to work or that others questioned the overall goals of rehabilitation suggests that not all men wanted to have their working capacity restored. Indeed, Perls's comments mirror those of Syrup in his analysis of the workplace re-integration of the disabled soldier – that the injured worker needed to be disciplined and monitored during his 'therapy' Moreover, clearly despite advances in technology which enabled them to resume their pre-war occupations, many preferred to take the so-called *Verlegenheitsberufe* of porters and messengers – precisely those positions from which they were being discouraged. For while the medical community found the work to be therapeutic and the industrial community clearly benefited from their labour, perhaps the simple fact is that many injured soldiers did not want to be returned to work. Perls's final comment recommending that those soldiers still under military jurisdiction be ordered to such 'therapy' if necessary only seems to confirm the sentiments about worker resistance originally set out in chapter 4.

The above section has outlined some of the ways in which one German industrial giant, the Siemens-Schuckert Works, re-used disabled soldiers in its factories during the war.[56] Imbued with a sense of responsibility toward the wounded, while also clearly benefiting from the fruits of their labour, engineers and doctors at the firm experimented with ways to return the severely injured soldier to work while also maximising his residual labour potential. Other firms did the same.[57] Thus orthopaedists' knowledge was incorporated into employment practices and industrial, organisation and many firms envisioned themselves as playing a crucial role in the medical project of rehabilitation while also contributing to the welfare of the entire nation. At the same time, by maintaining that the disabled be commandeered to work in factories if necessary, Perls' example suggests that at least one factory, Siemens, wanted even expanded control over these workers. Indeed, the firm soon looked directly to the military, bypassing orthopaedists completely, hoping to gain direct support from the state. On May 17, 1917, the Siemens-Schuckert Works office mailed to the Deputy War Office Bureau [*Kriegsamtstelle*] in Dresden an offprint of their photo-essay detailing the employment of the blind, remarking that 'we assume that these details will be of interest to you'.[58]

The German military recycles the disabled

As the programmes for recycling the disabled in the German industrial sector spread across the empire, news of the success in re-claiming the labour power of the wounded soldier within the war-time economy inevitably caught the attention of military authorities. Whereas initially the German army had been quick to discharge the severely injured soldier from military service and turn over the responsibility for his care and welfare to the civilian community, the growing crisis in labour convinced military officials to reconsider their hasty discharging of wounded men. Instead of releasing soldiers who would have previously been categorised as 'un-usable' [*nicht verwendbar*], military officials decided that rehabilitating the severely injured and re-mobilising their labour for the war effort might better serve the belligerent interests of the state.

By mid 1917 reforms to both the military draft and the Auxiliary Service law were being discussed among the war leaders. Under the original Auxiliary Service Law, every male German between the ages of seventeen and sixty who was not serving in the armed forces was required by law to perform Patriotic Auxiliary Service during the war. This patriotic service could include working in heavy industry to produce necessary war materials, working in the agricultural sector and food production, in the forestry service, or even caring for the sick.[59] Although the law restricted their labour by not allowing men to change jobs without certificates from their previous employers, the law did take into consideration men's ages, family status, place of residence, and pre-war occupation when procuring them a position in the war-time industrial economy. In addition to ensuring that the nation would have sufficient manpower for meeting its war-time needs, this sort of 'patriotic service' could also excuse certain men from military duty in the battlefields. That is, exemptions from military service could be requested for those men deemed absolutely crucial to industrial production – skilled workers especially were likely to be recalled from duty in occupying armies in order to return to their work in particular industries.[60] However, the heavy casualties at Verdun and the other 'killing fields' of the First World War made it clear to military leaders that they could no longer spare any man who was fit for battle duty. Consequently multiple revisions to both the military and civilian drafts were proposed in 1917 in order to enlarge the pool of human resources available for mobilisation.

These revisions included widening the age and bodily health limits at which men could be drafted. The OHL suggested lowering the age limit for compulsory work under the Auxiliary Service Law from seventeen to fifteen years old. In addition to lowering the age limit of the draft, the military leaders wanted to extend it to both women and those men who had been previously ruled 'unfit for duty'. Indeed as early as August 31, 1916 Hindenburg suggested that the 'wounded, prisoners of war, women, and minors' be drafted for war industry work.[61] Although this strategy was not immediately adopted, by then Colonel Max Bauer was caught mediating between industry demands and military needs. On the one hand Bauer promised industrial giants that those skilled workers already exempted from military duty would not be taken away from munitions production, but on the other, he insisted that these same industrialists make greater use of labour not liable to military service.[62] By 1916 the idea for re-using invalided soldiers in the labour force was already being discussed in the inner echelons of the German army. Therefore, when efforts to expand the Auxiliary Service Law to include the wounded and invalided failed,[63] military officials began looking for ways to re-mobilise these men within their own system. In order to free male bodies fit for military duty from crucial war-time industrial work, the army created a system for replacing exempted workers with recycled ones. They developed an internal system designed for re-mobilising and re-deploying the rehabilitated soldier according to war-time needs. It is this process I am calling the military's 'recycling of the disabled'.

Both the Kriegsamt and the War Ministry began to look for ways to use re-abled soldiers as 'replacement power' in industry and agriculture. Because the army needed more 'front-ready' troops, that is, men who were classified as *kv* and could be sent to the battlefield, its leaders created a system whereby fit workers previously exempted from military service due to their labour skills were gradually replaced by re-built, re-trained disabled soldiers. Mobilising the disabled, however, required that the armed forces revise the system of medical care and treatment of the injured soldier. Instead of simply discharging him and turning his care over to the civilian medical community (as was the norm), the Kriegsamt now took over the responsibility of medically assessing the disabled's injury, diagnosing his work potential, and even convincing future employers of his newly regained capacity for work. In accomplishing this take-over of the rehabilitation of the maimed soldiers, military administrators had to enlist the programmes and help of the civilian orthopaedic community in this process. Thus, in order to make these unfit men *wiederverwendungsfähig*, that is, 'recyclable', the military instituted its own structures for treating, training, and recycling the disabled soldier.[64]

First the Kriegsamt needed to identify which convalescing soldiers might be capable of being returned to work. As noted previously, the War Ministry had created a system of Medical Inspectorates in 1915 in order to more directly oversee and speed up the recovery of the nation's soldiers. However as manpower demands increased and the military sought to speed up soldier recovery, the Kriegsamtstelle were ordered to police their local reserve hospitals so that military recruiting officials – not doctors – could determine the fitness for work of Germany's wounded soldiers.[65] Moreover the number of War Medical Inspectorates was increased so that by 1918, there was generally one inspectorate based in each of the Corps districts.[66] Military officials were dissatisfied with the slow casualty recovery rate and put increasing pressure on medical officers and other doctors to speed things up.

In late June 1917, the Kriegsamt determined that the policy to recruit replacement labour power [*Austauschkräfte*] by having military hospital doctors register appropriate candidate-soldiers with its deputy offices had proved less successful than they had originally hoped. Indeed according to a directive from June 30, these notifications had been incomplete – when even submitted at all – and therefore the Kriegsamt was implementing changes to the system.[67] In order to meet both the labour needs of industry and the supply needs of the field army, the Kriegsamt had decided to dispense with its mustering lists and start conducting regular on-site bodily inspections of the recovering troops in order to determine locally and in person which soldiers were capable of work and which were not. Moreover, in order to accommodate this new policy of regular bodily inspections, the Kriegsamt decided to implement a few changes to the structure of the military hospital system. Whereas previous military policy had dispersed the various convalescing soldiers throughout the expanded reserve hospital system, the new policy was intended to funnel the disabled first through so-called Central-Lazarettes [*Zentrallazarette*] and personally evaluate their work potential from there.[68]

In addition to centralising selected wounded soldiers in these Central-Lazarettes and turning the evaluation of their bodily capacity over to military officials, the Kriegsamt announced its intention to bring industry officials into this evaluation process. Because written lists which described and ranked the recovering soldiers according to their bodily abilities had proved relatively ineffective for distributing the men, the Kriegsamt concluded that what was necessary was the creation of a facility to where ambulant and sick patients could be brought so that both the local war office bureaus and industry representatives could, together, personally inspect and evaluate them. An on-site evaluation in conjunction with prospective employers would not only ensure that suitable men were sent to the employers, but would, military officials argued, also save immensely on clerical work by dispensing with compiling lists, answering requests, and other communications. Clearly this was a process designed to both streamline and improve the system of re-evaluating the work-potential of the recovering soldiers.[69]

And indeed, according to an internal report, this new system was largely successful. The Kriegsamtstelle in Dresden did not hesitate to add that during a recent military hospital inspection of seventy-four convalescing soldiers, in fact seventy-one had been deemed fit enough to send off to industrial work.[70] Perhaps it is not surprising that, given the critical manpower needs after 1916, military administrators might evaluate some recovering soldiers as more capable of work than did their doctors, but eventually this need for fit healthy bodies would lead army officials to harness the project of Wiedereingliederung for the military's own war-time ends.

The War Ministry had also begun looking for ways to re-use the labour of disabled soldiers. Indeed by the turning point of the war, they published guidelines for accelerating the treatment and release of re-usable soldiers from the lazarettes. Although initially held as a speech at a meeting of the military medical inspectors and representatives from the army corps on July 1,1916, these ideas were also published by the War Ministry and circulated among the various reserve hospitals later that same month. In a 22-page booklet entitled, *Principles on the Question of Accelerating the Extraction of Troops Usable in the Military or War Industry from the Lazarette or Troop Formations,* General Schultzen pointed out the most common problems with and/or causes for delay in the release of recovering soldiers, and offered various suggestions for remedying them. Whether these delays were the result of medical conditions which escaped easy diagnosis (such as heart, kidney, or skin conditions which many field doctors did not immediately recognise), problems with coordinating paperwork, or conflicts between doctors and military officials, the pamphlet included suggestions for resolving these and other problems that confronted the various medical corps concerning the redistribution of recuperating soldiers.[71]

In addition to issuing empire-wide guidelines for regulating the activities, domain, and authority of military doctors, the War Ministry eventually took over control of convalescing troops directly – either through its own directives or those of the Kriegsamt. On February 2, 1917, General Marquard issued a decree specifically regarding the mustering of convalescing soldiers to the war economy. In order to ensure the absolute maximum 'extraction' of all available labour, he ordered that all *av* soldiers in the military hospitals, central mustering stations, reserve troops, and recuperating companies [*Genesendenkompagnien, Kriegsbeschädigtenkompagnien*] be organised and readied for war work. He emphasised that even those men just partially capable of work were to be mobilised. In addition he ordered the immediate relocation of all wounded men to the appropriate re-training hospitals and the accelerated release of all partially recovered soldiers from the infirmaries. Moreover, those war-disabled soldiers no longer fit for military service were to be sent to training hospitals for rehabilitation and eventual re-assignment in war industries. Those disabled soldiers who refused to cooperate or take up such work were to be commandeered to it under 'doctor's orders'.[72]

However, while the manpower shortage was most acute in munitions production and other war-related industry, it was not the only sector of the economy to which soldiers were being directed. In addition to sending the wounded and disabled soldiers into the factories, the Kriegsamt placed them in the countryside to help with domestic food production and other agricultural work. Orthopaedic medicine and rehabilitation technology had not just concentrated on returning disabled soldiers to industrial work and artisanal trades, they had also created programmes and artificial arms designed for returning the disabled to agricultural work. Indeed by 1917 the empire was facing an acute food shortage as the military draft, auxiliary service law, and high wages in war industry combined to drain nearly all available workers from the German countryside. Lack of agricultural labour in addition to the Allied blockade on imports had contributed to the widespread scarcity in foods – especially after the so-called 'turnip winter' of 1916/17, during which many Germans starved to death.[73]

None of this was lost on those in either the War Ministry or the Kriegsamt. In the spring of 1917, the Prussian War Minister Hermann von Stein ordered that all wounded and recuperating soldiers fit for agricultural labour were to be placed at the disposal of the empire's farmers. On March 21, 1917, the War Minister ordered that due to the shortage of labour in the countryside, soldiers recovering in military hospitals were to be made available for harvesting work. Moreover, he added that due to the widespread lack of awareness among Germany's farmers regarding the availability of soldiers for requisitioning, he also ordered the deputy generals [*Stellvertretende Generalkommandos*] to undertake a widespread campaign informing them of this possibility.[74]

Later that same year, Kühlwetter in the Kriegsamt revised von Stein's original decree by mandating that only war-disabled soldiers were to be made available for agricultural requisitioning. As an order of July 20, 1917 stated, not only was it crucial for food production that all war-disabled soldiers originally from rural areas be returned to the countryside, it was also a matter of national, even patriotic, duty. It seems that those soldiers no longer fit for war-duty [*kriegsunbrauchbar*] were now being commandeered to 'agricultural duty'.[75]

By 1918 the crisis in manpower had reached such drastic proportions that the War Ministry declared that the withholding of any *kv* soldier in the occupation army or war industry was to be considered treason. In justifying this decree, the directive noted, 'We do not lack men; it is only a matter of putting them in the right place and utilising them to their greatest capacity.'[76] By mid 1918, the war minister issued one of the more draconian measures which not only called for the bi-weekly re-evaluation of every soldier's potential for work and military service, but also forbade subsequent reversals or downgrading of this potential. Indeed, according to Stein's order of July 13, 1918, all soldiers were to report to the general mustering commission for bodily inspection. Once any soldier was declared *kv*, no military or troop doctor was allowed to revise or 'contradict' this evaluation. Moreover these mustering commissions were to re-evaluate all soldiers at the military hospitals and reserve lazarettes and send them immediately to the field.[77] By the end stages of the war, the German army had come to rely on the re-using [*Wiederverwendbarmachung*] of the labour of the severely and permanently injured in both the military and civilian economies – recycling the disabled had become an important, indeed crucial, component of the 'total mobilisation' of the German economy for war. However, while orders sent from above can reveal to us the intention of Germany's OHL regarding the use of the disabled soldier, a look at the implementation of these ideas on the local level reveals more concretely how these men were recycled.

Recycling the disabled in Saxony

Even before the above developments, officials in Saxony had been interested in how to maximise the labour of Germany's disabled soldiers. In 1915, the Saxon Minister of the Interior wrote to the Imperial War Ministry in Berlin informing them that local industrialists in Dresden had created a job placement service for disabled soldiers. In his letter of July 24, Minister von Vitzthum noted that the Association for the Protection of German Industry [*Deutsche Industrieschutzverband*] in Dresden had formed an employment agency for war-invalids. This agency had been designed to collect from its member firms and organisations lists of jobs and other assignments suitable for disabled soldiers in order to submit them to the Prussian War Ministry for publication in its newsletter. However, rather than encouraging the disabled veterans to apply directly to the hiring companies, this agency was being formed to act as a sort of clearinghouse for the war-invalids. This way the Association could centralise and distribute the workers in the most efficient manner possible – linking each disabled soldier with a post most suitable to his (and presumably each firm's) needs. Moreover, through the centralisation of job distribution, the association also aimed to keep the war-invalids firmly settled in their home regions by helping them find work nearby and thus mitigating against the 'un-economic [*unwirtschaftlich*] ebb and flow of job-seeking war-invalids from Saxony to Rhineland-Westphalia or from East Prussia back to Saxony'.[78] Although the creation of this job agency for the severely injured was intended to benefit the disabled soldier by finding him work, one cannot help but notice that the Association was also protecting the interests of its members, as well as looking to control the migratory patterns of the discharged veteran. Under the auspices of coordinating job placement for the disabled then, the local civilians had already been concerned with managing the labour economy of war-time Saxony since 1915. By 1917, this interest had extended to the Saxon Army, as well.

In response to the increasing pressure from Berlin to centralise and streamline the process for treating and evaluating wounded troops, General Georg von Broizem, the commanding general of the XII. Army Corps in Saxony, ordered the construction of two new soldier-patient institutions in Dresden: an Industry Lazarette and the Outpatient Employment Agency. The Industry Lazarette [*Industrielazarett*] was no ordinary recovery or convalescing hospital. Nor was it even a training school of the kind erected as part of the Berufsberatung programmes installed throughout the Empire. Rather, this industrial hospital was created expressly for collecting and centralising all convalescing soldiers already deemed fit for work (*av*) and parcelling them out to various industrial and trade concerns. Run by sympathetic doctors [*Chefärzte*] who were, as Broizem phrased it, 'on the side of the Kriegsamt', the industrial lazarette was placed under the administration of the Kriegsamtstelle in Dresden. Recovering soldiers from the surrounding military hospitals, civilian hospitals, and convalescent homes were relocated to this centralised military hospital where on-staff physicians evaluated their work capabilities. Whereas in the early years of the war, the military had been eager to relinquish responsibility for providing recovering soldiers with medical care and social welfare unless they could be returned to active service, by mid 1917, in response to orders from Berlin, the Saxon Army Corps was clearly more interested in recovering as many fit workers as possible. Moreover, in addition to sending them out to work, the Dresden Industry Lazarette provided its inmates with minimal medical care, housing, and other necessities so long as the wounded soldier could be made useful for industrial work.[79]

Once his bodily capacity was evaluated and graded, these medical and army officials of the Industry Lazarette distributed each recovering soldier among the nearby industries making sure each man's individual skills were allocated where necessary. In step with Berufsberatung guidelines in the civilian cripple-care community, these re-mobilised soldiers were to be returned to their pre-war occupations, however, only insofar as these were vocations or jobs necessary for war production.[80] Indeed, the needs of the Empire at war were eventually to take precedence over the soldier's own occupational interests – a point subsequently codified in the Saxon Army's own guidelines for Berufsberatung. In fact, by 1917 these guidelines clearly stated that 'during the war in addition to the personal interests of the war-disabled, vocational welfare (job placement) must also consider in the broadest way possible the needs of the war economy'.[81]

Moreover, those wounded soldiers whose occupations were not beneficial or 'useful' to the nation at war, were not to be brought to the Industry Lazarette. And on this point, von Broizem was especially clear – the Industry Lazarette was not conceived as a convalescing site or a rehabilitation school. That is, only those soldiers who had already been declared *av* were to be shipped and housed there. Those men who still needed certain bodily re-training were to be sent to the Central Lazarette for further treatment. Finally, even those wounded and disabled soldiers assigned to the Industry Lazarette were only to remain there until they were deemed once again *kv*, or discharged and returned to permanent work on the home front.[82] Clearly, as the war dragged on, the military was becoming increasingly interested in how recycling the disabled could enable wounded soldiers to continue to serve their country, instead of simply immediately discharging them.

In addition to building the Industry Lazarette, Broizem established an employment centre within the unit for managing the wounded's labour. Created on July 12, 1917, the Outpatient Employment Agency [*Arbeits- und Ambulatenzentrale Dresden*, AAZ] was the second institution constructed for recycling the Saxon army's disabled soldiers. The AAZ was an office designed specifically for regulating the recruitment of recovering soldiers. As such it encompassed three departments: an Industry Office, an Office for Lazarette Work, and an Office for Outpatient Inspections. All three offices were housed together and entrusted with monitoring and organising the distribution of wounded soldier's labour, and fell under the joint jurisdiction of the XII. Army's Medical Corps and the Kriegsamtstelle.[83]

The Industry Office, as its name suggests, was in charge of regulating the placement of injured soldiers in industrial work. This office handled the transfer and assignment of both those recovering soldiers already capable of work and those still undergoing treatment. Those soldiers still undergoing occasional treatment were to be sent to the above-mentioned Industry Lazarette which was subsequently placed under the watchful eye of the AAZ. Those soldiers already recovered were eventually commandeered to various industrial or commercial works according to their capabilities. Here, although their civilian employers managed their work, the soldiers were still technically on active duty in the military and thus the AAZ continued to monitor and evaluate their work progress, as well.[84]

The Office for Lazarette Work coordinated all employment within the various military hospitals of the XII. Army Corps. This office was responsible for ensuring that every home front hospital for soldiers (*Reservlazarett, Vereinslazarett, and Industrielazarett*) had sufficient facilities for employing those soldiers not yet fit enough to leave the hospital for work. That is, they were to make sure that enough craft shops and workrooms were available so that every recuperating soldier could engage in 'useful and profitable employment' – even if he could not leave the lazarette.[85] In this way, the AAZ ensured that a soldier's continuing treatment did not get in the way of employment, or provide an excuse for avoiding it.

In addition to facilitating the return to work of disabled soldiers by ensuring that they had the appropriate equipment, the Office for Lazarette Work was also responsible for managing all business and financial aspects of the hospitals. The AAZ was well aware that convalescents could not engage in truly 'productive work' without adequate resources and materials. Therefore in addition to negotiating the work and supply contracts for each lazarette, this office also was placed in charge of 'the procurement of raw materials, setting appropriate prices, bookkeeping, etc'.[86] In order to make certain that the inmates of the lazarette had enough raw goods and equipment to keep busy, each reserve hospital was to submit monthly reports to the head office of the AAZ updating officials there on the camp's production output, labour resources, and changes in its material needs.[87]

The third and final department of the AAZ was the Outpatient Office [*Ambulantenstelle*]. The Outpatient Office was responsible for the strict monitoring – and, when necessary, strict disciplining – of the convalescing and outpatient soldiers. Regulating these outpatient workers included issuing them with identification cards, creating work rosters, and placing the recovered in the appropriate post. Because this also included sometimes placing the injured soldier in industrial work, the Outpatient Office worked at times in cooperation with the Office for Industrial Work.

The creation of the AAZ was a clear attempt to centralise and regiment the evaluation and assignment of soldiers to war-related industry while also keeping them under strict military supervision. What is interesting is that not only did the AAZ seek to distribute those healed soldiers in nearby industrial works, but also to harness the labour of the recovering soldier by turning the lazarettes into a sort of 'cottage industry' in and of themselves. Like pre-industrial workers in the German countryside, injured soldiers soon found themselves engaged in basketry, wood-carving, brush-making, and other 'homework' that could be done from the hospital bed. And while these occupations may not have directly benefited the war economy, they did contribute to the goals of: keeping the wounded occupied; re-training him for future employment; providing future farmers with back up; working in out-of-season occupations, and even contributing to a civilian consumer economy slowed down due to the focus on munitions production and war materiel. By 1917 military doctors and the Kriegsamtstelle in Dresden were creating a way to meet the material needs of the military while also still contributing to the civilian labour and consumer economy.

Moreover, keeping the management of labour and raw materials for each lazarette under the auspices of military control clearly would have two distinct advantages. On the one hand military officials would have a more direct line of communication to the War Raw Materials Office (KRA) than their civilian counterparts, ensuring perhaps easier procurement of the raw goods necessary for hospital production. On the other, by using the labour of wounded and disabled soldiers who had not yet been discharged, military officials could bypass the labour problems and manpower shortages plaguing German industry by 1917. The AAZ did not have to negotiate with trade union officials or labour representatives in order to man its workshops; as soldiers, these recycled workers were still operating under military command.

The Saxon army's response to Berlin's commands did not stop with the creation of the AAZ, however. Two weeks later, von Broizem ordered the construction of a military School Lazarette [*Schul-lazarett*] in Dresden. Whereas the Industry Lazarette had been constructed as a way to make use of labour power *already* reclaimed through the new rehabilitative medicine and technology, the School Lazarette was erected precisely for the purposes of reclaiming the lost bodily capacity of the severely injured soldier and bolstering his 'will to work'. As part of the military's emerging interest in treating the wounded soldier, the School Lazarette was to provide routine orthopaedic follow-up care, physical therapy, and exercise drills – even 'mental intervention' – to those injured soldiers who needed such 're-education' [*Umschulung*] in order to be returned to work in industry, commercial trades, or farming.[88]

Additionally the construction of the Saxon army's new training lazarette did not seek to work alongside – or even in tandem with – those civilian rehabilitation programmes being run by local voluntary organisations. It was, in fact, designed to replace them. Indeed, the Saxon army's School Lazarette not only superseded the Central Workshop for War Wounded originally erected by local voluntary organisations in Dresden as part of the city's municipal Berufsberatung programme; it eventually took it over. General von Broizem's directive to construct the new military vocational training workshop included with it the repeal of all former legislation and decrees involving the Central Workshop. In addition to taking over the locally organised Berufsberatung School and incorporating its structures and equipment into the military's School Lazarette, von Broizem appointed a new leader to the renovated institution: General Professor Dr Theodor Kölliker. Both an army general and professor of orthopaedics, Kölliker had been assigned to an Army Corps in Bavaria where he had been the corps' expert medical advisor until he was transferred.[89] Now, according to von Broizem, Kölliker was being brought to Dresden to head up the transformation of Reserve Lazarette VII into an orthopaedic training school. In addition to re-designing the reserve hospital into an expert orthopaedic clinic which would be able to offer orthopaedic treatment, massage, physical therapy, hydro-therapeutic baths, and sport training, it was above all, being renovated to include special orthopaedic workshops for vocational and agricultural retraining.[90] With the creation of the XII. Army Corps' School Lazarette, the Saxon army was no longer simply managing the labour power of the disabled soldier; it had taken over the task of restoring it.

This re-orientation of the Saxon army's attitude toward the disabled soldier was in fact reflective of an important policy shift in the German military. Rather than being classified as useless or 'unfit for duty' [*kriegsunverwendbar – kr.u.*], disabled soldiers were now being considered re-usable – even re-deployable – by military leaders. The military had been impressed with the widespread success of civilian programmes of rehabilitation and obviously now sought to institute their own system of recycling the disabled. However, unlike civilian programmes that sought to return to the men to their pre-war vocations and social status, the military programmes for 'reclaiming' the work potential of the wounded soldier were interested in returning him to the war effort. Instead of being concerned with managing the post-war future of the disabled ex-serviceman, the German military rather concentrated on ways to immediately benefit from the recycled disabled soldier.

In Saxony the military administration ultimately became so concerned with maximising the recovered labour of the disabled soldier that it created special military units to increase the efficiency of their deployment. In 1917 the Saxon army began erecting *Wirtschafts-Battaillonen* (WB), so-called 'economic battalions' of disabled soldiers kept at the ready who could then be quickly mobilised to meet the specific needs of a particular war industry when necessary. According to the directive ordering the construction of these economic battalions, military officials had determined that 'the recruitment of convalescing soldiers and the construction of Industry Lazarettes has not only resulted in the bodily strengthening of the sick, but has also spoken volumes for the needs of the war economy'.[91] Indeed, by now the army had realised that the physical exercise and work regimens mandated by the new *Arbeitstherapie* as perfected by orthopaedists could also benefit the war effort directly. Not only would rehabilitating wounded soldiers into 'substitute-workers' [*Austauschkräfte*] increase the numbers of available men for the labour or military drafts, but individual programmes of rehabilitation could also be structured such that the work-therapy itself contributed to war munitions production. In fact, while military officials emphasised the importance of contributing to the wounded soldier's recovery, it is clear that their primary interest was not the disabled's welfare, but rather his potential availability to contribute to the war. A closer examination of the discussion surrounding Wirtschafts-Battaillonen reveals that they were clearly constructed with the goal of reconciling the manpower needs of both army and industry.

Creating economic battalions of skilled and unskilled workers to be deployed in factories not only provided war industries with much needed labour power, but also made it possible for these firms to release those fit men for whom they had previously obtained service exemptions. By healing and then returning wounded soldiers to the home front and into war industry, the German military could continue to draft men for the war effort without compromising munitions production. As the order explained it,

> The home front is currently being dominated by a shortage of labour – not just skilled workers, but also the unskilled. Moreover, not only can one no longer rely on the release of workers from the troops, but rather now one must contend with the withdrawal of substantial numbers of persons from firms in order that the replacement needs of the field army can be met – without any decline in the production of crucial war materials and equipment.[92]

As this excerpt from the WB order makes clear, the careful and efficient management of labour and military manpower was becoming crucial for meeting the needs of the German army.

Moreover, the Saxon army was becoming increasingly aware of the inefficient distribution and utilisation of 'soldier-power'. The same directive noted that due to the lack of widespread awareness of the dire labour situation, soldiers who were temporarily or even permanently unfit for duty were either 'lying idle' or not being used in the most important posts. In order to remedy this situation, the army had concluded that the expansion of the Industry Lazarette to include creating battalions of these injured men was necessary. Keeping them at the ready would allow for the quick evaluation of their work capability while also allowing for their easy deployment to various industries as necessary. *Wirtschafts-Bataillonen*, then, were meant to be independent military formations placed under the authority of the general army commander. In order to ensure that the labour of the disabled would be used in the most judicious and effective manner possible, a member of the Kriegsamtstelle as well as a battalion doctor was to be assigned to each WB. This way the men could be organised and distributed in direct response to military-industrial needs.[93] The creation of economic battalions, therefore, was a military solution specifically concerned with alleviating the labour shortage in war-time industry, *not* healing the wounded or carrying out battle strategy.

Conclusion

This chapter has examined how social reformers, industrial firms, and military circles harnessed medical programmes to heal and re-use the disabled soldier. In tracing the ways in which the labour of the rehabilitated soldier was manipulated by military and industrial sectors of the economy, I have demonstrated how the medical goal of making the disabled *wiederverwendbar*, that is, 'recyclable' was also related to the crisis in manpower and the greater war-time effort to exploit all the resources of the German Empire. As labour became scarce, industrial circles looked to the disabled, and developed guidelines for maximising their labour. The programmes and experiments developed at the Siemens-Schuckert Works are particularly illustrative of industry's recycling of the maimed.

Moreover, the evolving policy of the Kriegsamt reveals an increasing military interest in the disabled soldier. Initially discharged and shuffled into civilian care programmes, by the second half of the war, the German army was more interested in recycling the permanently wounded for its own ends, rather than releasing him from service. Whether deployed to desk duty, provided to factory managers, or loaned to farmers, by 1917 the disabled were in fact being re-mobilised – that is, recycled – by the German military, as well.

Notes

1 Friedrich Syrup, *Die Fürsorge für kriegsverletzte gewerbliche Arbeiter* (Schriften des Deutschen Werkmeister-Verbandes, 29) (Düsseldorf: Verlag der Werkmeister-Buchhandlung, 1916), 3. Copy in SHAD LVA 111.

2 BArch R1501/113089. Letter from von Stein to all Deputy War Generals, all Deputy War Economic Offices, the Navy, Ministry of the Interior, Ministry for Trade, and all Occupation Armies. September 6, 1918.

3 Syrup, *Die Fürsorge für kriegsverletzte gewerbliche Arbeiter*, 13.

4 There are plenty of battle and military histories of the First World War, but in the interests of space, I will refer to just a few. For more on the development of Falkenhayn's strategy, the development of a war of attrition, and the importance of Verdun as a turning point in the war, see Herwig, *The First World War*, 179–99. For more on the Battle of the Somme and the ensuing *Materialschlacht*, see Chickering, *Imperial Germany and the Great War*, 70; and Herwig, *The First World War*, 199–204.

5 Chickering, *Imperial Germany*, 79–80.

6 Chickering, *Imperial Germany*, 76.

7 Also known as the National Service Law. For more on the Auxiliary Service Law, see Chickering, *Imperial Germany*, 80–1. See also Feldman', *Army, Industry and Labor*, which exhaustively examines the evolution, implementation, and eventual failure of this law. As Feldman points out, despite attempts to regulate an efficient distribution of manpower and materials during the war, army officials, employers, and labour unions struggled against one another for most of the war, resulting in an inefficient – even wasteful – programme of resource management.

8 SHAD MdI 7417, fos. 35–44. See the letter from interior minister Vitzthum dated March 26, 1917 regarding the founding and purpose of the Landessiedlungsgesellschaft 'Sächsiches Heim'. See also the Constitution, Guidelines, and various other founding documents of the company, including the text of the 'Law for the Settlement of War Veterans'.

9 The *Kapitalabfindungsgesetz* was discussed in chapter 4.

10 SHAD MdI 7417, fol. 3. See the article 'Ansiedlung von Kriegsinvaliden durch die Siedlungsgesellschaft "Sachsenland"'.

11 BArch R3901/36098 (film). Advertisement for the 'Heimatdank-Siedlung Weinböhla'.

12 For more on the general policies and programmes developed during the war and designed for annexing territory to the east and re-settling it with Germans, see Vejas G. Liulevicius, *War Land on the Eastern Front: Culture, National Identity, and German Occupation in World War I* (Cambridge: Cambridge University Press, 2000).

13 SHAD AA 2377. See the article 'Verein "Ansiedlungshilfe für deutsche Krieger"' *Der Osten* (June 4, 1916), No. 22, 288.

14 See 'Verein " Ansiedlungshilfe für deutsche Krieger"', 287. Although the expan-

sionist policies of the members of the Settlement Help Society were clearly nationalist and aggressive in nature, they do not appear to have contained the same sort of racial agenda that later Nazi policies contained. They do however seem to presage the expansionist aims of the Third Reich. For more on Germany's goals of territorial expansion during WWI, see Fritz Fischer's classic (and controversy-stirring) study, Fritz Fischer, *Germany's War Aims in the First World War* (New York: W.W. Norton, 1967), especially pp. 429–43.

15 The Pan-Germanists and the Vaterlandspartei both actively supported annexation, too. See Diehl, 'The Organization of German Veterans, 1917–1919', 165–6. See also Liulevicius, *War Land on the Eastern Front.*

16 SHAD WM 1751. Kruschwitz, [no first name], 'Ländliche Siedlungspolitik in Sachsen' Speech held on January 28, 1916 by Regierungsbaumeister and Geschäftsführer der Zentralstelle für Wohnungsfürsorge in Saxony.

17 Kruschwitz, 'Ländliche Siedlungspolitik in Sachsen', 1–2.

18 BArch R86/2310. P. Wölbling, 'Der Stand der Kriegsbeschädigtenansiedlung,' excerpted article from undated edition of *Concordia: Zeitschrift der Zentralstelle für Volkswirtschaft* (1918), 222–4.

19 SHAD LVA 111. Syrup, *Die Fürsorge für kriegsverletzte gewerbliche Arbeiter,* 3.

20 Syrup, *Die Fürsorge für kriegsverletzte gewerbliche Arbeiter,* 9.

21 Syrup, *Die Fürsorge für kriegsverletzte gewerbliche Arbeiter,* 9–10.

22 Syrup, *Die Fürsorge für kriegsverletzte gewerbliche Arbeiter,* 10–12.

23 Syrup, *Die Fürsorge für kriegsverletzte gewerbliche Arbeiter,* 13.

24 Friedrich Heinrich Karl Syrup (1881–1945) is an interesting figure who deserves further study. After the war in the Weimar Republic, he served as president of the National Employment Bureau [Reichanstalt für Arbeitsvermittlung] from 1927 to 1939. He later served as Labour Minister during Kurt von Schleicher's brief chancellorship from December 1932 until Hitler was appointed chancellor. Under the Nazi regime, Syrup was a State Secretary in the Labour Ministry (Staatssekretär im Reichsarbeitsministerium) from 1938 to 1942. And although I have no direct evidence, it seems likely that Syrup's experience with factory and labour management during the First World War must have contributed to his later career.

25 Syrup, *Die Fürsorge für kriegsverletzte gewerbliche Arbeiter,* 13.

26 Syrup, *Die Fürsorge für kriegsverletzte gewerbliche Arbeiter,* 13–14. Whalen also notes the tensions between trade unions and employers regarding the use of disabled labour. See Whalen, *Bitter Wounds,* 100–1.

27 Felix Krais, *Die Verwendungsmöglichkeiten der Kriegsbeschädigten in der Industrie, in Gewerbe, Handel, Handwerk, Landwirtschaft, und Staatsbetrieben* (Stuttgart: Krais Verlag, 1916). Krais noted on the title page that his work was produced in 'cooperation with the medical authorities'.

28 Siemens Archive (Munich). LM 330. Paul H. Perls, 'Kriegsblindenbeschäftigung im Kleinbauwerk der Siemens-Schuckert-Werke: Beschäftigung, Schutzmaßnahmen, Entlohnung' (Berlin, Siemens-Schuckert-Werke: 1921), 2.

29 Wilfried Feldenkirchen, *Siemens: Von der Werkstatt zum Weltunternehmen* (Munich: Piper, 1997), 107–8.

30 For more on this see Feldman, *Army, Industry and Labor,* 469. For a discussion of how the industrial giant Krupp also benefited from the war, see William Manchester, *The Arms of Krupp: The Rise and Fall of the Industrial Dynasty that Armed Germany at War* (Back Bay Books, 2003).

31 Feldenkirchen, *Siemens,* 108–9.

32 For more on the war-time struggle between military leaders and industrial representatives, see Feldman, *Army, Industry and Labor,* especially pp. 301–48.

33 SHAD KA (P) 18189. Paul H. Perls, 'Kriegsblindenbeschäftigung in der Werkstatt: Arbeitsmöglichkeiten bei der Massenherstellung elektrischer Installationsmaterialien'. Sonderausdruck aus *Werkstattstechnik* 2 (1917).

34 Perls, 'Kriegsblindenbeschäftigung in der Werkstatt', 1.

35 Perls, 'Kriegsblindenbeschäftigung in der Werkstatt', 1–4.

36 Perls, 'Kriegsblindenbeschäftigung in der Werkstatt', 3.

37 Perls, 'Kriegsblindenbeschäftigung in der Werkstatt', 4.

38 Perls, 'Kriegsblindenbeschäftigung in der Werkstatt', 4.

39 Perls, 'Kriegsblindenbeschäftigung in der Werkstatt', 5.

40 Perls, 'Kriegsblindenbeschäftigung in der Werkstatt', 5.

41 Perls, 'Kriegsblindenbeschäftigung in der Werkstatt', 5.

42 Paul H. Perls, 'Wiederertüchtigung schwerbeschädigter Kriegsteilnehmer in der Werkstatt'. Reprint from the *Elektrotechnische Zeitschrift* 16 (1917). A copy can be found in SHAD KA (P) 18189.

43 Perls, 'Wiederertüchtigung schwerbeschädigter Kriegsteilnehmer'.

44 Perls, 'Wiederertüchtigung schwerbeschädigter Kriegsteilnehmer', 1.

45 Perls, 'Wiederertüchtigung schwerbeschädigter Kriegsteilnehmer', 4.

46 See the cases of the metalsmith R, the construction worker F, the carpenter K, and the factory worker. K. Perls, 'Wiederertüchtigung schwerbeschädigter Kriegsteilnehmer', 4–6.

47 Perls, 'Wiederertüchtigung schwerbeschädigter Kriegsteilnehmer', 6.

48 In the article, Perls describes twelve cases; however, the sixth case actually discusses two men. Perls, 'Wiederertüchtigung schwerbeschädigter Kriegsteilnehmer', 1–6.

49 Siemens Archive (Munich). LM 330. 'Die Kriegsbeschaedigtenarbeit im Kleinbauwerk der Siemens-Schuckert- Werke GmbH' [no publishing information], 113–57 The employment statistics are from p. 131.

50 Siemens Archive (Munich). LM 330. 'Die Kriegsbeschaedigtenarbeit im Kleinbauwerk der Siemens-Schuckert- Werke GmbH'. The labour efficiency studies are found under 'Untersuchungen über die Arbeitsleistung kriegsinvalider Industriearbeiter an Hand der Stundenverdienst- und Stundenzahlleistung zahlreicher Kriegsbeschädigten aus dem Kleinbauwerk', 132–52.

51 Perls, 'Wiederertüchtigung schwerbeschädigter Kriegsteilnehmer', 6.

52 Perls, 'Wiederertüchtigung schwerbeschädigter Kriegsteilnehmer', 7

53 The Elektrotechnische Verein Berlins established guidelines for the re-use of

disabled veterans in 1916. See 'Leitsätze für die Wiederertüchtigung im Krieg schwerbeschädigter Industriearbeiter', *ETZ* (1916), 447.

54 Indeed there was widespread fear among disabled veterans that returning to work and earning a wage would reduce their pensions; Perls was not wholly correct when he argued that pensions would not be reduced upon employment. In 1914, the German armed forces were still using the disability pension system established in 1906/1907 under the Mannschaftsversorgungsgesetz. This system determined pension amounts according to the wounded soldier's rank, not his injury. So soldiers of differing ranks could be awarded vastly different pensions – regardless of whether they suffered from exactly the same injury. In this sense, the military's pension system was meant to reinforce its own internal social order, not dispense any restitution for an injured body. The National Pension Law [Reichsversorgungsgesetz, RVO] of 1920 changed things. Upon its passage, the pension that a disabled WWI soldier received became a combination of a variety of allowances dependent upon an individual soldier's circumstances. These could include a 'mutilation allowance' [*Verstümmelungszulage*], a 'war allowance' [*Kriegszulage*], and an 'age allowance' [*Alterszulage*]; once determined, these were fixed. However, the primary pension for disabled soldiers remained the 'injury pension' which was determined according to the degree of his physical debility. And, in keeping with the German welfare tradition, this was determined not by some standard definition of the 'worth' of a body part or injury, but rather according to the degree by which his ability to practise his craft, trade, or profession was hindered. That is, a soldier's pension amount was dictated by the degree to which his earning capacity was limited. Therefore, if a doctor determined that a disabled soldier – through rehabilitation, medicine, and prosthetic devices – could be 're-abled' and sent back to work, then it is easy to see how his 'disability pension' would be lowered accordingly. So while the supplementary allowances for rank, amputation, war-related injury, and age were stable, a disabled soldier's main pension was in fact open to negotiation and re-evaluation. For more on pensions see, Whalen, *Bitter Wounds*, 88–9, 131–9, 142–7; and Biesalski, 'Die ethische und wirtschaftliche Bedeutung der Kriegskrüppelfürsorge'.

55 Perls, 'Wiederertüchtigung schwerbeschädigter Kriegsteilnehmer', 8

56 Perls published other studies on his experiences with the war-disabled in the factory. These include Siemens Archive (Munich). LM 330 [Sammelhefte on Schwerbeschädigter]. Paul H. Perls, 'Kriegsblindenbeschäftigung im Kleinbauwerk der Siemens-Schuckert-Werke (Beschäftigung – Schutzmaßnahmen – Entlohnung)' (Siemens-Schuckert-Werke: 1921).

57 Perls noted the following firms AEG (Apparatefabrik II); Bergmann Elektricitätwerke AG, E. Zweitusch & Co., GmbH; Dr Paul Meyer AG; Deutsche Telefonwerke GmbH; H. Aron Elektrizitätszählerfabrik GmbH; Ehrich & Graetz. Perls, 'Kriegsblindenbeschäftigung', 2. Krais's volume also includes notes of firms and other concerns using disabled labour. Krais, *Die Verwendungsmöglichkeiten der Kriegsbeschädigten.*

58 SHAD KA (P) 18189. Letter from the Siemens-Schuckert-Werke to Kriegsamtstelle XII (Dresden) dated May 7, 1917, which included a Sonderdruck of 'Kriegsblindenbeschäftigung in der Werkstatt: Arbeitsmöglichkeiten bei der Massenherstellung elektrischer Installationsmaterialien'. *Werkstattstechnik*, Vol. 2, 1917.

59 Feldman's book includes a translated copy of the Auxiliary Service Law. See the appendix, 'The Auxiliary Service Law of December 5, 1916', in Feldman, *Army, Industry, and Labor*, 535–41.

60 Herwig, *The First World War*, 260.

61 Herwig, *The First World War*, 260.

62 Feldman, *Army, Industry, and Labor*, 163–4.

63 Feldman, *Army, Industry, and Labor*, 409–20.

64 The Kriegsamt issued guidelines and suggestions for recycling the disabled in the department's official newsletter. See for instance 'Vom Krankenbett zur Kriegsarbeit' *Kriegsamt: Amtliche Mitteilungen und Nachrichten* 4 (1917): 18; and 'Beschäftigung und Entlohnung kriegsbeschädigter sowie gv. und av. Facharbeiter und Handwerker', *Kriegsamt: Amtliche Mitteilungen und Nachrichten* 4 (1917): 8. Copies in BA-MA. PHD 6/205. Several military doctors also wrote war-time articles documenting their personal experience with creating and running orthopaedic workshops and curative stations in the military lazarettes as part of the army's revolutionised response to treating disabled soldiers. See for example Dr R. Burmeister (Marine-Stabsarzt), *Eine mediko-mechanische Abteilung von Leichtverwundeten kostenlos hergestellt* [Veröffentlichungen aus dem Gebiete des Militär-Sanitätswesens, 67] (Berlin: August Hirschwald, 1918) and Oberstabsarzt Dr W. Halberling, *Entwicklung der Kriegsbeschädigtenfürsorge von den ältesten Zeiten bis zur Gegenwart* (Veröffentlichungen aus dem Gebiete des Militär-Sanitätswesens, 73) (Berlin: August Hirschwald, 1918), 138–9. Copies of both found in BA-MA PHD 6. 163/11.

65 SHAD KA (P) 18189. Directive from the Kriegsamtstelle XII. Dresden to the Sanitätsamt XII. Dresden. June 30, 1917.

66 Cron, *Imperial German Army*, 293.

67 SHAD KA (P) 18189. Directive from the Kriegsamtstelle XII. Dresden to the Sanitätsamt XII. Dresden. June 30, 1917.

68 SHAD KA (P) 18189, fol. 14r. Directive from the Kriegsamtstelle XII. Dresden to the Sanitätsamt XII. Dresden. June 30, 1917.

69 SHAD KA (P) 18189, 14r–v. Directive from the Kriegsamtstelle XII. Dresden to the Sanitätsamt XII. Dresden. June 30, 1917.

70 SHAD KA (P) 18189, 14r–v. Directive from the Kriegsamtstelle XII. Dresden to the Sanitätsamt XII. Dresden. June 30, 1917.

71 BA-MA PHD 6/197. Schultzen [no first name], *Gesichtspunkte zur Frage der beschleunigten Herausziehung militärisch oder in der Kriegswirtschaft verwendbarer Mannschaften aus den Lazaretten und Truppenteilen* (Kriegsministerium: Berlin, 1916) No. 3422/7.16.M. A. Original archivist markings indicate that this pam-

phlet was initially archived at the Reservelazarett Meiningen suggesting that military hospitals throughout the empire received copies of it.

72 SHAD KA (P) 18189, fos. 107–8. Erlass des Kriegsministeriums (Kriegsamt) from February 2, 1917 (copy), 'Heranziehung genesender Mannschaften zur Kriegswirtschaft' No. 110/1.17. AZS 6.

73 For more on the decline in agricultural production, scarcity of food, the British 'hunger blockade' and the 'turnip winter' of 1916/17 see Herwig, *The First World War*, 283–93.

74 SHAD KA (P) 18189, fol. 117. Order of the War Ministry (von Stein) to all deputy generals (Königliche Stellvertretende Generalkommandos) dated March 21, 1917. No. 5603/3. 17.

75 SHAD KA (P) 18189, fos. 114–15. Order of the Kriegsamt (v. Kühlwetter) to all deputy generals (including the War Economics Office, Office of the Interior and other offices) dated July 20, 1917. No. 130/7. 17. AZS 6.

76 SHAD KA (P) 18189, unnumbered. Order of the War Ministry dated June 29, 1918. No. 1504/6.18 C 1 b.

77 SHAD KA (P) 18189, unnumbered. Order of the War Ministry dated July 13, 1918. No. 1926/6.18 C 1 b.

78 SHAD AAA 2379, fos. 4–6. Carbon copy of a letter from Vitzthum to the Kriegsministerium July 24, 1915.

79 SHAD KA (P) 18189, fol. 20. 'Heranziehung genesender Lazarettkranker zur Arbeit' K.V.Bl. 1917, No. 2095 V v. 7.7.17 (Abschrift). Von Broizem also issued orders to construct a second 'Industrielazarett' for the XII. Army Corps in Zittau (in southeast Saxony), once construction on the Dresden one was complete.

80 SHAD KA(P) 18189, fol. 20. 'Heranziehung genesender Lazarettkranker zur Arbeit' K.V.Bl. 1917, No. 2095 V v. 7.7.17. (Abschrift).

81 SHAD KA (P) 18189, fos. 60–3. 'Berufsberatung' 'Während des Krieges muss diese Berufsfürsorge (Vermittlung von Arbeitsstellen) neben den persönlichen Interessen der Kriegsbeschädigten in weitem Umfang den Bedürfnissen der *Kriegswirtschaft* Rechnung tragen [emphasis in original]'. The quote is on fol. 60.

82 SHAD KA (P) 18189, fos. 20r–v. 'Heranziehung genesender Lazarettkranker zur Arbeit' (Abschrift) K.V.Bl. 1917, No. 2095 V v. 7.7.17.

83 SHAD KA (P) 18189, fol. 19r. 'Arbeits- und Ambulantenzentrale Dresden' (Abschrift) No. 2095 V.v.12.7.17.

84 'Arbeits- und Ambulantenzentrale Dresden', fol. 19r.

85 'Arbeits- und Ambulantenzentrale Dresden', fol. 19r.

86 'Arbeits- und Ambulantenzentrale Dresden', fol. 19r.

87 'Arbeits- und Ambulantenzentrale Dresden', fol. 19v.

88 SHAD KA (P) 18189, fol. 21r. 'Kriegsbeschädigtenfürsorge' (Abschrift) No. 2266 V v. 31.7.17.

89 SHAD KA (P) 18189, fol. 21r. 'Kriegsbeschädigtenfürsorge' (Abschrift) No. 2266 V v. 31.7.17.

90 SHAD KA (P) 18189, fos. 21r–v. 'Kriegsbeschädigtenfürsorge' (Abschrift) No. 2266 V v. 31.7.17.

91 SHAD KA (P) 18188. 'Begründung der Errichtung von Wirtschafts-Bataillonen (WB)'.

92 SHAD KA (P) 18188. 'Begründung der Errichtung von Wirtschafts-Bataillonen (WB)'.

93 SHAD KA (P) 18188. 'Begründung der Errichtung von Wirtschafts-Bataillonen (WB)'.

Conclusion

MOBILISATION, MILITARISATION, AND MEDICALISATION IN WWI GERMANY

> The war and its effects, as well as the new Prussian disabled law, have so fundamentally changed the foundations of disabled welfare that a new edition of this handbook was unavoidable (*Handbook of Disability Welfare*, 2nd ed., 1922).[1]

Imperial Germany lost the Great War. In the midst of revolution, her people starving, her armies retreating, and her resources exhausted, the German Empire collapsed. After Kaiser Wilhelm II abdicated, the government of the newly formed Weimar Republic signed an armistice with the Entente Powers on November 11, 1918. This might prompt some scholars to conclude, then, that the recycling of disabled soldiers in war-time Germany was ineffective.

But this study was never intended to be a history of how Germany lost (or might have won) the war. Rather, this book has concentrated on revealing the unique medical processes which were set in motion in Germany as a direct result of the First World War. The specialisation of orthopaedics, the revolution in artificial limb design, the creation of modern rehabilitation, and the re-conceptualisation of the disabled body were all phenomena which – in Germany – were inextricably tied to the impact and experience of war. Furthermore, regardless of the war's outcome, these processes were themselves successful in that they carried over into post-war Germany and became factors in the organisation of society in the new Weimar Republic.

Take for instance the case of German orthopaedists. Though imbued with a patriotic commitment to healing the disabled soldier, orthopaedists also saw in this project the opportunity to demonstrate the importance of their medical specialty. In taking on their war-time mission to restore the physical health and bodily integrity of the wounded warrior, they seized the chance to show how their expertise could not just rescue the long-term future of the severely injured veteran, but also mitigate the economic and social consequences of the war. As they revolutionised artificial limbs, modernised therapeutic regimens, and created the institutional structures of modern rehabilitation in Germany, they were simultaneously demonstrating their central significance to the long-term health of the nation. Furthermore, over the course of the war, they were able to position themselves as authorities in rehabilitation-related fields, such as prostheses design and disability welfare, which previously had been dominated by other experts (in this case engineers and social workers). Most importantly, however, not only did they carve out this new area of orthopaedic expertise in medical and social fields, they also became indispensable to industrial and army officials *during* the war. And for this, orthopaedists were rewarded, receiving precisely those markers of specialisation which had eluded them before 1914.

A quick look at the immediate post-war period illustrates the success of specialisation nicely. In 1922 Fritz Lange updated the *Handbook of Orthopaedics*, and, though by today's standards six years might seem a long time in between revisions of a medical text, Lange felt compelled to explain to his readers why he was publishing a second edition so closely on the heels of the first. The recent war, he informed them, had so fundamentally influenced orthopaedics that it was now crucial to ensure that this dearly acquired knowledge not be lost. As Lange pointed out,

> everyone who experienced the same profound helplessness upon realising that our peacetime preparations were wholly insufficient to meet the demands of this war feels now compelled to demand that these war-time advances not be lost, but rather be preserved for future generations of doctors – and not just in case of future conflicts, but also in the interests of those casualties of peace: accident victims.[2]

Indeed, a comparison of the two editions also supports the claim that the specialty had developed significantly during the war. In the revised text one finds new chapters on artificial limbs, war orthopaedics, and disability care – topics which could be found nowhere in the 1914 edition of the manual, and whose inclusion underscores both their recent development and shifting centrality to the field.[3] Moreover, the publication of other orthopaedic manuals on the heels of war also attests to the expansion of the field due to war-time developments and discoveries.[4]

Just as importantly, however, the war impacted the institutional and professional development of orthopaedics. Lange informed his readers that across the nation there now existed no less than sixty-four orthopaedic institutes in Germany – ten more than in 1914 – and they were not only engaged in healing the disabled, but also continuing the clinical research that had begun in the war. He also advocated creating more university polyclinics and out-patient facilities in order to achieve these goals while also reaching more patients.[5] Indeed, clearly others agreed with this sentiment because between 1914 and 1927, German universities founded three more orthopaedic clinics and five additional professorships, with more appearing in the following years. Moreover, in 1924 orthopaedics became a required subject (*Pflichtfach*) in German medical schools – decades before it did in Britain.[6] Thus whereas Roger Cooter discounts the impact of the war years on orthopaedic specialisation in Great Britain, for orthopaedists in Germany, the First World War was of central significance to specialisation.[7] By first re-orienting their disciplinary focus to include injured soldiers, and then expanding their medical practices to include rehabilitation therapies and disabled welfare, orthopaedists established a specialised professional niche for themselves which could not only further the interests of a nation plunged into 'total war', but also deal with its aftermath a decade later. Only in proving their usefulness to the modern, belligerent state were Germany's orthopaedists able to attain what had eluded them in peacetime – specialisation.[8]

Orthopaedic specialisation was not the only successful medical process in Germany which can be linked directly to the First World War. The 'cultural invention of disability' is another important war-related transformation in German society. Before the war, the disabled were a largely marginalised population with varying degrees of access to medical care or social welfare. To be sure, the empire-wide social insurance system established in the 1880s had guaranteed all injured or invalided citizens the financial support of a pension, but this was a sum determined largely not by injury, but rather by socio-economic status. That is, members of the working and middle classes received different compensation amounts – even if they had suffered the same bodily injury. The disabled working poor in Germany generally still relied on voluntary aid from charity groups or, worse, they were institutionalised and thus doubly 'hidden' from society. Moreover, before the war there was no standardised system of medical treatment or therapeutic rehabilitation available to most Germans. Those elements which were available – hand-crafted artificial limbs or the care of a private physician – were extremely expensive and thus remained accessible largely only to the wealthier, upper-class patients. As this study has revealed, modern physical rehabilitation in Germany was essentially invented during the First World War specifically for treating the disabled soldier – a man whose bodily sacrifice was considered so great that he deserved something *better* than what had been previously available. Thus the war itself created the conditions necessary in the German Empire for inspiring this medical re-invention of the so-called 'crippled' body

– a large population of 'deserving' injured coupled with colossal financial drain.

But the story does not end there. In 1920 the Prussian government passed the *Law for the Severely Disabled*. This law extended the medical and rehabilitative services created for disabled veterans to *all* citizens. Moreover in drafting this legislation, the authors pointed specifically to the rapid developments in 'cripple care' made during the war when justifying the expansion of these treatments to the entire population.[9] At the same time, in defining this new disability care and outlining its parameters, the law also clearly stated that only those doctors thoroughly trained *in orthopaedics* were deemed qualified to treat or evaluate the disabled patient. Thus what had been initially developed specifically for soldiers trickled down to the civilian population, effectively granting thousands of other Germans access to modern rehabilitation – something they did not have before the war. Furthermore the law simultaneously acknowledged this field as the medical domain of orthopaedists.[10]

In 1922, the same year that Lange updated his textbook, Konrad Biesalski published a volume carefully outlining the goals and objectives of the new disability care. The updated *Guidelines for Disability Care* [*Leitfaden der Krüppelfürsorge*] gathered together the various developments and medical innovations from the war while also outlining how to use them for improving the care and welfare of *all* Germany's disabled persons – 'war cripples' and 'peace cripples' alike. To paraphrase Biesalski, the impact of the war on medical practice, the experiences gained from treating disabled soldiers, and above all the recent passage of the new disability law had culminated in a veritable revolution in 'cripple welfare' in Germany.[11] By positioning themselves as leaders in the transformation and administration of the new disability care, Germany's orthopaedists had in effect *medicalised* what had until 1914 been understood by most Germans as a component of poor relief. By re-casting physical impairment as a medical condition which could be ameliorated, improved, perhaps even 'cured' – the nation's orthopaedists had convinced both legislative and political circles not just to create an organised system of medical welfare for Germany's disabled, but also to place them in charge of it.[12] That is, over the course of the war, orthopaedists had simultaneously medicalised both the system of rehabilitation as well as the disabled body itself; they had fostered a society-wide re-conceptualisation of what had been previously considered the permanently 'crippled' body into one that modern medicine could heal.[13] And consequently German attitudes regarding the disabled shifted, as well.[14]

In addition to the medical benefits that disabled Germans gained, however, perhaps more importantly they also – to borrow a phrase – 'became visible'.[15] The war had generated scores of public lectures, exhibitions, popular publications, and consumer items all geared toward improving the life of the disabled soldier. Whether through facilitating his return to work via new prosthetic aids or increasing his acceptance in society by re-educating his able-bodied compatriots, the result of all this work was that – veterans or not – disabled Germans became more visible as consumers, as workers, and as members of the public sphere. Thus this medicalisation of disability and its simultaneous healing helped permanently injured Germans reclaim their place in civil society.

During the war, city, state, and eventually the federal governments began formulating policy in order to regulate public interactions with disabled soldiers and standardise civic treatment of these newly reclaimed citizens. For instance, signs were posted in public spaces urging fellow citizens to 'make allowances for the war-invalid' by allowing him to go to the head of long queues or giving up their seats in trams. In Berlin and Aachen, special train compartments were reserved especially for the war-disabled, thus ensuring they had easy access to transportation to and from work.[16] In 1918 officials began proposing the introduction of hiring quotas [*Einstellungszwang*], which would regulate the employment of the disabled by federal mandate – a law eventually passed in the newly formed Weimar Republic. The recycling of disabled bodies had therefore important, long-term repercussions for both orthopaedists and their patients.[17]

Still, beyond the unique story of how the First World War impacted post-war German medicine and society, this book has also shed new light on the significance of modern medicine to the waging of war in modern Germany. Whereas previous historians have concentrated upon the impact of war on developments in modern medicine, this study highlights rather the impact of medical developments on the organisation of German army and society for war. That is, it has shown how orthopaedists and their rehabilitation programmes became central to two other important war-time processes in Imperial Germany – the *militarisation of the body* and the *medicalisation of war*.

For years, historians of medicine have contended that one of the unintended consequences of war is medical innovation. This conventional thesis suggested that due to the massive physical destruction and human cost of war, medical practitioners were often forced to 'rise to the challenge' of bodily injury and disease brought on by organised conflict. Thus, the medical innovations forged by quick-thinking doctors or field nurses in times of great crisis were counted among the 'good' by-products or outcomes of war. This school of thought clearly echoes the ancient Hippocratic sentiment that 'war is the only proper school for the surgeon'.[18]

But recently medical historians, most notably Roger Cooter, have challenged this notion that war is good for medicine and that there is medical 'progress through bloodshed'.[19] Indeed, in his book on orthopaedics in Great Britain, Cooter holds that the Great War marked not innovation in the discipline so much as a rupture in their professional and organisational development.[20] Other historians have shown how the brutal conditions of war resulted rather in much greater instances of malnutrition, infectious disease, and infant mortality among civilian populations – especially in instances where the majority of available medical resources were diverted to the military.[21] This study has clearly demonstrated specific ways in which the war not only mobilised Germany's orthopaedists, but also inspired medical innovation within their ranks.

However, this study reveals how developments in German medicine became also constitutive elements of modern warfare.[22] The story I have traced here demonstrates how the re-orientation of German orthopaedists to create sturdy workers from 'crippled soldiers' was not simply the story of war-time advances in biomedical technology. Nor did it end with the buttressing of Imperial Germany's crumbling social order via class-based rehabilitation programmes and prosthetic devices – although, as I have demonstrated, each of these goals was certainly at play in medical and rehabilitation circles during the war. Rather, this book has revealed that the medical mission to 'recycle the disabled' eventually became an organising component of total war.

The medicalisation of war

The incorporation of orthopaedic knowledge and authority into the structures and practices of war-time mobilisation is clear evidence of the medicalisation of war taking place in Imperial Germany. The most dramatic examples of this phenomenon were the programmes instituted in German military and industrial circles to recycle the disabled soldier in the war effort. As the last chapter pointed out not only did Siemens, for instance, experiment with using disabled soldiers as munitions workers, but the German army, too, discovered the advantages that rehabilitation could offer a beleaguered army plagued by an increasingly desperate manpower shortage. Through harnessing the project of *Wiedereingliederung*, building their own system of rehabilitation workshops, and directing the disabled soldier into specific industries, the German army could essentially re-deploy the severely injured soldier from the trenches at the front, to surgery and hospital beds behind the lines, and eventually to work spaces in industry – ultimately freeing up able-bodied men working on the home front to replace those lost in battle. In consciously directing some recovering soldiers into agricultural production, military authorities attempted to mitigate the severe food shortage paralysing the nation after the winter of 1916–1917. And though the military and industrial programmes for recycling the disabled were ones created and administered by authorities in those sectors of society, Germany's orthopaedists were right by their side – offering advice and direction on how to accomplish these goals. Indeed these programmes would not have been possible without men like Fritz Lange or Konrad Biesalski. Thus as orthopaedists demonstrated their success in rehabilitating the disabled, the German army found ways to incorporate these innovations into their strategies for modern war – the management of manpower resources, the management of materiel production, the management of food resources, and the management of raw materials.

Moreover German military authorities were well aware of how fundamentally important these medical innnovations had become to the waging of modern war. This is illustrated nowhere more compellingly than in the repeated attempts by the German government to censor the dissemination of war-time medical discoveries to their enemies. By 1915 the War Ministry began trying to control the spread of any information regarding the health or medical treatment of Germany's soldiers as a matter of protecting national security.[23] However, in response to news that the British government was showing an increasing interest in German prosthetic designs and manufacturing, in 1917 the Supreme War Office issued an order specifically outlawing the distribution of any information pertaining to the recent innovations in artificial limbs.[24] Clearly by 1917 orthopaedic strategies to treat, heal, and recycle the disabled had become critical elements in modern Germany's organisation for and management of 'total war'.

Militarising the disabled

Indeed orthopaedists became rather powerful organising authorities during the war. They successfully parlayed their medical expertise not only into professional recognition, but also into directing nearly all aspects of the severely injured soldier's life. Through rehabilitation therapies and the re-integration programmes created alongside them, orthopaedists exercised significant control over his medical treatment, vocational training, professional placement, and geographical re-location. Once orthopaedists were assigned to military lazarettes and reserve hospitals, they could influence a soldier's duty status by determining his degree of 'usability' [*Verwendbarkeit*], that is, his bodily capacity for work.[25] In fact what the new orthopaedics eventually made possible was the creation of a perpetual relay of useful bodies, an assembly line system of bodily repair and redistribution, what we might consider the militarisation of the disabled within a larger war-time 'economy of the body'.

The militarisation of Germany in the First World War is a much studied subject. When the war radicalised in 1916, German military and civilian authorities implemented those more familiar policies of 'total war' – extension of compulsory military conscription for men, the civilian labour draft at the home front, the organisation and distribution of all available war materiel, the total mobilisation of all elements of German society for the organised production of violence. The emergent war-time 'economy of the body' was the systematic classification, ranking, and efficient re-distribution of the state's *human resources* in order to support the nation-at-war. Calculating an individual's usefulness to the nation – or the *Volksgemeinschaft*, as many Germans were already calling it – meant, therefore, evaluating each individual's potential for making a bodily contribution to the nation's war effort. Or, as Biesalski phrased it, it meant knowing his or her *körperliche Leistungsfähigkeit*.

Bodily capability could be measured in various ways and include multiple, even overlapping, capacities. It might mean being fit for military duty of some kind – as in one of the several *verwendungs* categories used by the German military (kv, gv, av). It might also mean producing war materiel by working in the munitions industries. It could also mean working in the nation's hinterlands, for instance in farming, animal husbandry, or the forest service – all employment sectors for which *Berufsberäter*, incidentally, found the disabled especially suitable. In fact, this sort of 'productive work' was exactly the kind of bodily capability that orthopaedists were trying to restore to the disabled soldier; and, clearly the physical re-building of male bodies became especially crucial to the military-industrial project of continuing the war.

Other historians have shown that this bodily capability was not defined strictly in terms of its combat value. Bodily utility might also be defined in terms of its potential for human reproduction. As Elisabeth Domansky has argued, in WWI Germany the belligerent state was also particularly interested in organising and controlling women's reproductive behaviour as a means of managing the nation's ravaged population during the war.[26] However, her study of the 'militarisation of reproduction' focused on the control and subjugation of German sexual behaviour – men's and women's reproductive 'service to the nation'.[27] In addition, Cornelie Usborne's study of pronatalist policies in WWI Germany has documented how state concerns about (male) military fighting power became linked with the control of women's sexuality and fertility. Nonetheless she, too, focuses on what we might call the 'reproductive body'.[28] Therefore, what is important to understanding my idea of an economy of the body is the way in which the material body itself was considered useful to the state.

Thus, in this war-time 'economy of the body', the body's value to the state was determined from a matrix of possibilities – and nearly every German could eventually be deemed useful or fit for the war effort in some way – however minor. Women could be employed in munitions factories, children could collect scrap metal, and retired workers might supervise and train the disabled in recovery homes. Furthermore, a person's bodily utility might increase or decrease over the course of the war – reflecting as it did changes in war-time needs. Skilled workers and child-bearing women increased in value as the war continued; and, once they could be healed and returned to the workforce, so, too, did disabled soldiers. In this sense bodies themselves came to be perceived as war materiel – a kind of raw resource to be deployed and used where needed. Whether cannon fodder, war industry workers, or recycled soldiers, the establishment of an economy of the body was part of the war-time state's attempt to organise and mobilise all its resources.

Furthermore, given the centrality of modern war to my argument, it is important to understand this system as a *militarised* economy of the body. Here I want to stress that I do not understand these militarised bodies to be the heroic, warrior image of man which has been typically included in such designations. That is, the militarised body to which I refer does not denote the sort of embodied soldierdom characterised in studies by George Mosse or Klaus Theweleit. The bodies of the disabled are not the 'fallen soldiers' erected across the nation in an effort to re-write the memory of a lost war.[29] Nor are these 'Red Badge of Courage'-bodies, male identities transformed through the somatic experience of battle.[30] Finally, neither are these proto-fascist bodies – forged in the bloody battles of the First World War and trying in a post-war home front to re-create their front experiences.[31] Rather, here I find most useful the concept of militarisation as Michael Geyer has defined it, that is, as 'the complex process of organizing civil society to produce violence.'[32] However, whereas Geyer focuses on the processes of militarising society – its social groups and cultural institutions – what has interested me in this study is the organisation of these material bodies themselves.

Therefore what this book has laboured to illustrate is how, through the intricate web of army, medicine, and society, the disabled body itself became regimented, rationalised, centralised – even industrialised – during the war in order to achieve the state's belligerent goals. By turning soldiers into war materiel with cheap, interchangeable parts, German orthopaedists fundamentally became part of the war machine itself, enlisted not simply as healers of violence, but rather as wagers, or producers, of war. Recycling the disabled, then, perhaps tells us as much about the 'goodness' of medicine for war, as it does about the history of rehabilitation in WWI Germany. Moreover, the pivotal role that German orthopaedists played in making the disabled soldier *wiederverwendbar* begs the question: In what other ways did German medicine support or enable the war effort? Perhaps it is now time to re-examine our understandings and definitions of 'total mobilisation' and consider more centrally the role of doctors and other medical professionals in the organisation of modern societies for 'total war'. It was, after all, the extreme conditions of the Great War that encouraged Germany's orthopaedists to re-orient their field in the first place.

Notes

1 Konrad Biesalski, *Leitfaden der Krüppelfürsorge* (Leipzig: Leopold Voß, 1922), 3.
2 Lange, *Lehrbuch* (1922), v.
3 Lange, *Lehrbuch* (1922), 543–92.
4 Hermann Gocht, *Die Orthopädie in der Kriegs- und Unfallheilkunde* (Stuttgart: Enke, 1921).
5 Lange, *Lehrbuch* (1922), 590–1.
6 Hans-Heinz Eulner, *Die Entwicklung der medizinischen Spezialfächer an den Universitäten des deutschen Sprachgebietes* (Stuttgart: Ferdinand Enke, 1970), 394–5. Full professorships were created in Heidelberg (1919), Leipzig (1922), Freiburg (1924), Berlin (1927), and Würzburg (1929). Clinics were founded in Berlin (1915), Heidelberg (1919), and Würzburg (1916). Moreover, a professorship in Vienna was also established, thus suggesting that in Austria a similar development was also occurring. The majority of professorships and university clinics in Germany are founded after the Second World War which might lead some to see the period after 1945 as more significant to orthopaedics. However, one must also consider the rupture in German university expansion and development caused by the worldwide depression (1929) and the Nazi seizure of power (1933) as well as WWII. It is not surprising that in these times of extreme financial duress that university expansion would be hampered. For example Eulner notes the major expansion of university orthopaedics in the years 1945–1970, however, his is primarily an institutional history of medical specialties which does not locate these developments within any political, social or economic context. Eulner, *Die Entwicklung der medizinischen Spezialfächer*, 387–96.
7 Eulner, *Die Entwicklung der medizinischen Spezialfächer*, 394–5. For more on the integration of orthopaedics into the medical curriculum in Great Britain, see Cooter, *Surgery and Society*, 234–49.
8 Just as Elizabeth Lunbeck has argued that American psychiatry was able to achieve authority through the redefinition of their conceptual frameworks, so too, did German orthopaedists rise in both professional prestige and expand their medical purview by re-orienting their field. This re-orientation, however, was also fundamentally dependent upon the medicalisation of physical disability which occurred during the war, as well. For more on Lunbeck's argument see Elizabeth Lunbeck,

The Psychiatric Persuasion: Knowledge, Gender, and Power in Modern America (Princeton: Princeton University Press, 1994).

9 'Gesetz, betr. die öffentliche Krüppelfürsorge. Vom 6. Mai 1920' *Volkswohlfahrt: Amtsblatt und Halbmonatsschrift des Preussischen Ministeriums für Volkswohlfahrt.* Vol. 1, No. 9: 179.

10 'Gesetz, betr. die öffentliche Krüppelfürsorge. Vom 6. Mai 1920', 180.

11 Biesalski, *Leitfaden der Krüppelfürsorge,* 3. For another volume detailing the extension of the war-time innovations to civilian accident victims, see chapter 5 'Die orthopädische Übungsbehandlungen auf Grund der Erfahrungen des Krieges,' in Gocht, *Die Orthopädie in der Kriegs- und Unfallheilkunde.*

12 'Gesetz, betr. die öffentliche Krüppelfürsorge. Vom 6. Mai 1920', 179, 180.

13 This medicalisation of disability was discussed in chapter 4.

14 For another perspective on the emerging visibility of disabled persons in German culture, see Carol Poore, *Disability in Twentieth-Century German Culture* (Ann Arbor: University of Michigan Press, 2007).

15 This phrase is borrowed from the title of an early European women's history text. See Renate Bridenthal and Claudia Koonz, eds, *Becoming Visible: Women in European History* (Boston: Houghton Mifflin, 1977).

16 Prof. F. Schwalbe, 'Kriegsbeschädigtenfürsorge', *Europäische Staats und Wirtschaftszeitung,* (December 30, 1918), 138–44.

17 Although I argue that these developments in disability welfare ultimately benefited the civilian disabled, scholars such as Deborah Cohen, Christopher Jackson, and Robert Whalen have focused on how they alienated the war-disabled, who ultimately felt slighted by laws which forced them to 'work' for their pensions and subsumed them into the larger disabled community. For more on the social programmes developed in the Weimar Republic for the war-disabled, see Cohen, *The War Come Home.*

18 For more on the historiography of the place of war in the history of medicine and the centrality of this thesis, see Roger Cooter, 'War and Modern Medicine', in W.F. Bynum and R. Porter, eds, *Companion Encyclopedia of the History of Medicine* (1994), 1536–73, especially pp. 1541–6.

19 In addition to Cooter's historiographical piece 'War and Modern Medicine', see also his earlier piece, Roger Cooter, 'Medicine and the Goodness of War', *Canadian Bulletin of Medical History/Bulletin canadien d'histoire de la médecine,* Vol. 7, No. 2: 147–59.

20 Roger Cooter, *Surgery and Society in Peace and War: Orthopaedics and the Organization of Modern Medicine, 1880–1948* (London: Macmillan, 1993).

21 See Cooter, 'War and Modern Medicine', 1548–50.

22 Mark Harrison has recently suggested that the relationship between medicine and warfare should be examined more closely, as well, arguing that medicine has contributed to the 'rationalisation' of war. See Mark Harrison, 'Medicine and the Management of Modern Warfare', *History of Science* Vol. 34 (1996), 379–410.

23 BayHStA/Abt. IV, Stv GenKdo I, AKSanAm 459. Directives of Kriegsministerium July 9, 1915 and June 17, 1916.

24 BayHStA/Abt. IV, Stv GenKdo I, AKSanAm 459. Directive from the Kriegsamt Kriegsministerium May 12, 1917 to all Deputy Corps Headquarters and all Sanitation Offices.

25 Whalen also notes the important role played by doctors in the evaluation of a soldier's 'fitness for duty' and the overall important role of physicians in the lives of the war-disabled – especially with regard to determining the extent to which they were physically disabled, and thus the size of their pensions. See Whalen, *Bitter Wounds*, 59–67.

26 See Elisabeth Domansky, 'Militarization and Reproduction in World War I Germany', pp. 427–63 in Geoff Eley, ed., *Society, Culture, and the State in Germany 1870–1930* (Ann Arbor: University of Michigan Press, 1997).

27 Elisabeth Domansky has argued that the industrialisation of warfare necessitated the re-organisation of gendered relationships of production, reproduction, and destruction. The most significant of these re-organised relationships was the militarisation of reproduction and the reconstitution of patriarchy via the ascendancy of the 'male-soldier' who replaced the 'male-father' as supreme social authority. By controlling the private, reproductive behaviour of both German men and women, the state was able to simultaneously intervene into the familial (private) sphere, thus dissolving the European bourgeois family which had dominated nineteenth-century society. See Domansky, 'Militarization and Reproduction'.

28 See Cornelie Usborne, '"Pregnancy is the Woman's Active Service": Pronatalism in Germany during the First World War', pp. 389–416 in Richard Wall and Jay Winter, eds, *The Upheaval of War: Family, Work, and Welfare in Europe, 1914–1918* (New York: Cambridge University Press, 1988).

29 See George L. Mosse, *Fallen Soldiers: Reshaping the Memory of the World Wars* (New York: Oxford University Press, 1990); George L. Mosse, *The Image of Man: The Creation of Modern Masculinity* (New York: Oxford University Press, 1996); and George L. Mosse, *Nationalism and Sexuality: Respectability and Abnormal Sexuality in Modern Europe* (New York: H. Fertig, 1985).

30 Stephen Crane, *The Red Badge of Courage* (London: Everyman, 1993). I thank Roger Cooter for this reference.

31 For more on the fascist bodies and masculinity of Freikorps soldiers, see Klaus Theweleit, *Male Fantasies*(2 vols). Trans by Stephen Conway and Erica Carter (Minneapolis: University of Minnesota Press, 1985–1989).

32 Michael Geyer, 'The Militarization of Europe, 1914–1945', in John R. Gillis, ed., *The Militarization of the Western World* (New Brunswick, N.J.: Rutgers University Press, 1989).

Bibliography

Primary sources

Archival sources

Bundesarchiv Berlin-Lichterfelde (BArch)

R86 Reichsgesundheitsamt (National Health Office)
1272 Deutsche Vereinigung für Krüppelfürsorge
2310 Berufsberatung
2320

R1501 Reichsamt des Innen (Department of the Interior)
113045 Fürsorge für die Kriegsinvaliden, 1914–1919
113089 Die Kriegsbeschädigten
113089/6 Zentralstelle für Berufsberatung heimkehrender Kriegern und Internierten

R3901 Reichsarbeitsministerium (RAM, Labour Ministry)
8730 Orthop. Werkstätten und Versorgungsstellen im Allgemeinen, 1921–1922
8866 Vereine und Stiftungen für Kreigsbeschädigte und deren Hinterbliebenen, Juli 1916–
9334 Fürsorge für Verstummelte und Sieche
36098 (film)
36070 (film) Reichsausschuss der Kriegsbeschädigtenfürsorge (8866)

Bundesarchiv Militärarchiv Freiburg (BA-MA)

Preussisches Heer (Drucksachen) (PHD)
6/197
6/163/11
6/205 Kriegsministerium

Bundesarchiv Filmarchiv (Berlin)
Ansichten aus dem Lazarett Jakobsberg, orthopädisches Lazarett des XX.A.K., Allenstein O.pr. (1918)
Reserve-Lazarett Ettlingen i. Baden, Turnübungen der Amputierten (Gehschule) (1918)

Bayerisches Hauptstaatsarchiv (BayHSta) Abteilung IV: Kriegsarchiv
Stv GenKdo I. AK
San A 308
San A 413
San A 459

Sächsische Hauptstaatsarchiv Dresden (SHAD)

Amt der auswärtigen Angelegenheiten (Foreign Office) (AAA)
2376
2377
2389 Verschiedenes

Kriegsamtstelle Dresden (files from Potsdam) (KA (p))
18188 Errichtung von Wirtschaftsbattaillonen und die Kriegsbeschädigtenfürsorge
18189 Die Beschäftigung von Kriegsbeschädigte und die KBfürsorge

Landesversicherungsamt (National Insurance Office) (LVA)
111 Fürsorge für verkrüppelte Kriegsteilnehmer 1915

Ministerium des Innen (Ministry of the Interior) (MdI)
7417
17742 Aufgaben der Kriegswohlfahrtspflege, 1917–1919

Wirtschaftsministerium (Economics Ministry) (WM)
1751 Errichtung von Rentengütern bez. Heimstätten

Dresden Stadtarchiv

Schulamt III
813 Einarmigerschule, uberhaupt Unterricht an Kriegsverletzte, 1914–1919

Deutsche Hygiene-Museum Dresden (DHMD)
837 Jahresbericht 1912–1918

Siemens Archive (Munich)
LM 330 Sammelhelfte zur Schwerbeschädigten

Journals and newspapers
Concordia: Zeitschrift der Zentralstelle für Volkswirtschaft, 1914–1919
Deutsche Illustrirte Zeitung [*sic*]
Feldärztliche Beilage zur Münchener medizinische Wochenschrift, 1916–1917
Illustrirte Zeitung [*sic*], 1914–1917
Kriegsamt: Amtliche Mitteilungen und Nachrichten
Münchener medizinische Wochenschrift, 1915–1920
Der Osten, 1916–1917
Zeitschrift für orthopädische Chirurgie, 1916–1918
Zentralblatt für chirurgische und mechanische Orthopädie, 1916

Published primary sources

Aereboe, Friedrich. *Der Einfluss des Krieges auf die landwirtschaftliche Produktion* [Carnegie Endowment for International Peace. Division of Economics and History]. New Haven: Yale University Press, 1927.

'Bericht der ausserordentlichen Tagung der Deutschen Orthopädischen Gesellschaft', *Zeitschrift für orthopädische Chirurgie*. Vol. 37 (1916): 209–671.

Biesalski, Konrad. 'Die ethische und wirtschaftliche Bedeutung der Kriegskrüppelfürsorge und ihre Organisation im Zusammenhang mit der gesamten Kriegshilfe' [Vortrag im Rahmen der Ausstellung für Verwundeten- und Krankenfürsorge im Sitzungssaale des Reichstags gehalten am Januar 13. 1915]. Leipzig: Leopold Voss Verlag, 1915.

——. *Die Kunstglieder der Versuchs- und Lehrwerkstätte des Oskar-Helene-Heims*. Stuttgart: Ferdinand Enke, 1917.

——. *Kriegskrüppelfürsorge: Ein Aufklärungswort zum Troste und zur Mahnung*. Leipzig: Leopold Voss Verlag, 1915.

——. *Leitfaden der Krüppelfürsorge*. Leipzig: Leopold Voß, 1922.

——. 'Das neue Modell der aktiven Fischerhand und Arbeitsklaue', *Münchener medizinische Wochenschrift*. Vol. 65, No. 39 (1918): 1078–9.

——. 'Praktische Vorschläge für die Kriegskrüppelfürsorge', Sonderabdruck aus der *Zeitschrift für Krüppelfürsorge*. Leipzig: Leopold Voss Verlag, 1915.

——. 'Über Prothesen bei Amputationen des Armes insbesondere des Oberarmes'. *Münchener medizinische Wochenschrift*. Vol. 44 (1915): 1492–6.

——. *Umfang und Art des jugendlichen Krüppeltums und der Krüppelfürsorge in Deutschland*. Leipzig: Voss, 1909.

Böhm, Max. 'Ueber den Armersatz bei Landwirten', *Münchener medizinische Wochenschrift*, Vol. (1918): 65: 99–100.

Borchardt, M. et al., *Ersatzglieder und Arbeitshilfen für Kriegsbeschädigte und Unfallverletzte*. Berlin, Springer, 1919.

Burmeister, Dr R. (Marine-Stabsarzt), *Eine mediko-mechanische Abteilung von Leichtverwundeten kostenlos hergestellt* [Veröffentlichungen aus dem Gebiete des Militär-Sanitätswesens, 67]. Berlin: August Hirschwald, 1918.

Castendyck, M. 'Ein Vorschlag zur Verbesserung der künstlichen Hand'. *Zentralblatt für chirurgische und mechanische Orthopädie, Einschliesslich der gesamten Heilgymnastik und Massage*. Vol. 10 (1916): 137–9.

Dietrich, Eduard. 'Eröffnungsansprache zur konstituierenden Versammlung', *Zeitschrift für Krüppelfürsorge*. Vol. 2, No. 1 (1909/10): 7–8.

Devine, Edward T. *Disabled Soldiers and Sailors: Pensions and Training* [Preliminary Economic Studies of the War, 12]. New York: Oxford University Press, 1919.

du Bois-Reymond, R. 'Physiologie des Armes und des Beins', in M. Borchardt et al., eds, *Ersatzglieder und Arbeitshilfen für Kriegsbeschädigte und Unfallverletzte*. Berlin, Springer: 1919.

Ehrenfest-Egger, Arthur and Siegfried Neutra. 'Die Carnesarmprothese', *Zeitschrift für orthopädische Chirurgie*. Vol. 38 (1918): 695.

'Gesammelte Arbeiten ueber die Prothesenbau' Vol. 37, a special edition of *Zeitschrift für orthopädische Chirurgie*. Stuttgart: Ferdinand Enke, 1917.

Gocht, Hermann. *Die Orthopädie in der Kriegs- und Unfallheilkunde*. Stuttgart: Enke, 1921.

Gocht, Hermann, R. Radike, and F. Schede, eds. *Künstliche Glieder* [Deutsche Orthopädie 2], 2nd ed. Stuttgart: Ferdinand Enke, 1920.

Guradze, P. 'Über Amputationsstumpf und Prothesen', *Zeitschrift für orthopädische Chirurgie*. Vol. 37 (1917): 83–93.

Halberling, Oberstabsarzt Dr W., *Entwicklung der Kriegsbeschädigtenfürsorge von den ältesten Zeiten bis zur Gegenwart* (Veröffentlichungen aus dem Gebiete des Militär-Sanitätswesens, 73.) Berlin: August Hirschwald, 1918.

Hartmann, Konrad. 'Die Prüfstelle für Ersatzglieder', in M. Borchardt et al., eds, *Ersatzglieder und Arbeitshilfen für Kriegsbeschädigte und Unfallverletzte*. Berlin, Springer: 1919.

Hartwell, Edward M. 'Peter Henry Ling, the Swedish Gymnasiarch', *American Physical Education Review*. Vol 1, No.1 (1896): 1–13.

Heeres-Sanitätsinspektion des Reichskriegsministeriums, *Gliederung des Heeressanitätswesens im Weltkriege 1914/1918. Sanitätsbericht über das Deutsche Heer, Vol. I.* Mittler und Sohn: Berlin, 1935.

Heimatdank Ausstellung für Kriegsbeschädigten-Fürsorge [Exhibition Catalogue]. Leipzig, 1917.

Hoffa, Albert. *Lehrbuch der Fracturen und Luxationen für Aerzte und Studierende*. 2nd ed. Würzburg: Stahel, 1891.

——. *Lehrbuch der orthopädischen Chirurgie*. Stuttgart: Ferdinand Enke, 1905.

Hoffmann, W., et al. *Die deutschen Ärzte im Weltkriege; ihre Leistungen und Erfahrungen*. Berlin: E.S. Mittler und Sohn, 1920.

'Industrielle Kriegsbeschaedigten-Fuersorge', *Meissner Tageblatt* (192) August 19, 1916.

Janssen, Peter. 'Was muss der Lazarettarzt von der Prothese wissen?', *Feldärztliche Beilage zur Münchener medizinische Wochenschrift*. No. 12 (1917): 398–401.

Koehler, A. *Die Kriegschirurgie des Jahres 1917* [Veröffentlichungen aus dem Gebiete des Militär-Sanitätswesens, No. 76]. Berlin: August Hirschwald, 1921.

Krais, Felix, ed. *Die Verwendungsmöglichkeiten der Kriegsbeschädigten in der Industrie, in Gewerbe, Handel, Handwerk, Landwirtschaft, und Staatsbetrieben*. Stuttgart: Krais Verlag, 1916.

Lange, Fritz. 'Eine neue Kunst-und Arbeitshand'. *Feldärtzliche Beilage zur Münchener medizinische Wochenschrift*. No. 20 (1917): 661–4.

——. *Ein Leben für die Orthopädie: Erinnerungen von Fritz Lange*. Stuttgart: Ferdinand Enke, 1959.

Lange, Fritz, ed. *Lehrbuch der Orthopädie*. Jena: Gustav Fischer, 1914.

——. *Lehrbuch der Orthopädie*. 2nd ed. Jena: Gustav Fischer, 1922.

——. *Lehrbuch der Orthopädie*. 3rd ed. Jena: Gustav Fischer, 1928.

Lange, Fritz, and J. Trumpp, *Kriegs-Orthopädie* [Taschenbuch des Feldarztes, Vol. III]. Munich: J.F. Lehmann Verlag, 1915.

Lange, Fritz, and Hans Spitzy, eds. *Chirurgie und Orthopädie im Kindesalter*. Leipzig: Vogel, 1910.

Lau, Konrad, et al., 'Die Organisationen für die Versorgung des Heeres', Part 2 in *Der grosse Krieg, 1914–1918: Volume 9: Die Organisationen der Kriegsführung*. Leipzig: Barth, 1923.

Lovett, Robert W., 'Editorial', *J Bone Joint Surg Am*. 1910; s 2–7: 556–7.

Mietens, Theodor. 'Eine künstliche Hand für einen Klaviertechniker', *Münchener medizinische Wochenschrift*. Vol. 67 (1920): 1055.

——. 'Ein willkürlich beweglicher Arbeitsarm'. *Feldärtzliche Beilage zur Münchener medizinische Wochenschrift*. No. 3 (1917): 100–3.

Möhring, P. 'Die orthopädische Übungsbehandlung auf Grund der Erfahrungen des Krieges' in Hermann Gocht, ed. *Die Orthopädie in der Kriegs- und Unfallheilkunde* [Deutsche Orthopädie, 4]. Stuttgart: Ferdinand Enke, 1921.

Mollenhauer, P. 'Bericht über die ausserordentliche Tagung der Deutschen Vereinigung für Krüppelfürsorge', *Zentralblatt für chirurgische und mechanische Orthopädie* Vol. 10 (1916), 74–81.

[National Hygiene Museum.] *Ausstellung für Verwundeten- und Krankenfürsorge im Kriege*. Berlin: J.J. Weber, 1915.

——. *Führer durch das Gesamtgebiet der Kriegsbeschädigtenfürsorge*. Dresden: National Hygiene Museum, 1917.

——. *Die Kriegsbeschädigtenfürsorge in Deutschland*. Exhibit Catalogue. Dresden: National Hygiene Museum, 1917.

Nieny, Karl. 'Die Behandlung und Ausrüstung der Amputierten im Marinelazarett Hamburg', *Zeitschrift für orthopädische Chirurgie*. Vol. 37 (1917): 302–22.

Neustätter, Otto. 'Kriegsbeschädigtenfürsorge in früherer Zeit', in Artur Baumgarten-Crusius, ed. *Geschichte der Sachsen im Weltkrieg* [Sachsen in Grosser Zeit, 3]. Leipzig: Max Lippold, 1920.

Paal, [Hermann]. *Kriegsbeschädigten-Fürsorge und Ärzte*. Münster: Universitätsbuchdruckerei Johannes Bredt, 1915.

Paalzow, Generalarzt Dr, [no first name]. 'Das Sanitätswesen im Kriege' in [Ausstellung für Verwundeten- und Kranken-Fürsorge im Kriege], *Die Sanitäre Kriegsrüstung Deutschlands: 14 Vorträge gehalten in der Ausstellung für Verwundeten- und Kranken-Fürsorge im Kriege, Berlin 1914/1915*. Berlin: Oehmigke Verlag, 1915.

Perls, Paul H. 'Kriegsblindenbeschäftigung in der Werkstatt: Arbeitsmöglichkeiten bei der Massenherstellung elektrischer Installationsmaterialien'. Sonderausdruck aus *Werkstattstechnik*. 2 (1917).

——. *Kriegsblindenbeschäftigung im Kleinbauwerk der Siemens-Schuckert-Werke: Beschäftigung – Schutzmaßnahmen – Entlohnung*. Siemens-Schuckert-Werke: 1921.

——. 'Wiederertüchtigung schwerbeschädigter Kriegsteilnehmer in der Werkstatt (Arbeitstherapie)'. Erweiterter Sonderabdruck aus der *Elektrotechnischen Zeitschrift*. 16 (1917).

Radike, R. 'Künstliche Arme und Hände', in Hermann Gocht, et al., eds. *Deutsche Orthopädie*. Vol. 2: *Künstliche Glieder*. Stuttgart: Ferdinand Enke, 1920.

Remarque, Erich Maria. *All Quiet on the Western Front* [*Im Westen nichts neues*, 1929]. Trans. by A.W. Wheen. New York: Ballantine Books, 1982.

[Reichsarbeitsministerium]. *Deutsche Sozialpolitik 1918–1928: Erinnerungsschrift des Reichsarbeitsministeriums*. Berlin: Mittler und Sohn, 1929.

Riedinger, J. 'Zur Frage der Arbeitsarme', *Feldärztliche Beilage zur Münchener medizinische Wochenschrift*. No. 35 (1916): 1280–1.

Roeseler, Hans. 'Deutsche Kriegsfürsorge'. *Wegweiser für das werktätige Volk* 5, No. 1 (January 1918): 1–16.

Salzmann, Walter. *Der sorgenfreie Kriegsinvalide: Die Hinterbliebenenversorgung*. Cassel: Friedr. Lometsch, 1915.

Sauerbruch, F. 'Willkürlich bewegbare Arbeitsklauen'. *Münchener medizinische Wochenschrift*. Vol. 10 (1918): 257–8.

Schede, Franz. 'Zur Mechanik deskünstlichen Kniegelenks. Ein aktives Kunstbein', *Münchener medizinische Wochenschrift*.Vol. 6 (1918): 616–19.

Schlesinger, G. 'Die Mitarbeit des Ingenieurs bei der Durchbildung der Ersatzglieder'. *Zeitschrift des Vereins deutscher Ingenieure* (1917).

Schultzen, [no first name]. *Gesichtspunkte zur Frage der beschleunigten Herausziehung militärisch oder in der Kriegswirtschaft verwendbarer Mannschaften aus den Lazaretten und Truppenteilen*. Kriegsministerium: Berlin, 1916.

Silberstein, Adolf. 'Bein- und Armersatz im Kgl. Orthopädischen Reservelazarett zu Nuernberg'. *Zeitschrift für orthopädische Chirurgie*. Vol. 37 (1917): 350–84.

———. *Ergebnisse der Kriegsinvalidenfürsorge im Reserve-Lazarett Nürnberg*. Würzburg: Curt Kabitzsch, 1916.

———. *Kriegsinvalidenfürsorge* [Würzburger Abhandlungen aus dem Gesamtgebiet der praktischen Medizin, 15]. Würzburg: Curt Kabitzsch, 1915.

Steinthal, [no first name]. 'Wege und Ziele zum Problem der künstlichen Hand' *Bruns' Beiträge zur klinischen Chirurgie*. Vol. 106 (1917):725–31.

Stocker, August. *Kriegshinterbliebenenfürsorge: Ein Handbuch der sozialen Fürsorge für die Hinterbliebenen der im Kriege Gefallenen*. Karlsruhe: Macklot, 1918.

Syrup, Friedrich. *Die Fürsorge für kriegsverletzte gewerbliche Arbeiter*. (Schriften des Deutschen Werkmeister-Verbandes, 29.) Düsseldorf: Verlag der Werkmeister-Buchhandlung, 1916.

[Ulmer Verwundetenschule], *Die Ulmer Verwundetenschule: Ihre Werkstätten, Kurse, und Einrichtungen der Beratungsstelle für Kriegs-Invaliden*. Ulm, Verwundetenschule, 1918.

von Aberle, Rudolf (Ritter). 'Künstliche Gliedmassen fuer Kriegsverwundete', *Zeitschrift für orthopädische Chirurgie*. Vol. 35 (1916): 584–610.

von Baeyer, [Hans]. 'Prothesen aus Weissblech', *Münchener medizinische Wochenschrift*. Vol. 44 (1915): 1496–9.

von Bissing, Alice (Freifrau). *Die Frau in der Kriegsbeschädigtenfürsorge*. Leipzig: Leopold Voss, 1917.

von der Osten-Sacken und von Rhein, Ottomar (Freiherrn). *Preussens Heer von seinen Anfaengen bis zur Gegenwart. Vol. III.*. Berlin: Mittler und Sohn, 1914.

Wiener, Kurt. 'Fingerbesteck für Einhändige', *Münchener medizinische Wochenschrift*. Vol. 93 (1916): 1442.

Witzel, O. 'Die Aufgaben und Wege für den Hand- und Armersatz der Kriegsbeschädigten', *Münchener medizinische Wochenschrift*. Vol. 44 (1915): 1491–2.

Wollmann, LAB. Generalleutnant z.D. 'Neuzeitliche Kriegsbeschädigten-Fürsorge durch Turnen und Sport'. *Illustrirte Zeitung* (2/1917: 3864), 107–8.

Würtz, Hans. *Der Wille Siegt!* [Beiträge zur Invalidenfürsorge 1]. Berlin: Reichsverlag Hermann Kalkoff, 1916.

Secondary sources

Aly, Götz. *Cleansing the Fatherland: Nazi Medicine and Racial Hygiene*. Baltimore: Johns Hopkins University Press, 1994.

Anderson, Julie. 'Rehabilitating Blind Bodies: St Dunstan's 1918–1939'. Unpublished paper, 2003.

——, *War, Disability, and Rehabilitation in Britain: 'Soul of a Nation'*. Manchester: Manchester University Press, 2011.

Angetter, Daniela Claudia. *Dem Tod geweiht und doch gerettet: Die Sanitätsversorgung am Isonzo und in den Dolomiten 1915–1918* [Beiträge zur Neueren Geschichte Österreichs, 3]. Frankfurt: Peter Lang, 1995.

——, *Krieg als Vater der Medizin: Kriege und ihre Auswirkungen auf den medizinischen Fortschritt anhand der 2000-jährigen Geschichte Österreichs*. Wien: Österreichischer Kunst- und Kulturverlag, 2004.

Bajohr, Frank. *Zwischen Krupp und Kommune*. Essen: Klartext Verlag, 1988.

Biwald, Brigitte. *Von Helden und Krüppeln: Das Österreichisch-Ungarische Militärsanitätswesen im Ersten Weltkrieg*. ÖBV & hpt Verlag: Vienna, 2002.

Bessel, Richard. *Germany After the First World War*. Oxford: Oxford University Press, 1993.

Blackbourn, David and Geoff Eley. *The Peculiarities of German History*. New York: Oxford University Press, 1984.

Bleker, Johanna. 'To Benefit the Poor and Advance Medical Science: Hospitals and Hospital Care in Germany, 1820–1870', in Manfred Berg and Geoffrey Cocks, eds. *Medicine and Modernity: Public Health and Medical Care in Nineteenth- and Twentieth-Century Germany*. Washington, D.C.: German Historical Institute, 1997.

Bourke, Joanna. *Dismembering the Male: Men's Bodies, Britain, and the Great War*. Chicago: University of Chicago Press, 1996.

Braun, Arnim. *Oscar Vulpius: Leben und Werk: Ein Wegbereiter der Orthopädie und orthopädischen Chirurgie in Heidelberg*. Heidelberg: Guderjahn, 1997.

Bridenthal, Renate and Claudia Koonz, eds, *Becoming Visible: Women in European History*. Boston: Houghton Mifflin, 1977.

Burhenne, Karl. *Werner Siemens als Sozialpolitiker*. Munich: C.H. Beck, 1932.

Burleigh, Michael. *Death and Deliverance: 'Euthanasia' in Germany c. 1900–1945*. New York: Cambridge University Press, 1994.

Campbell, Joan. *Joy in Work, German Work: The National Debate, 1800–1945*. Princeton: Princeton University Press, 1989.

Carden-Coyne, Ana. *Reconstructing the Body: Classicism, Modernism, and the First World War*. Oxford: Oxford University Press, 2009.

Chickering, Roger. *Imperial Germany and the Great War*. New York: Cambridge University Press, 1998.

Chickering, Roger and Stig Förster, eds. *Great War, Total War: Combat and Mobilization on the Western Front, 1914–1918*. New York: Cambridge University Press, 2000.

Cohen, Deborah. *The War Come Home: Disabled Veterans in Britain and Germany, 1914–1939*. Berkeley: University of California Press, 2001.

——. 'Will to Work: Disabled Veterans in Britain and Germany after the First World War', in David A. Gerber, ed. *Disabled Veterans in History*. Ann Arbor: University of Michigan Press, 2000.

Conrad, Peter, *The Medicalization of Society: On the Transformation of Human Conditions into Treatable Disorders*. Baltimore: Johns Hopkins University Press, 2007.

Cooter, Roger. 'Medicine and the Goodness of War', *Canadian Bulletin of Medical History/Bulletin canadien d'histoire de la médecine*. Vol. 7, No.2: 147–59.

——. *Surgery and Society in Peace and War: Orthopaedics and the Organization of Modern Medicine, 1880–1948*. London: Macmillan, 1993.

——. 'War and Modern Medicine', in W.F. Bynum and R. Porter, eds. *Companion Encyclopedia of the History of Medicine*. London/New York: Routledge, 1993), 1536–73.

Cooter, Roger, Mark Harrison, and Steve Sturdy, eds. *Medicine and Modern Warfare*. Atlanta: Rodopi, 1999.

——. *War, Medicine, and Modernity*. Stroud: Sutton, 1998.

Craig, Gordon A. *Germany 1866–1945*. New York: Oxford University Press, 1978.

Crane, Stephen. *The Red Badge of Courage*. London: Everyman, 1993.

Cron, Hermann. *Imperial German Army 1914–18. Organization, Structure, Orders of Battle*. Solihull: Helion & Co, 2002.

Crouthamel, Jason. 'Invisible Traumas: Psychological Wounds, World War I, and German Society, 1914–1945'. Dissertation: Indiana University, 2001.

——. *The Great War and German Memory: Society, Politics, and Psychological Trauma*. Exeter: University of Exeter Press, 2009.

Dawson, William Harbutt. *Social Insurance in Germany 1883–1911: Its History, Operation, Results, and a Comparison with the National Insurance Act 1911*. London: T. Fisher Unwin, 1912.

Diehl, James M. 'The Organization of German Veterans, 1917–1919', *Archiv für Sozialgeschichte*. Vol. 11 (1971): 141–84.

——. *Paramilitary Politics in Weimar Germany*. Bloomington: Indiana University Press, 1977.

——. *The Thanks of the Fatherland: German Veterans after the Second World War.* Chapel Hill: University of North Carolina Press, 1993.

Domansky, Elisabeth. 'Militarization and Reproduction in World War I Germany', in Geoff Eley, ed. *Society, Culture, and the State in Germany 1870–1930.* Ann Arbor: University of Michigan Press, 1997.

Eckart, Wolfgang U. and Christoph Gradmann, eds. *Die Medizin und der Erste Weltkrieg.* Pfaffenweiler: Centaurus, 1996.

Eckart, Wolfgang U. and Alexander Neumann. *Medizin im Zweiten Weltkrieg: militärmedizinische Praxis und medizinische Wissenschaft im 'Totalen Krieg'.* Paderborn: Schöningh, 2006.

Eghigian, Greg. *Making Security Social: Disability, Insurance, and the Birth of the Social Entitlement State in Germany.* Ann Arbor: University of Michigan Press, 2000.

Engelstein, Stefani, *Anxious Anatomy: The Conception of the Human Form in Literary and Naturalist Discourse,* Albany, NY: SUNY Press, 2008.

——. 'Out on a Limb: Military Medicine, Heinrich von Kleist, and the Disarticulated Body', *German Studies Review.* Vol. 23, No. 2: 225–44.

Eulner, Hans-Heinz. *Die Entwicklung der medizinischen Spezialfächer an den Universitäten des deutschen Sprachgebietes.* Stuttgart: Ferdinand Enke, 1970.

Feldenkirchen, Wilfried. *Siemens: Von der Werkstatt zum Weltunternehmen.* Munich: Piper, 1997.

Feldman, Gerald. *Army, Industry and Labor in Germany, 1914–1918.* Providence: Berg, 1992.

Fischer, Fritz. *Germany's War Aims in the First World War.* New York: W.W. Norton, 1967.

Figg, Laurann and Jane Farrell-Beck, 'Amputation in the Civil War: Physical and Social Dimensions', *Journal of the History of Medicine and Allied Sciences.* Vol. 48: 454–75.

Förster, Stig. 'The Armed Forces and Military Planning', in Roger Chickering, ed. *Imperial Germany: A Historiographical Companion.* Westport, Conn.: Greenwood, 1996.

Gerber, David. 'Disabled Veterans: Why Are They Different? What Difference does It Make?' *Disability History Association Newsletter.* Vol. 3, No. 1 (2007): 14–26.

Gerber, David A., ed. *Disabled Veterans in History.* Ann Arbor: University of Michigan Press, 2000.

Geyer, Michael. 'The Militarization of Europe, 1914–1945', in John R. Gillis, ed. *The Militarization of the Western World.* New Brunswick, N.J.: Rutgers University Press, 1989.

Gilbert, Martin. *The First World War: A Complete History.* New York: Holt and Company, 1994.

Gregory, Adrian. 'Lost Generations: The Impact of Military Casualties on Paris, London, and Berlin', in Jay Winter and Jean-Louis Robert, eds, *Capital Cities at War: Paris, London, Berlin 1914–1919* [Studies in the Social and Cultural History of Modern Warfare]. New York: Cambridge University Press, 1997.

Gumprecht F. and G. Pfarrius. *Lehrbuch der Arbeiter-Versicherungsmedizin*. Leipzig: Barth, 1913.

Hale, Matthew. *Human Science and Social Order: Hugo Munsterberg and the Origins of Applied Psychology*. Philadelphia: Temple University Press, 1980.

Harrison, Mark. *The Medical War: British Military Medicine in the First World War*. Oxford: Oxford University Press, 2010.

——. 'Medicine and the Management of Modern Warfare', *History of Science*. Vol. 34 (1996): 379–410.

——. *Medicine and Victory: British Military Medicine in the Second World War*. Oxford: Oxford University Press, 2004.

Hau, Michal. *The Cult of Health and Beauty in Germany: A Social History, 1890–1930*. Chicago: University of Chicago Press, 2003.

Heipertz, W. 'Geschichte der Krankengymnastik', in August Rütt, ed., *Geschichte der Orthopädie im Deutschen Sprachraum*. Stuttgart: Enke, 1993.

Hennock, E. P. *The Origin of the Welfare State in England and Germany, 1850–1914: Social Policies Compared*. Cambridge: Cambridge University Press, 2007.

Herwig, Holger H. *The First World War: Germany and Austria-Hungary, 1914–1918*. New York: Arnold, 1997.

Hobsbawm, Eric and Terence Ranger, eds. *The Invention of Tradition*. Cambridge: Cambridge University Press, 1983.

Hofer, Hans-Georg, Cay-Rüdiger Prüll, and Wolfgang U. Eckart, eds. *War, Trauma, and Medicine in Germany and Central Europe (1914–1939)* [Neuere Medizin und Wissenschaftsgeschichte, 26]. Freiburg: Centaurus Verlag, 2011.

Howard, Michael. *The Franco-Prussian War: The German Invasion of France*. New York: Collier Books, 1969.

Huerkamp, Claudia. 'The Making of the Modern Medical Profession, 1800–1914: Prussian Doctors in the Nineteenth Century', in Geoffrey Cocks and Konrad H. Jarausch, eds, *German Professions, 1800–1950*. New York: Oxford University Press, 1990.

Jackson, Christopher R. 'Infirmative Action: The Law of the Severely Disabled in Germany'. *Central European History*. Vol. 26 (1993): 417–55.

Jeschal, Godwin. *Politik und Wissenshaft deutscher Ärzte im Ersten Weltkrieg* [Würzburger medizinhistorische Forschungen, 13]. Hannover: Horst Wellm Verlag, 1977.

Kienitz, Sabine. *Beschädigte Helden: Kriegsinvalidität und Körperbilder 1914–1923* [Krieg in der Geschichte, 41]. Paderborn: Schöningh, 2008.

——. 'Body Damage: War Disability and Constructions of Masculinity in Weimar Germany', in Karen Hagemann and Stefanie Schüler-Springorum, eds., *Home/front: The Military, War, and Gender in Twentieth-Century Germany*. Oxford: Berg, 2002.

Kliche, Christian. *Die Stellung der deutschen Militärärzte im Ersten Weltkrieg* (Dissertation: FU-Berlin, March 20, 1968).

Koven, Seth. 'Remembering and Dismemberment: Crippled Children, Wounded Soldiers, and the Great War in Britain'. *American Historical Review*. Vol. 99 (1994): 1167–202.

Larsson, Marina. *Shattered Anzacs: Living with the Scars of War*. Seattle: University of Washington Press, 2009.

Leed, J. *No Man's Land: Combat and Identity in World War I*. Cambridge: Cambridge University Press, 1979.

Lerner, Paul. *Hysterical Men: War, Psychiatry, and the Politics of Trauma in Germany, 1890–1930*. Ithaca: Cornell University Press, 2003.

Lifton, Robert Jay. *The Nazi Doctors: Medical Killing and the Psychology of Genocide*. New York: Basic Books, 1986.

Linker, Beth. 'Feet for Fighting: Locating Disability and Social Medicine in First World War America'. *Social History of Medicine*. Vol. 20, No. 1 (April 2007): 91–109.

———. *War's Waste: Rehabilitation in World War I America*. Chicago: University of Chicago Press, 2011.

Linton, Derek. 'The Obscure Object of Knowledge: German Military Medicine Confronts Gas Gangrene during World War I'. *Bulletin of the History of Medicine*. Vol. 74 (2000): 291–316.

Liulevicius, Vejas G. *War Land on the Eastern Front: Culture, National Identity, and German Occupation in World War I*. Cambridge: Cambridge University Press, 2000.

Lunbeck, Elizabeth. *The Psychiatric Persuasion: Knowledge, Gender, and Power in Modern America*. Princeton: Princeton University Press, 1994.

McClelland, Charles E. *The German Experience of Professionalization: Modern Learned Professions and their Organizations from the Early Nineteenth Century to the Hitler Era*. New York: Cambridge University Press, 1991.

Magri, Susanna. 'Housing', in Jay Winter and Jean-Louis Robert, eds, *Capital Cities at War: Paris, London, Berlin 1914–1919*. Cambridge: Cambridge University Press, 1997.

Manchester, William. *The Arms of Krupp: The Rise and Fall of the Industrial Dynasty that Armed Germany at War*. London: Back Bay Books, 2003.

Marx, Karl and Frederick Engels. *Manifesto of the Communist Party*. New York: International Publishers, 1948.

Micale, Marc and Paul Lerner. *Traumatic Pasts: History, Psychiatry, and Trauma in the Modern Age*. Cambridge: Cambridge University Press, 2001.

Michl, Susanne. *Im Dienste des 'Volkskörpers': deutsche und französische Ärzte im Ersten Weltkrieg*. Göttingen: Vandenhoeck & Ruprecht, 2007.

Mosse, George L. *Fallen Soldiers: Reshaping the Memory of the World Wars*. New York: Oxford University Press, 1990.

———. *The Image of Man: The Creation of Modern Masculinity*. New York: Oxford University Press, 1996.

———. *Nationalism and Sexuality: Respectability and Abnormal Sexuality in Modern Europe*. New York: H. Fertig, 1985.

Nash, D.B. *Imperial German Army Handbook 1914–1918*. London: Ian Allan, 1980.

Natt, Hugo. *Zwischen Schützengraben und Skalpell: Kriegstagebuch eines Arztes, 1914–1918*, edited by Heinrich Hesse and Bernhard Natt. Gutenberg: Computas Druck Satz & Verlag, 2010.

Naujoks, Horst, ed. *Äskulap in Kurland und Wolhynien, 1914–1919: Feldpostbriefe und Tagebuchseiten von Hans Naujoks, kgl.preuss. Feldunterarzt* [Archiv der Zeitzeugen, 20.] Münster: Monsenstein und Vannerdat OHG, 2012.

Neumann, H.W. '100 Jahre Orthopädie in Deutschland'. *Zeitschrift für Orthopädie und ihre Grenzgebiete*. Vol. 139, No. 5 (2001): 373–4.

Nicosia, Francis R. *Medicine and Medical Ethics in Nazi Germany: Origins, Practices, Legacies*. New York: Berghahn Books, 2002.

Oskar-Helene-Heim: 80 Jahre Feier. [Oskar-Helene-Heim]. Berlin: Freie Universität, 1994.

Panchesi, Roxanne. 'Reconstructions: Prosthetics and the Rehabilitation of the Male Body in World War I France'. *Differences*. Vol. 7, No. 3 (1995): 109–40.

Paul, Johann. *Alfred Krupp und die Arbeiterbewegung*. Düsseldorf: Schwann, 1987.

Perry, Heather R. 'Re-Arming the Disabled Veteran: Artificially Rebuilding State and Society in World War One Germany', in Katherine Ott et al., eds, *Artificial Parts, Practical Lives: Modern Histories of Prosthetics*. New York: New York University Press, 2002.

——. 'The Thanks of the Fatherland? WWI and the Orthopaedic Revolution in Disability Care', in Hans-Georg Hofer, Cay-Rüdiger Prüll, and Wolfgang Eckart, eds, *War, Trauma, and Medicine in Germany and Central Europe (1914–1939)* [Neuere Medizin und Wissenschaftsgeschichte, 26]. Freiburg: Centaurus Verlag, 2011.

Poore, Carol. *Disability in Twentieth-Century German Culture*. Ann Arbor: University of Michigan Press, 2007.

Povacz, Franz. *Geschichte der Unfallchirurgie*. Heidelberg: Springer, 2007.

Proctor, Robert. *Racial Hygiene: Medicine under the Nazis*. Cambridge: Harvard University Press, 1988.

Prüll, Cay-Rüdiger. 'Pathology at War', in Cooter, et al., eds. *Medicine and the Management of Modern Warfare*. Amsterdam: Rodopi, 1999.

Rabinbach, Anson. *The Human Motor: Energy, Fatigue and the Origins of Modernity*. New York: Basic Books, 1990.

Reznick, Jeffrey S. *Healing the Nation: Soldiers, Caregivers and British Identity During World War I*. Manchester: Manchester University Press, 2005.

——. 'Work-Therapy and the Disabled British Soldier in Great Britain in the First World War: The Case of Shepherd's Bush Military Hospital, London', in David A. Gerber, ed., *Disabled Veterans in History*. Ann Arbor: University of Michigan Press, 2000.

Ring, Friedrich. *Zur Geschichte der Militärmedizin in Deutschland*. Berlin: Deutscher Militärverlag, 1962.

Ring, Friedrich and H.W. Hackenberg. *Zur Geschichte der Militärmedizin in Deutschland*. Berlin: Deutsche Militärverlag, 1962.

Risse, Guenter B. *Mending Bodies, Saving Souls: A History of Hospitals*. New York: Oxford University Press, 1999.

Rosenthal, Anton. 'The Arrival of the Electric Streetcar and the Conflict over Progress in Early 20th-Century Montevideo'. *Journal of Latin American Studies.* Vol. 27, No. 2 (1995): 319–42.

Schneider, William H. 'Blood Transfusion between the Wars'. *Journal of the History of Medicine and Allied Sciences.* Vol. 58, No. 2 (2003): 187–224.

Schwarzmann-Schafhauser, Doris. *Orthopädie im Wandel: Die Herausbildung von Disziplin und Berufsstand in Bund und Kaiserreich(1815–1914).* Stuttgart: Franz Steiner, 2004.

Shephard, Ben. *A War of Nerves: Soldiers and Psychiatrists in the Twentieth Century.* Cambridge: Harvard University Press, 2001.

Showalter, Dennis. 'Mass Warfare and the Impact of Technology', in Roger Chickering and Stig Förster, eds., *Great War, Total War: Combat and Mobilization on the Western Front, 1914–1918.* New York: Cambridge University Press, 2000.

Theweleit, Klaus. *Male Fantasies.* (2 vols). Trans by Stephen Conway. Minneapolis: University of Minnesota Press, 1985–1989.

Thomann, Klaus-Dieter. *Das behinderte Kind: 'Krüppelfürsorge' und Orthopädie in Deutschland 1886–1920.* Stuttgart: Gustav Fischer, 1995.

———.'Die medizinische und soziale Fürsorge für die Kriegsversehrten', in Wolfgang U. Eckart and Christoph Gradmann, eds, *Die Medizin und der Erste Weltkrieg.* Pfaffenweiler: Centaurus, 1996.

Urlanis, Boris. *Bilanz der Kriege.* Berlin: VEB Deutscher Verlag der Wissenschaften, 1965.

Usborne, Cornelie. '"Pregnancy is the Woman's Active Service": Pronatalism in Germany during the First World War', in Richard Wall and Jay Winter, eds, *The Upheaval of War: Family, Work, and Welfare in Europe, 1914–1918.* New York: Cambridge University Press, 1988.

van Bergen, Leo. *Before My Helpless Sight: Suffering, Dying, and Military Medicine on the Western Front, 1914–1918.* Burlington, VT: Ashgate, 2009.

Wall, Richard and Jay Winter, eds. *The Upheaval of War: Family, Work, and Welfare in Europe, 1914–1918.* New York: Cambridge University Press, 1988.

Ward, Stephen R., ed. *The War Generation: Veterans of the First World War.* Port Washington, N.Y.: Kennikat Press, 1975.

Weindling, Paul M. *Health, Race, and German Politics Between National Unification and Nazism, 1870–1945.* New York: Cambridge University Press, 1989.

Weisz, George. *Divide and Conquer: A Comparative History of Medical Specialization.* New York: Oxford University Press, 2006.

Wessinghage, D. 2001. 'Die Gesellschaften deutscher Orthopäden in den ersten 20 Jahren'. *Der Orthopäde.* Vol. 30, No. 10 (2001): 675-84.

Wetz, H.H. 'Zur Geschichte der Armprothetik', in *Geschichte operativer Verfahren an den Bewegungsorganen.* [Jahrbuch des Deutsches orthopaedisches Geschichts- und Forschungsmuseum, 2], Darmstadt: Steinkopff, 2000.

Whalen, Robert Weldon. *Bitter Wounds: German Victims of the Great War, 1914–1939.* Ithaca: Cornell University Press, 1984.

Winter, Jay and Jean-Louis Robert, eds. *Capital Cities at War: Paris, London, Berlin 1914–1919*. New York: Cambridge University Press, 1997.

Wood, Nathan D. 'Becoming Metropolitan: Cracow's Popular Press and the Representation of Modern Urban Life, 1900–1915'. Dissertation: Indiana University, 2004.

——. *Becoming Metropolitan: Urban Selfhood and the Making of Modern Cracow*. DeKalb: Northern Illinois University Press, 2010.

Zelizer, Viviana A. *Pricing the Priceless Child: The Changing Social Value of Children*. Princeton: Princeton University Press, 1985.

Internet sources

www.medtech.tu-berlin.de/menue/forschung/schwerpunkte/hilfsmittelforschung/
www.schoen-kliniken.de/ptp/kkh/okm/klinik/profil/geschichte/
www.wdl.org/en/item/250/

Index